The Social Psychology of Stigma

The Social Psychology of Stigma

Edited by

Todd F. Heatherton
Robert E. Kleck
Michelle R. Hebl
Jay G. Hull

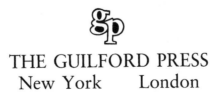

THE GUILFORD PRESS
New York   London

©2000 The Guilford Press
A Division of Guilford Publications, Inc.
72 Spring Street, New York, NY 10012
www.guilford.com

Paperback edition 2003

This book is printed on acid-free paper.

Last digit is print number: 9   8   7   6   5   4   3

Library of Congress Cataloging-in-Publication Data

The social psychology of stigma/edited by Todd F. Heatherton . . . [et al.].
    p. cm.
  Includes bibliographical references and index.
  ISBN 1-57230-573-8 (hard)   ISBN 1-57230-942-3 (paper)
    1. Stigma (Social psychology). I. Heatherton, Todd F.

HM1131 .S63 2000
305—dc21   00-022356

About the Editors

Todd F. Heatherton received his BSc from the University of Calgary and his PhD in experimental psychology from the University of Toronto. Following a 1-year period as a postdoctoral fellow at Case Western Reserve University, he joined the Harvard Psychology Department in 1990. He left Harvard in 1994 to join the faculty at Dartmouth College, where he is currently Associate Professor of Psychology. His main research examines the situational, individual, motivational, and affective processes that interfere with self-regulation. Dr. Heatherton has authored or coauthored more than 60 journal articles and chapters and has published two books. He has been on the executive committees of the Society of Personality in Social Psychology, the Association of Researchers in Personality, and the International Society of Self and Identity.

Robert E. Kleck is a professor in the Department of Psychology at Dartmouth College. He received his BA from Denison University and his PhD from Stanford University in 1964. His research has focused on the interaction of facial appearance and facial expression in determining both emotional attribution and person perception outcomes, awareness of the information that people transmit to each other in face-to-face interactions, and the conditions or individual characteristics that one either is or is not a target of social discrimination. Dr. Kleck has been Associate Editor for the *Journal of Personality and Social Psychology* and the *Journal of Nonverbal Behavior*. He is also a Charter Fellow of the American Psychological Society.

Michelle R. Hebl is currently an assistant professor in the Department of Psychology at Rice University. She received her BA at Smith College in

1991, her MS at Texas A&M University in 1993, and her PhD at Dartmouth College in 1997. She was a Visiting Assistant Professor for 1 year at Dartmouth College before joining the Department of Psychology at Rice in 1998. Her research focuses on workplace discrimination and the barriers stigmatized individuals face in the hiring process, business settings, and medical community. In 1999, she received an American Psychological Foundation Grant for her research on discrimination in the workplace, and she received a Rice University Women's Resource Center Impact Award for her research on gender issues and service to women in the community. Dr. Hebl is also passionate about teaching and recently coedited the second volume of the *Handbook for Teaching of Psychology*.

Jay G. Hull received his BA from the University of Texas at Austin in 1974. He was a National Science Foundation Graduate Fellow at Duke University and received his PhD in experimental social psychology in 1979. Following graduate school, he spent 3 years as a postdoctoral fellow in Sheldon Stryker's program on Self, Identity, and Mental Health in the Department of Sociology at Indiana University. He joined the faculty at Dartmouth College in 1982 and is currently a professor in the Department of Psychological and Brain Sciences. Although Dr. Hull has published articles on personality and health, the application of structural equation modeling to issues in personality measurement, and the effects of social support on depression in elders, his main interests remain the structure of self-knowledge and the function of self-regulation.

Contributors

Terrilee Asher, MA, Department of Psychology, Arizona State University, Tempe, Arizona

Monica Biernat, PhD, Department of Psychology, University of Kansas, Lawrence, Kansas

Jim Blascovich, PhD, Department of Psychology, University of California at Santa Barbara, Santa Barbara, California

Celina Chatman, PhD, Research Center for Group Dynamics, Institute of Social Research, University of Michigan, Ann Arbor, Michigan

Delia Cioffi, PhD, New York, New York

Christian S. Crandall, PhD, Department of Psychology, University of Kansas, Lawrence, Kansas

Jennifer Crocker, PhD, Research Center for Group Dynamics, Institute of Social Research, University of Michigan, Ann Arbor, Michigan

John F. Dovidio, PhD, Department of Psychology, Colgate University, Hamilton, New York

Todd F. Heatherton, PhD, Department of Psychological and Brain Sciences, Dartmouth College, Hanover, New Hampshire

Michelle R. Hebl, PhD, Department of Psychology, Rice University, Houston, Texas

Sarah B. Hunter, PhD, Department of Psychology, University of California at Santa Barbara, Santa Barbara, California

Lee Jussim, PhD, Psychology Department, Rutgers University, New Brunswick, New Jersey

Robert E. Kleck, PhD, Department of Psychological and Brain Sciences, Dartmouth College, Hanover, New Hampshire

Brian Lickel, BA, Department of Psychology, University of California at Santa Barbara, Santa Barbara, California

Stephanie Madon, PhD, Department of Psychology, Iowa State University, Ames, Iowa

Brenda Major, PhD, Department of Psychology, University of California at Santa Barbara, Santa Barbara, California

Wendy Berry Mendes, MA, Department of Psychology, University of California at Santa Barbara, Santa Barbara, California

Carol T. Miller, PhD, Department of Psychology, University of Vermont, Burlington, Vermont

Joann M. Montepare, PhD, Psychology Program, School of Communication Sciences and Disorders, Emerson College, Boston, Massachusetts

Steven L. Neuberg, PhD, Department of Psychology, Arizona State University, Tempe, Arizona

Polly Palumbo, MA, Psychology Department, Rutgers University, New Brunswick, New Jersey

Diane M. Quinn, PhD, Department of Psychology, University of Connecticut, Storrs, Connecticut

Laura Smart, PhD, New England Research Institutes, Watertown, Massachusetts, and Department of Psychology, Brandeis University, Waltham, Massachusetts

Alison Smith, PhD, Psychology Department, Rutgers University, New Brunswick, New Jersey

Dylan M. Smith, PhD, Department of Psychology, University of Kansas, Lawrence, Kansas

Charles Stangor, PhD, Department of Psychology, University of Maryland, College Park, Maryland

Jennifer Tickle, BA, Department of Psychological and Brain Sciences, Dartmouth College, Hanover, New Hampshire

Daniel M. Wegner, PhD, Department of Psychology, University of Virginia, Charlottesville, Virginia

Leslie A. Zebrowitz, PhD, Department of Psychology, Brandeis University, Waltham, Massachusetts

Preface

Dartmouth College owns a mansion on a lake—and not just any lake, but Squam Lake, the location in New Hampshire where they filmed the movie *On Golden Pond*. Our social group is fortunate to have funds available, provided by the Lincoln Filene Chair at Dartmouth College, to host a small gathering of colleagues at this wonderful spot, which is known as the Minary Center. Typically, we identify a topic of interest to us and invite a dozen or so of the world's leading experts to join us for in-depth, focused discussions. Perhaps not surprisingly, very few people have turned down our invitations over the past few years. The setting is tranquil, the scenery spectacular, the facilities glorious, the food and wine of gourmet quality, the intellectual atmosphere superb, and we pay all expenses. This is not a hard sell.

The meetings are anything but your typical conference proceedings. We do not allow formal papers, and most of the program involves guided discussion. Issues of particular significance are identified in advance, in consultation with our guests, and then we discuss the most pressing issues in six or seven sessions. We make sure to allow plenty of leisure time for informal discussions, with additional large gaps in the program to allow for enjoyment of the recreational amenities. It is as idyllic as it sounds.

Over the last 4 years, we have had leading social, personality, clinical, and developmental psychologists join us at the Minary Center. For the topic of stigma we were able to attract a stellar group of academics, including (alphabetically) Monica Biernat, Jim Blascovich, Chris Crandall, Jennifer Crocker, Jack Dovidio, Lee Jussim, Brenda Major, Carol Miller, Steve Neuberg, Dan Wegner, Bernie Weiner, and Leslie

Zebrowitz. The Dartmouth faculty were Jay Hull, Delia Cioffi, Robert Kleck, and Todd Heatherton. This volume comes out of this meeting, but it is quite different from traditional conference proceedings. Indeed, many hours were spent at the meeting discussing just exactly how a book on stigma should be organized and put together. However, our planning for this volume started many months earlier.

In the year before the Minary Conference on Stigma, a working group was formed to plan the program for the meeting. Robert Kleck and Todd Heatherton chaired a weekly discussion session that consisted of faculty, graduate students, honors students, and interested undergraduates. We developed a list of potential attendees and then invited them to come. We were pleased that all but one of our invitees were able to join us in New Hampshire; the unidentified other was already booked, and unable to wiggle out of that commitment. In advance of the Minary Center meeting, we asked the participants to identify the 5–10 most important questions that they believed needed to be addressed in the stigma/social stereotypes literature. Each contributor took our task to heart and we ended up with more than 10 pages of thoughtful, evocative questions. We then organized the questions into a smaller group of central themes, and asked the invitees to help us lead discussions of those themes at the meeting. This served as the initial plan for the organization of this volume.

During the first meeting, the group discussed the goal of producing a coherent and integrated volume of chapters on stigma and social stereotyping. The group worked through the themes and issues and set out the view of stigma articulated in the opening chapter, as thoughtfully expressed by Jack Dovidio, Brenda Major, and Jennifer Crocker. The group spent the final day determining who would write each chapter, with the proviso that authors could include their personal interests in their chapters. Contained in this book are 14 chapters that represent the state of the art in terms of the social psychological processes involved in stigmatization.

Stigma is not inherently an enjoyable topic. The stigmatized are ostracized, devalued, rejected, scorned, shunned, discriminated against, insulted, attacked, and even murdered. Those who perceive themselves to be members of a stigmatized group, whether it is obvious to those around them or not, often experience psychological distress and may even view themselves contemptuously. To be discussing such issues "on Golden Pond" was paradoxical—removed as it is from the harsh realities of bearing stigma. Yet, the setting allowed us to really think about stigma in a way that few of us had been able to do individually. We were able to discuss important ideas and findings that have emerged over the last two decades on the social consequences of stigma. For instance, the group believed that an insufficient amount of attention had been paid to the motives, cognitions, and emotional reactions of those being stigmatized, and even less attention had been devoted to analyzing interactions between those who are stigmatized and those doing the stigmatizing. The chapters in this volume represent our shared view on the topics of importance to the social psychological understanding of stigma.

Acknowledgments

We would like to acknowledge a number of individuals who assisted with the Minary Conference on Stigma. Primary thanks goes to George Wolford, the Lincoln Filene Chair at Dartmouth College. George, a cognitive psychologist by training but a social psychologist at heart, provided the funding for the entire meeting from his chair's endowed funds. We also thank Laura and Drew Hinman, the gracious and patient hosts of the Minary Center, for making everything run so smoothly and for arranging everything, from the wonderful meals, to the endless refreshments, to the boat tours of Squam Lake. The Dartmouth College social graduate students were instrumental in planning the conference and also in keeping the guests talking during the meeting. This group included Mikki Hebl, Jennifer Tickle, Kathleen Vohs, Kris Koepsel, and Lauren Wittenberg. Minutes for the meeting were capably taken by Julie McGuire, an honors student at Dartmouth completing her thesis on stigma.

We are also grateful to Seymour Weingarten at The Guilford Press for his support of this project. Carolyn Graham has shown patience and persistence in guiding the editorial process. The authors, of course, are to be thanked not only for their excellent chapters, but also for helping us spend a wonderful weekend "on Golden Pond."

Contents

1

Stigma: Introduction and Overview

JOHN F. DOVIDIO
BRENDA MAJOR
JENNIFER CROCKER

Stigmatization, at its essence, is a challenge to one's humanity—for both the stigmatized person and the stigmatizer. Crocker, Major, and Steele (1998) explain that "a person who is stigmatized is a person whose social identity, or membership in some social category, calls into question his or her full humanity—the person is devalued, spoiled, or flawed in the eyes of others" (p. 504; see also Goffman, 1963; Jones et al., 1984). From the perspective of the stigmatizer, stigmatization involves dehumanization, threat, aversion, and sometimes the depersonalization of others into stereotypic caricatures. Thus stigmatization is personally, interpersonally, and socially costly.

Classic treatments of stigmatization have tended to view the processes and consequences of stigma in highly dispositional terms, reflecting, or being reflected in, individual differences. Stereotyping and prejudice, which are central to stigmatizing others, were once seen as reflections of a constellation of personality characteristics (authoritarianism, political and economic conservatism, ethnocentrism, and anti-Semitism), and hence as problems located in specific individuals (Adorno, Frenkel-Brunswik, Levinson, & Sanford, 1950). Similarly, it was assumed that the experience of being stigmatized, or being the target of stereotypes and prejudice, resulted in distortions of the personality of the

1

stigmatized person—most often in low self-esteem (e.g., Allport, 1954/ 1979). For instance, Allport (1954/1979) posed this question: "What would happen to your personality if you heard it said over and over again that you are lazy and had inferior blood?" (p. 42). And then he answered, "Group oppression may destroy the integrity of the ego entirely, and reverse its normal pride, and create a groveling self-image" (p. 152). (See Crocker & Major, 1989, for a review.)

The past half-century has seen a dramatic transformation in social-psychological views of stereotyping and prejudice. Rather than regarding prejudice as a reflection of problematic personality traits resulting from deep-seated, often unconscious inner conflicts, social psychologists now consider stereotyping to be a normal (if undesirable) consequence of people's cognitive abilities and limitations, and of the social information and experiences to which they are exposed. Similarly, views of the consequences of being the target of stigma have also been transformed over the past half-century. Rather than assuming that the experience of being stigmatized inevitably results in deep-seated, negative, and even pathological consequences for the personality of a stigmatized individual, researchers in this area now assume that people who are stigmatized experience a set of psychological predicaments, which they cope with using the same coping strategies as those used by nonstigmatized people when they are confronted with psychological challenges such as threats to self-esteem (e.g., Crocker et al., 1998; Goffman, 1963; Miller & Major, Chapter 9, this volume). As a consequence, there is considerable individual variation within stigmatized groups, just as there is within nonstigmatized groups (e.g., Major, Barr, Zubek, & Babey, 1999). Thus current views of stigma, from the perspectives of both the stigmatizer and the stigmatized person, consider the processes of stigma to be highly situationally specific, dynamic, complex, and nonpathological.

The responses of people to members of stigmatized groups are not consistently negative. Negative feelings toward persons with physical disabilities are frequently accompanied by sympathy; attitudes toward Blacks often involve sympathy and a desire to be fair and egalitarian, as well as negative affective reactions (Dovidio & Gaertner, 1998; Gaertner & Dovidio, 1986; Jones et al., 1984; Katz, 1981). This ambivalence, under some conditions, can produce more positive reactions to members of stigmatized groups than to people who are not stigmatized. Likewise, the responses of people to being stigmatized by others are not consistently negative. Although the experience of being devalued, stereotyped, and targeted by prejudice may take a toll on self-esteem, academic achievement, and other outcomes, many people with stigmatized attributes have high self-esteem, perform at high levels, are happy, and appear to be quite resilient despite their negative experiences. And just as contemporary research on stereotyping and prejudice indicate that the processes and expression of stereotypes are highly dependent on the situational context (e.g., Gaertner & Dovidio, 1986), the experience of being devalued is also highly dependent on social context (Crocker et al., 1998).

Because stigma is largely a social construction, a characteristic may be stigmatizing at one historical moment but not at another, or in one given situation but not in another within the same period. Context is also a critical determinant of the psychological consequences of stigmatization. Crocker and Quinn (in press) propose that "the consequences of social stigma emerge in the situation, as a function of the meaning that situation has for people with valued and devalued identities" (p. 2). These views illustrate the fundamentally social nature of stigma.

This volume focuses on the social psychology of stigma. Like theorists who take traditional approaches, the chapter authors in this volume uniformly view stigma as a social construction, shaped by cultural and historical forces. Moreover, what makes the present approach more uniquely social-psychological is the consistent emphasis on the effects of the immediate social and situational context on the stigmatizer; on the stigmatized; on their interaction; and ultimately on the personal and social affective, cognitive, and behavioral consequences of these transactions. However, the authors of this volume's chapters also recognize that stigma is more than an interpersonal process: It is determined by the broader cultural context (involving stereotypes, values, and ideologies), the meaning of the situation for participants, and the features of the situation that influence this meaning. In the remainder of this chapter, we define "stigma," consider different types of stigmas, explore potential functions of stigmatization, sketch a framework for viewing the range of phenomena involved in the study of stigma, and present an overview of the other chapters in this volume.

WHAT IS STIGMA?

Stigma is a powerful phenomenon, inextricably linked to the value placed on varying social identities. It is a social construction that involves at least two fundamental components: (1) the recognition of difference based on some distinguishing characteristic, or "mark"; and (2) a consequent devaluation of the person. Goffman (1963) described stigma as a sign or a mark that designates the bearer as "spoiled" and therefore as valued less than "normal" people. Stigmatized individuals are regarded as flawed, compromised, and somehow less than fully human. More recent definitions have focused on the contextual and dynamic nature of stigma. Jones and colleagues (1984) observed that "the stigmatizing process is relational. . . . [A] condition labeled as discrediting or deviant by one person may be viewed as benign and a charming eccentricity by another" (p. 5). Likewise, Crocker and colleagues (1998) have argued that "stigmatized individuals possess (or are believed to possess) some attribute, or characteristic, that conveys a social identity that is devalued *in some particular social context*" (emphasis added; p. 505). As Hebl and Kleck illustrate in Chapter 14 of this volume, aspects of the natural and constructed physical environment (e.g., steeply graded terrain or the absence of elevators) can also facilitate the stigmatization process in subtle and not-so-subtle ways. The social context and the physical environment thus fundamentally influence whether a characteristic of an individual will become stigmatizing or will be attended to at all.

The concept of stigma is related to, but not synonymous with, other negative evaluations of personal and social characteristics. With regard to personal qualities and individual identity, stigma is similar to the concepts of "marginality" (Frable, 1993) and "deviance" (Archer, 1985). Archer (1985) defines deviance as "a perceived behavior or condition that is thought to involve an undesirable departure in a compelling way from a putative standard" (p. 748). Frable (1993) defines marginality as belonging to a social group that is both statistically unusual and centrally defining. Like a person who is deviant or marginalized, a stigmatized person is perceived to represent a departure from normative expectations. However, people can be deviant or become marginalized because of unusual positive characteristics (e.g., extreme wealth) as well as negative ones (see Crocker et al., 1998; Frable, 1993), whereas people are stigmatized for having some undesirable characteristic. Moreover, even when deviance is associated with a negative quality, it may not involve stigmatization unless the distinguishing mark is associated with generalized inferences about the bearer's identity—attributions that "discredit the bearer" (Jones et al., 1984, p. 8). Thus, although stigma involves perceptions of deviance, it is more than that.

Stigma is also related to prejudice, in the sense that the person who is stigmatized is almost always the target of prejudice. "Prejudice" is widely defined as a negative attitude. Some researchers have asserted that *any* negative attitude toward a group represents prejudice (e.g., Ashmore, 1970, p. 253). However, other researchers have argued that a prejudicial attitude, by definition, is necessarily inaccurate or overgeneralized. Allport (1954/1979) defined prejudice as "an antipathy based on faulty and inflexible generalization. It may be felt or expressed. It may be directed toward a group as a whole, or toward an individual because he is a member of that group" (p. 9). Brigham (1971) defined prejudice as a negative attitude that (by whatever criterion) is seen as unjustified by an observer, whereas Jones (1986) used the term to refer to "a faulty generalization from a group characterization (stereotype) to an individual member of that group irrespective of either (1) the accuracy of the group stereotype, or (2) the applicability of the group characterization to the individual in question" (p. 288). Although stigmatization involves these elements of prejudice and, like prejudice, involves pervasive cultural ideologies about the worth of different groups, stigma is a more encompassing term.

In summary, stigma is a term that involves both deviance and prejudice but goes beyond both. Stigma involves perceptions of deviance but extends to more general attributions about character and identity. Stigma is more inclusive than prejudice because it involves individual-based responses to deviance, as well as group-based reactions as a function of category membership. Because stigma is socially defined, there is considerable variation across cultures and across time about what marks are stigmatizing (e.g., homosexuality—see Archer, 1985; being fat—see Archer, 1985; Crandall, 1994; Hebl & Heatherton, 1998). Thus the major negative impact of stigmatization normally resides not in the physical consequences of the mark, but rather in its social and psychological consequences. Although some stigmatizing conditions (e.g., AIDS) do involve direct threats to one's health, most do not. Rather, most potentially stigmatizing conditions (e.g., facial disfigurement) lead to social avoidance or rejection, and, through mechanisms such as these, threaten psychological health. Stigma can pose a direct threat to physical well-being, however, as illustrated by the recent murders of Blacks and gays in the United States. Furthermore, even when stigma and social rejection do not jeopardize physical well-being directly, they can do so indirectly—for example, through limiting access to health care, education, employment, and housing (see Miller & Major, Chapter 9, this volume), as well as through increasing stress and creating anxiety (see Cioffi, Chapter 7, this volume). Jones and colleagues (1984) noted, "It is the dramatic essence of the stigmatizing process that a label marking the deviant status is applied, and this marking process typically has devastating consequences for emotions, thought, and behavior" (p. 4). The psychological and social consequences of stigma involve the responses both of the perceivers and of stigmatized people themselves.

TYPES AND DIMENSIONS OF STIGMA

Researchers have long sought to organize stigmas into meaningful categories. In his classic monograph *Stigma: Notes on the Management of Spoiled Identity*, Goffman (1963) distinguished three different varieties of stigma or stigmatizing conditions: "abominations of the body" (e.g., physical deformities), "blemishes of individual character" (e.g., mental disorders, addictions, unemployment), and "tribal identities" (e.g., race, sex, religion, or nation). Using a different approach, Jones and colleagues (1984) identified six dimensions of stigmatizing conditions: (1) "concealability," which involves the extent to which the stigmatizing characteristic is necessarily visible (e.g., facial disfigurement vs. homosexuality); (2) "course of the mark," relating to whether the mark may become more salient or progressively debilitating over time (e.g., multiple sclerosis vs. blindness); (3) "disruptiveness," which refers to the degree to which the stigmatizing characteristic (e.g., stuttering) interferes with the flow of interpersonal interactions; (4) "aesthetics," which relates to subjective reactions to the unattractiveness of the stigma; (5) "origin" of the stigmatizing mark (such as congenital, accidental, or intentional), which can also involve the person's responsibility for creating the mark; and (6) peril, which involves the perceived danger of the stigmatizing conditions to others (e.g., having a highly contagious, lethal disease vs. being overweight). Scholars have also used an empirical approach to identify the dimensions of stigma (e.g., Deaux, Reid, Mizrahi, & Ethier, 1995; Frable, 1993). The dimensions that emerge as most central in this approach are the perceived danger of the stigma (peril), the visibility of the stigma (concealability), and the controllability of the stigma (origin) (Deaux et al., 1995; Frable, 1993).

In contrast to the distinctions made by Jones and colleagues (1984), Crocker and colleagues (1998) argue that "visibility" and "controllability" are the most important dimensions of stigma for the experience of both the stigmatizer and the stigmatized person. Crocker and colleagues (1998) propose that because visible stigmas are readily apparent, "the stigma can provide the primary schema through which everything about them is understood by others" (p. 507). The visibility of the stigma determines how aware stigmatized people are that reactions to them may be due to the stigma (Kleck & Strenta, 1980). A visible stigmatizing mark can create attributional ambiguity for outcomes, causing a stigmatized person to be uncertain whether negative outcomes are deserved or stem from others' prejudice (Crocker, Voelkl, Testa, & Major, 1991). In addition, the visibility of a stigmatizing mark can influence how people cope with stigma (Miller & Major, Chapter 9, this volume), how much of their effort they devote to concealing a stigma (Smart & Wegner, Chapter 8, this volume), and the extent to which they socially compare with stigmatized others. Those whose stigmas are invisible may be spared social rejection, but may suffer other costs that can ultimately affect well-being, such as a loss of social comparisons with and social support from similar others (Frable, Platt, & Hoey, 1998; Major & Gramzow, 1999).

The controllability of stigma directly involves the person's responsibility for having the stigmatizing mark in the first place, as well as for maintaining or eliminating the mark. Controllability is important because people with stigmas that are perceived to be controllable are less liked and more rejected than those whose stigmas are perceived to be uncontrollable (Weiner, Perry, & Magnusson, 1988; see also Crandall, Chapter 5, this volume). Perceptions of controllability for the same stigma (e.g., homosexuality, being overweight) can vary substantially among observers. These perceptions shape reactions in fundamental ways—cognitively (e.g., the amount of blame ascribed), emotionally (e.g., responding with anger or sympathy), and behaviorally (e.g., choosing to help) (Weiner et al., 1988). The perceived controllability of stigma is also an important dimension from the perspective of stigmatized persons. The perceived controllability of the stigma, for example, affects how stigmatized people construe others' reactions to them, as well as the impact of stigma on self-esteem (Crocker & Major, 1994).

FUNCTIONS OF STIGMATIZING OTHERS

Whereas the perspectives described above seek common defining features of stigma, an alternative perspective is to consider what functions stigmatization serves. Social stigma is ubiquitous and is observed in virtually every society. Crocker and colleagues (1998) observe: "The universality of social stigma suggests that it may have some functional value for the individual who stigmatizes, for the group from which he or she comes, for the society, or all of these" (p. 508). Stigmatizing others can serve several functions for an individual, including self-esteem enhancement, control enhancement, and anxiety buffering. Stigmatization can produce self-esteem enhancement through downward-comparison processes (Wills, 1981). According to downward-comparison theory, comparing oneself to less fortunate others can increase one's own subjective sense of well-being and therefore boost one's self-esteem. Downward comparison can be relatively passive (e.g., seeking out others who are less well off in some relevant dimension) or more active (e.g., creating a condition of disadvantage of others through discrimination). Stigmatization can involve both passive and active forms of downward comparison.

Stigmas arouse anxiety (see Hebl, Tickle, & Heatherton, Chapter 10, this volume) and feelings of threat in perceivers (see Blascovich, Mendes, Lickel, & Hunter, Chapter 11, this volume). Stigmatizing others can then enhance the stigmatizer's perceived and actual control to the extent that it leads to differential treatment, systematic avoidance, segregation, and marginalization of others who are threatening to the stigmatizer's personal well-being (e.g., criminals) or values (e.g., adherents of certain religions). In addition, to the extent that stigmatization elicits stereotypic associations for that "type" of target, the perceiver's feelings of control may be enhanced, because stereotypes create a larger context that enables the perceiver to go beyond the immediate information and make inferences about the character and future behavior of the target (Mackie, Hamilton, Susskind, & Rosselli, 1996).

Stigmas may also arouse a particular type of anxiety in others—an existential anxiety originating from awareness of their mortality. According to terror management theory (Solomon, Greenberg, & Pyszczynski, 1991), perceptions of difference and deviance are often sufficient to arouse existential anxiety; however, it is especially likely to occur when these differences generate concerns in people about their own vulnerability, such as when these stigmas involve physical disability and disfigurement. Existential anxiety, in turn, motivates people to reinforce their cultural world view. One way of doing so is to reject those who are different or who deviate from cultural norms or standards. This rejection of difference is likely to be particularly strong for stigmas based on abominations of the body, for which the mark is the source of the existential anxiety.

Stigmatization can also enhance self-esteem by motivating favorable intergroup comparisons. Social identity concerns become important when a mark represents a category of people (such as a racial, ethnic, or national group), rather than reflecting primarily on an individual. According to social identity theory (Tajfel & Turner, 1979), social categorization of people into outgroups (different from the self) and an ingroup (including the self) stimulates a motivation to perceive or achieve a sense of positive group distinctiveness. Like downward comparison, this motivation can initiate a search for dimensions on which the ingroup is favored over the outgroup (and to placing greater emphasis on these dimensions), and it can also motivate active discrimination against outgroups. Enhancement of one's own group relative to outgroups, then, reflects positively on collective as well as personal self-esteem.

In addition, stigmatization may arise from motivations to justify or rationalize the status quo in society, which often involves institutional forms of discrimination and segregation that serve both individual and group functions. Individually, this type of stigmatization can increase personal opportunity by limiting opportunities of potential competitors.

Stigmatization of this form serves a group justification function (see also system justification; Jost & Banaji, 1994), providing a rationale that explains and excuses disparate social treatment of identifiable groups of people. Also, through systematic discrimination and residential, occupational, and social segregation, it reinforces the collective control of one group over another. Historically, for example, White Americans developed racial ideologies that helped to justify the laws enabling them to achieve two important types of economic exploitation: slavery and the seizure of lands from native tribes (Klinker & Smith, 1999). Thus, although the belief that race is a biological construct is fundamental to racism, race (like other stigmatizing marks) is actually a social construction that permits the exploitation of one group over another with the development of the ideology that justifies it (Fields, 1990). What particular groups become stigmatized (e.g., Blacks or Italians) depends upon the function stigmatization serves for the dominant group. For instance, during the period of significant immigration from southern Europe to the United States during the early 1900s that generated social and economic threats to many Americans, Italians were characterized as racially and intellectually inferior. In Nazi Germany, Jews were stigmatized in the service of economic and political gain. Although the type of anxiety described by terror management theory is uniquely personal, threats to the integrity and future of one's group also exacerbate intergroup bias, conflict, intolerance for difference, and stigmatization (Brewer & Brown, 1998).

Perhaps because of the broad range of marks that provide a basis for stigmatization, the contextual and relational nature of stigma, and the conceptual breadth of the term, any attempt to summarize the essential elements of stigma either structurally or functionally will inevitably fall short. Nevertheless, in the next section we present a perspective for approaching stigma that helps to provide an organizing framework for the book.

A CONCEPTUAL FRAMEWORK

Rather than describing stigma in terms of its key structural elements or functions, we propose an alternative, complementary perspective that attempts to locate the study of stigma within the larger context of general social-psychological processes. As illustrated in Figure 1.1, there are three fundamental dimensions within this model: (1) "perceiver–target," (2) "personal–group-based identity," and (3) "affective–cognitive–behavioral response."

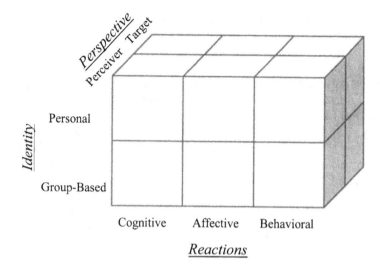

FIGURE 1.1. Three dimensions in the study of stigma.

The Perceiver–Target Dimension

As is evident from our foregoing discussion, one of the most basic issues in understanding stigma and stigmatization involves recognizing the different perspectives and experiences of those who are stigmatizing others and those who are being stigmatized. We have termed those who are stigmatizing others "perceivers." Some researchers have referred to these people as "nonstigmatized" or as "normals." We note, however, that people who are involved in stigmatizing others may also be stigmatized in some way themselves. This may occur on a different dimension (e.g., deaf people stigmatizing others on the basis of race); on the same dimension, such as race (e.g., Asians stigmatizing Blacks); or within one's own racial group (e.g., lighter-skinned Blacks stigmatizing darker-skinned Blacks; Russell, Wilson, & Hall, 1992). We also acknowledge, however, that "perceivers" are not simply "observers": They participate actively in perceptual, memorial, interpretational, and attributional processes, and in the behavioral processes that can perpetuate and exacerbate stigmatization. Similarly, "targets" are not passive recipients of stigmatization: They too are active perceivers who interpret, cope, and respond to stigmatization (see Hebl & Kleck, Chapter 14, this volume). We have adopted the terms "perceiver" and "target" because, however imperfect, they best apply to the broader range of work in social psychology.

Differences in perspective between perceivers and targets, such as those between actors and observers, have a great impact on the types of attributions (e.g., situational or dispositional) that people make for the same behaviors (Jones & Nisbett, 1971). In addition, perceivers and targets have different needs, goals, and motivations, which can further shape how they perceive and interpret information in different ways (Deaux & Major, 1987; Swann, 1987). These different perspectives influence the social roles of stigmatizers and stigmatized persons, influence how they adapt to and cope with those roles, and ultimately affect the development of personal and group identities.

A recognition of the distinct perspective and experiences of perceivers and targets suggests that a truly comprehensive understanding of stigma requires studying the *interaction* of perceivers and targets (see Jussim, Palumbo, Chatman, Madon, & Smith, Chapter 13, this volume). Unfortunately, we know considerably more about perceivers and targets separately than we do about their actions together. With respect to prejudice, Devine and Vasquez (1998) have observed:

> Somewhat symptomatic of the limitations of existing theory is that the previous work has examined majority group members (e.g., whites and heterosexuals) and minority group members (e.g., blacks and homosexuals) separately. . . . As a result, the literature has had very little to offer to help us understand the nature of the interpersonal dynamics of intergroup contact. . . . We have not yet examined carefully and fully the nature of interpersonal dynamics that emerge between majority and minority group members when they are brought together in a specific interpersonal situation. In other words, we do not know what happens when interaction begins. (pp. 240–241)

Furthermore, when interaction is studied, it is often not interaction with others who are *actually* stigmatized, but with others who are *believed* to be stigmatized. For example, one common paradigm that has been used in studies of the self-fulfilling prophecy is to lead perceivers to believe that the person with whom they are interacting has a particular characteristic (e.g., is attractive or unattractive; Snyder, Tanke, & Berscheid, 1977), whereas the target is another naive participant who is randomly assigned to the condition and is unaware that he or she is being stigmatized. How these participants behave may not closely resemble the responses of people who are aware that they are being stigmatized, who have been chronically stigmatized, who have internalized (although they do not necessarily endorse) aspects of the stigmatization, and who have made the consequent adjustments and developed the coping styles that enable them to adapt daily to being stigmatized (see Crocker, 1999; Miller & Myers, 1998; Steele & Aronson, 1995).

In summary, we believe that the distinction between perceivers and targets is fundamental to understanding stigma and stigmatization. The distinction between perceivers and targets is at least as important for understanding stigma as, and probably more important than, the distinction between actors and observers is for understanding the fundamental attribution error. Nonetheless, as we have noted earlier, stigma is not only an interpersonal phenomenon but also a collective and cultural one, and its effects are observable in the absence as well as the presence of social interaction. Consequently, a full understanding of stigma will require going beyond studying targets, perceivers, and their interactions. We return to this issue later in the chapter.

The Personal–Group-Based Identity Dimension

The second fundamental dimension of our framework involves the distinction between personal and social identity. The distinction between interpersonal and intergroup processes is a prevalent one in social psychology. Although some theorists have focused on the similarities in the processes that govern these phenomena (see Hamilton & Sherman, 1996), others have emphasized that different modes of processing are involved. These different modes critically influence cognitive representations and affective, or evaluative, responses.

Taking the perspective of the perceiver, Fiske and Neuberg (1990) propose that "people form impressions of others through a variety of processes that lie on a continuum reflecting the extent to which the perceiver utilizes a target's particular attributes" (p. 2). At one end of the continuum are category-based processes, in which category membership determines impressions with minimal attention to individual attributes. At the other end of the continuum are individuating processes, in which individual characteristics, but not group membership, influence impressions. Brewer (1988) has similarly proposed a dual-process model of impression formation, with the primary distinction in this model being person-based and category-based responding. Person-based processing is bottom-up and data-driven, beginning "at the most concrete level and stops at the lowest level of abstraction required by the prevailing processing objectives" (Brewer, 1988, p. 6). Category-based processing, in contrast, proceeds from global to specific; it is top-down. Like Fiske and Neuberg (1990), Brewer proposes that category-based processing is more likely to occur than person-based processing, because social information is typically organized around social categories.

From the perspective of the target as well as of the perceiver, the distinction between personal identity and social identity is a critical one. Self-categorization theory (Turner, Hogg, Oakes, Reicher, & Wetherell,

1987; see also social identity theory, Tajfel & Turner, 1979) proposes that these are two ends of a continuum, and that where a person is on this continuum determines his or her responses. When personal identity is salient, an individual's needs, standards, beliefs, and motives primarily determine behavior. In contrast, when people's social identity is activated, "people come to perceive themselves more as interchangeable exemplars of a social category than as unique personalities defined by their individual differences from others" (Turner et al., 1987, p. 50). Under these conditions, collective needs, goals, and standards are primary (Verkuyten & Hagendoorn, 1998). Thus whether a person's personal or collective identity is more salient is a factor that critically shapes how the person perceives, interprets, evaluates, and responds to situations and to others.

In summary, because stigma is both an interpersonal and an intergroup phenomenon, understanding it requires a knowledge of both (1) personal processes, reactions, and identity; and (2) collective processes, action, and identity. The distinction between individual and categorical responses is a fundamental one for considering the behaviors of targets as well as of perceivers. It affects how people process information, how they interpret information and make attributions, and what motives are most salient. We have avoided the term "versus" in describing this dimension because, as other theorists have argued, we believe that the personal–group-based identity dimension represents a continuum rather than totally discrete, mutually exclusive states.

The Affective-Cognitive-Behavioral Dimension

Affective, cognitive, and behavioral elements reflect the basic components of the tripartite view of attitudes in general and intergroup attitudes in particular (Harding, Proshansky, Kutner, & Chein, 1969). Some researchers (e.g., Zajonc, 1980) have argued that the distinction between affective and cognitive systems is a basic one. The affective system is hypothesized to be more primitive and fundamental, faster, but more diffuse than the cognitive system. The cognitive system, in contrast, may be slower but is more deliberative, elaborative, and goal-directed. Behavioral reactions may precede emotional experience or full cognitive deliberation (as the James–Lange theory proposed), or they may be consequences of affective reactions or cognitive effort, or they may stem from the joint effects of both. However, as with our other two dimensions, we propose that the affective–cognitive–behavioral distinction does not represent necessarily separate processes. Instead, stigmatization reflects a blend of these processes and their interactions, with the primacy of the factors being a function of the nature of the stigma, the context in which it is encountered, and individual differences among the interactants.

Affective reactions may play a primary role in stigmas involving people with facial disfigurements or other "abominations of the body" (Siller, Ferguson, Vann, & Holland, 1968; see also Jones et al., 1984). Stigmas of this type commonly produce dominant, affective negative reactions of an "untutored, primitive quality" (Jones et al., 1984, p. 226) and immediate behavioral aversion. These responses may have a genetic, evolutionary basis. Consistent with this notion, these reactions occur cross-culturally (Douglas, 1966), early in development (Jones et al., 1984), and across species (Hebb & Thompson, 1968; Wilson, 1975). Nevertheless, cognitive factors can also play an important (if secondary) role. Despite potentially genetic predispositions, these reactions may be altered by learning and experience (e.g., among members of the medical community; see Jones et al., 1984). In addition, cognitive consideration of social standards and personal standards can elicit a subsequent and quite different emotion—sympathy. Thus, as a consequence of cognitive consequences of initial negative reactions, attitudes toward people with physical deformities or disabilities may be strongly ambivalent (Katz, 1981).

Although the negative affective reaction to people with physical disfigurements and disabilities is unusual in its spontaneity and intensity, overall ambivalent responses can occur for other types of stigma as well. For instance, with respect to tribal stigmas, Katz (1981) suggested parallels between the reactions of "normal" persons to people with physical disabilities and the responses of many Whites to Blacks. Many Whites initially experience feelings of anxiety, discomfort, fear, and aversion in the presence of Blacks (Kovel, 1970; Gaertner & Dovidio, 1986). Their behavior is spontaneously avoidant. Nevertheless, many Whites also develop feelings of sympathy for Blacks. The simultaneous existence of negative and positive feelings among Whites characterizes the nature of the ambivalence hypothesized to be central to many forms of contemporary racial attitudes (see Dovidio & Gaertner, 1998).

Whereas affective reactions may be more likely to dominate initial reactions to stigmas that are more individually oriented, reactions to those that are more collective may initially be "cooler" and more cognitive. For instance, collective stigmas are often associated with well-learned, consensual stereotypes. These stereotypic schemas, which may be spontaneously accessible, significantly influence how information is encoded, stored, and retrieved: "Once cued, schemas affect how quickly we perceive, what we notice, how we interpret what we notice, and what we perceive as similar and different" (Fiske & Taylor, 1991, p. 122). They also influence how the perceiver behaves toward the target, and ultimately how the target responds. Affect may be secondary in these types of situations.

An association between personal–group-based identity and affective–cognitive reactions may be common, but these dimensions do not necessarily coincide. For example, emotional reactions (e.g., anger, sympathy) to a person with AIDS (largely an individual-level mark) may be determined largely by the attributions a perceiver makes about the cause of the condition (e.g., drug use, blood transfusion)—a basic cognitive activity (see Weiner et al., 1988). With respect to "blemishes of individual character," criminals may elicit both affective and cognitive reactions. Which is the preponderant response, however, may be determined by the specific nature of the crime. A murderer may be likely to elicit particularly strong negative affective reactions (fear, anger, revulsion) and aversion; attributions and stereotypes may be secondary. In contrast, an embezzler may primarily bring to mind stereotypic associations of "white-collar criminals"; the affective reaction is likely to be less intense and less negative. Nevertheless, stereotypes may produce further affective reactions. The activation of stereotypes can make other affective information accessible (Fiske, 1982; Fiske, Neuberg, Beattie, & Milberg, 1987; Fiske & Pavelchak, 1986). Affective responses involve a "range of preferences, evaluations, moods, and emotions" (Fiske & Taylor, 1991, p. 410).

In summary, stigmatization is associated with affective, cognitive, and behavioral reactions. These may occur in any order, and their effects are not necessarily independent. For example, affective reactions may occur initially, but subsequent cognitive responses can temper, modify, or justify these affective responses, sometimes producing other emotions that create psychological ambivalence. Alternatively, cognitive activity (e.g., attributions) may occur first; the consequence of the attributional process then determines the affective reaction (e.g., sympathy or disgust), which ultimately motivates action. We propose that which type of response occurs first or foremost is conditional upon the type of stigma involved; the context in which it is encountered; and individual differences in experiences, beliefs, values, goals, and roles.

Advantages of the Three-Dimensional Framework

Overall, we believe that the three-dimensional framework we have outlined has three main advantages. First, it may help to suggest links to fundamental processes that are of general interest to social psychology—for example, to stereotyping, prejudice, threat, and coping. Thus research on this topic not only can be viewed in terms of its unique contribution to understanding the phenomenon of stigma, but also can be appreciated for its contribution to our knowledge of more general psychological processes. Second, this framework provides a way to organize and integrate research. For example, research on stigma and stereotypes has largely focused on the perceptions of the perceiver, on cognitive responses, and on collective stigmas. Research on responses to facial disfigurement have focused both on reactions of perceivers (generally affective and occurring at the individual level) and on adjustments made by targets (both cognitive and affective, but also focusing largely on individual identity; see Lefebvre & Munro, 1986). Mapping out the areas for which considerable research and conceptual understanding exist may also help us recognize the areas that are underresearched and not well understood. Third, considering stigmatization along multiple dimensions such as these may encourage a greater emphasis on the complex, iterative, and dynamic relationships between stigmatizers and people being stigmatized.

Limitations of the Framework

Any attempt to organize a topic as broad and complex as stigma will involve oversimplification, which may obscure critical distinctions or exclude important points. We have presented our framework as an organizing one, not necessarily as a comprehensive perspective. The approach has its limitations, and here we acknowledge two of the most significant. First, the perceiver–target dimension implies that stigma occurs only in social interaction. This is consistent with the approach of Jones and colleagues (1984), which emphasizes stigma in social transactions— and primarily in one-on-one interactions. Nevertheless, as we have noted earlier, it is important to emphasize that stigma is a collective and cultural phenomenon, not simply an interpersonal one. Many of the consequences of stigma occur in the absence of interactions with a perceiver. Crocker (1999) has argued that the interaction between the collective representations one brings to a situation and the nature of the situation, rather than the interaction between a target and perceiver, is what shapes stigmatization. Cultural representations are stereotypes, ideologies, values, and beliefs that are widely known, often widely shared, and widely communicated in the mass media, whether or not people actually endorse them. Stigmatized people, either through direct experience or through awareness of cultural representations, know that their social identity is devalued by others (Crocker et al., 1998). Awareness that one's social identity is devalued can threaten both collective esteem and personal self-esteem, although it does not necessarily lead either to low personal self-esteem or to low collective esteem. In addition to knowing that their social identity is generally devalued by others, stigmatized persons may also be cognizant of specific stereotypes of their group. Awareness of negative stereotypes associated with one's group, in turn, can produce a particular vulnerability that Steele and Aronson (1995; see also Steele, 1997) have identified as "stereotype threat." In contrast to the potentially general reactions to the devaluation of one's group, stereotype threat leads to self-threat only when the specific content of a negative stereotype is salient and directly relevant to one's behavior or attributes in a given situation. For example, emphasizing that a test is diagnostic of one's ability can increase the salience of stereotypes about the intellectual limitations of African Americans, which can produce poorer performance on the task for African American but not for European American students (Steele & Aronson, 1995). These findings illustrate that the negative consequences of stigma do not require an interaction between a target and perceiver, or even the presence of a perceiver. Although this perspective is not emphasized in the social interaction framework presented here, it does not preclude it.

Second, the identification of separate levels of the dimensions may imply a discrete difference, when actually the dimensions are continuous and responses may reflect a blend of reactions. With respect to the personal–group-based identity dimension, for instance, self-categorization theory (Turner et al., 1987) views individual and collective identity as a continuum. Which is salient, and the degree to which each is salient, are functions of the social context. In terms of the cognitive–affective–behavioral distinction, all of these types of reactions are typically inextricably involved and linked. Nearly all stigmas involve some affective reaction, and beliefs, values, and meanings (if not clear stereotypes) are implicated in stigmatization. Behavioral responses may be consequences of these responses or may precede and shape cognitive and affective reactions.

Nevertheless, despite its obvious limitations, the three-dimensional framework we have presented here can help to illustrate how the chapters in this volume relate to one another; beyond that, it may be useful for identifying areas that are currently underresearched but are potentially theoretically and pragmatically productive. In the next section we consider the implications of this framework as an integrating theme, as we provide an overview of the each of the chapters within this volume.

CHAPTER OVERVIEWS

Part I of this volume includes four chapters that focus on stigmatization from the perspective of the perceiver. Neuberg, Smith, and Asher (Chapter 2) approach the issue of why people stigmatize from a "biocultural" orientation. These authors acknowledge that stigmatization may serve valuable proximate functions by improving the psychological welfare of the stigmatizer, and they recognize the importance of immediate social forces in the development and expression of stigmatization (see Stangor & Crandall, Chapter 3). However, they propose, more broadly and fundamentally, that stigmatization "is rooted primarily in the biologically based need to live in effective groups" (p. 33).

Specifically, Neuberg, Smith, and Asher argue that stigmatization is a response to factors that threaten the effectiveness and efficiency of group functioning, which is an essential aspect of human existence. Stigmatization occurs when basic principles of group living—reciprocity, trust, common values, and group welfare—are violated. With respect to the first principle, people who take more than they give by intention (e.g., by thievery) or by limited ability to reciprocate (e.g., by disability) are likely to be stigmatized. In terms of trust, cheaters and traitors (e.g., "Benedict Arnolds") are also targets of stigmatization because they threaten group welfare. Because effective group functioning depends on common values and ideals, people (e.g., homosexuals) who are seen by others as undermining the socialization of mainstream group values become stigmatized. Whereas the first three principles apply mainly to responses to members of one's own group who threaten group functioning from within, the fourth principle recognizes that outgroup members will also be stigmatized if their actions are seen to be threatening to the welfare of one's group. Neuberg and colleagues suggest that this biocultural approach helps to explain the ubiquity of stigmatization in terms of both process and content across time and culture.

Stangor and Crandall (Chapter 3) also examine the origins of stigmatization. They first consider why some attributes appear to be universally stigmatized (e.g., mental illness), whereas others (e.g., fatness) show substantial variability across cultures. In their attempt to answer the question about why people stigmatize others, Stangor and Crandall next review a range of theories of psychological processes in other domains. These theories involve the functions of stigmatization, the development of new beliefs or accentuation of existing beliefs based on group categorization and differentiation, and the role of social consensus in the origin and maintenance of stigmatization. The authors offer an integrative analysis of the etiology of stigmas and stigmatization that centers on stigma as threat. Threat may be realistic and involve tangible outcomes, or it may be symbolic and associated with challenges to one's world view. Thus, whereas Neuberg, Smith, and Asher emphasize the more distal causes of stigmatization, Stangor and Crandall focus on more proximate psychological forces. As Neuberg and his colleagues articulate, these may be viewed as complementary rather than competing perspectives.

Biernat and Dovidio, in Chapter 4, also focus on the perceiver in the process of stigmatization. However, whereas the previous two chapters emphasize general processes and conditions that facilitate the development of stigmatization, Biernat and Dovidio examine how specific cultural associations with stigmatized groups and members of those groups, once established, can either influence affective, cognitive, and behavioral responses to the stigmatized or arise as justifications for the negative treatment of these groups. Within the three-dimensional framework, this chapter emphasizes the perceiver, group-based identities, and cognitive processes. The authors argue that "although stereotyping and stigmatization are closely related terms, they are not identical. Stigmatization can sometimes occur in the absence of consensual stereotypes" (p. 89). The importance of stereotyping is hypothesized to be greater for socially identifiable groups (e.g., groups bearing tribal stigmas, or people with common defects of character), to rationalize negative group-based attitudes and discrimination, than it is for people with more idiosyncratic stigmas that may generate more immediate and readily explained reactions. Biernat and Dovidio propose that stereotypes help to justify stigmatization, but these authors view stereotypes as potential consequences as well as causes of negative reactions to stigmatized people.

In Chapter 5, the final chapter of Part I, Crandall further explores the consequences of stigmatization for the perceiver. Crandall proposes that general "justification ideologies" precede and thus shape reactions to stigmatized individuals. He asks this question: "Do people experience a near-total collapse of empathy, unaware of the pain of exclusion while willingly excluding the stigmatized?" (p. 126). He answers, "This is unlikely," and instead proposes that people adopt beliefs that justify stigmatization and "allow, release, or even *promote* stigmatization responses" (original emphasis, p. 128). Crandall identifies two categories of justification ideologies. One is an "attributional" approach, in which attributions of causality, responsibility, and blame justify stigmatization. The other is a "hierarchical" approach, in which superior–inferior relations are accepted as good, inevitable, or "natural." This distinction corresponds roughly to the personal–group-based distinction in our three-dimensional framework: Attributions generally involve explanations for an individual's actions or condition, whereas hierarchical ideologies relate to the social order of groups. Moreover, both attributional and hierarchical justifications shape the affective, cognitive, and ultimately the behavioral reactions to stigmatized people and groups. For example, attributing responsibility for a mark to the stigmatized target can produce anger rather than empathy, can influence the salience of consonant cognitions, and can determine whether the stigmatized will be responded to with assistance or aversion (see Weiner, 1986). Crandall concludes that these justification beliefs "provide cognitive and emotional cover for negative treatment of stigmatized individuals" (p. 144).

Part II of this volume focuses on the responses of the stigmatized. The four chapters in this section emphasize the active role that stigmatized persons play in reacting to coping with stigmatization.

In Chapter 6, Crocker and Quinn consider the consequences of social stigma for the self-esteem of stigmatized individuals. They begin by considering the historical context of research on social stigma and self-esteem, and the way in which the established wisdom of social psychology came to suggest that social stigma creates low self-esteem for those who are stigmatized. They then "briefly consider the empirical evidence for this claim, which is at best inconsistent and at worst contradictory" (p. 153). According to Crocker and Quinn, this contradiction is related to a basic problem in the way self-esteem is defined in much of this literature—as a stable trait consistent across social situations and contexts. Instead, they argue that self-esteem is a judgment about the worth of the self "constructed at the moment, in the situation, as a function of the meanings that individuals bring with them to the situation, and features of the situation that make those meanings relevant or irrelevant" (pp. 153–154).

Cioffi, in Chapter 7, discusses what she calls "the 'social token,' who navigates the commute between public acts and private self-views" (p. 185). A social token is a notable representative of a social category (by virtue of his or her distinctiveness) who believes that others hold negative attitudes about him or her because of social category membership. The target's perspective; group-based identity; and cognitions, expectations, and behaviors are central themes in this chapter. Specifically, Cioffi outlines a model of how feelings of social distinctiveness intensifies feelings of being scrutinized by others, which affect how people manage their public behaviors. How people behave in front of others then influences the actor's (in this case, the stigmatized person's) self-definition. Cioffi's model resembles the "looking-glass self" metaphor—the idea the people come to see themselves as others see them (Cooley, 1902/1956). However, she expands upon this perspective by emphasizing, first, the importance of a stigmatized person's perceptions of what others "see"; and, second, the person's interpretations of his or her own public behavior as reflections of identity.

Smart and Wegner, in Chapter 8, pursue Goffman's (1963) observation that people experience physical strain in the process of attempting to conceal "invisible" stigmas. Within the three-dimensional framework we have presented, this chapter emphasizes the cognitive responses of targets to their social identity as potentially stigmatized persons. The authors' analysis is guided by the "preoccupation model of secrecy" (Lane

& Wegner, 1995), which proposes that strategies employed to maintain secrecy, such as thought suppression, often activate cognitive processes that produce excessive thinking about the secret. In particular, attempts at thought suppression lead to intrusive thoughts about the secret, which result in renewed efforts to keep the thoughts out of consciousness, and ultimately to a preoccupation with the secret and its suppression. Smart and Wegner review research on stigmatization that is consistent with this model; they also describe their own research, which provides direct support for the preoccupation model as it applies to invisible stigmas (eating disorders). They conclude the chapter by considering strategies for the mental control of invisible stigmas.

In Chapter 9, Miller and Major address the ways in which stigmatized targets cope with prejudice and stigma-related stress. Within the three-dimensional framework presented here, this chapter emphasizes the target; personal identity concerns; and affective, cognitive, and behavioral responses to stigma. Framing their analysis within theories of stress and coping, Miller and Major argue that the implications of stigma for the psychological well-being of stigmatized individuals depend on how these individuals appraise their predicament and on the coping strategies they use to deal with it. Miller and Major address two broad, overlapping categories of coping strategies the stigmatized may adopt. "Problem-focused" coping strategies attempt to reduce problems associated with the stigma, and can include coping efforts targeted at the self (e.g., dieting), at the perceivers (e.g., eliminating their prejudice), or at the situation (e.g., avoidance). "Emotion-focused" coping strategies attempt to regulate stressful emotions associated with the stigma and seek to protect self-esteem from threat. Group identity, stigma concealability, and perceived control are discussed as moderators of these coping strategies. Miller and Major conclude with a discussion of the costs of different coping strategies, and with the observation that no one strategy is likely to be effective for all individuals across all situations.

The four chapters in Part III of the volume offer a close examination of the nature and consequences of interactions between perceivers and targets—the "social interface." Hebl, Tickle, and Heatherton explore "awkward moments" in social transactions between nonstigmatized and stigmatized individuals in Chapter 10. These authors define such moments as disruptions in the flow of interaction. Two themes emerge from their examination of firsthand accounts of awkward moments by both nonstigmatized and stigmatized individuals. First, anxiety, which is defined as physiological arousal accompanied by apprehension, "is present as a precursor or as a concomitant to each awkward moment" (p. 280). Second, both stigmatized and nonstigmatized individuals "arrange their lives so as to minimize or altogether avoid [these interactions]" (p. 281).

Hebl et al. expand upon the notion of anxiety to consider the role of fear, lack of experience, concern about violating norms, thought suppression, misinterpretations, hostility, and ambivalence in accounting for the awkward moments of nonstigmatized individuals. These reactions involve both personal and category-based identity, as well as relate to cognitive, affective, and behavioral responses. The authors further identify fear of rejection, awareness of being "on stage," and social expectations as factors underlying the awkward moments of stigmatized individuals. Hebl et al. conclude by highlighting the importance of attenuating awkward moments and suggesting specific strategies for reducing the awkwardness of these interactions.

In Chapter 11, Blascovich, Mendes, Lickel, and Hunter examine how and why stigma increases the likelihood of "antisocial interaction." They explore affective, cognitive, and behavioral responses, but suggest the overarching influence of motivation, which involves these responses but is "more than simply the sum or even the interaction of these components" (p. 308). From the perspective of perceivers, the authors propose that threat, involving "the perception of possible physical or psychological harm" (p. 309), motivates either flight or fight in interactions involving stigmatized individuals. This threat may be a reaction to negative stereotypes (associated group-based identities) or unlearned affective cues (often person-based). The targets, the stigmatized persons, also experience threat in terms of negative reactions and the experience of prejudice and discrimination. Blascovich et al. draw on their previous work on challenge and threat as general motivational states, and they review physiological markers of these states. They then apply this framework, both theoretically and empirically, to understanding the nature, processes, and consequences of interactions between stigmatized and nonstigmatized individuals.

Zebrowitz and Montepare explore the operation of a particular type of stigmas, age stigmas, in Chapter 12. Specifically, they "examine the stigmatizing experiences of those who are 'too young' or 'too old,' the ways in which age-stigmatized people cope with those experiences, and the possible functions of age stigmas" (p. 334). The course of age stigmas is also relatively unique: People typically mature from one stigmatized category (adolescence) to the nonstigmatized and then to another stigmatized category (the elderly). Zebrowitz and Montepare also explore the importance of cultural and situational context for age-based schemas. They observe, "The social–developmental framework of this chapter emphasizes that no individual who achieves his or her full life expectancy can avoid being a member of a stigmatized group" (p. 361). Like Biernat and Dovidio in Chapter 4, these authors focus on a group-based identity. However, more than the previous chapters, this chapter emphasizes both the perceiver and the target. Zebrowitz and Montepare document negative stereotypes, prejudice, and discrimination toward adolescents and the elderly; discuss people's awareness of and immediate reactions to these biases; and consider longer-term coping and compensation mechanisms—affective, cognitive, and behavioral.

In Chapter 13, Jussim, Palumbo, Chatman, Madon, and Smith extend Blascovich and colleagues' and Hebl and colleagues' analyses of the nature of interaction between nonstigmatized and stigmatized individuals into the area of self-fulfilling prophecies. A self-fulfilling prophecy occurs when initially erroneous social beliefs lead to their own fulfillment—that is, when the targets of these beliefs come to behave in a manner that is consistent with and actually confirms the erroneous beliefs. This chapter thus focuses on the dynamics of social interactions between targets and perceivers, and on how group-based identities can shape the nature and behavioral consequences of these interactions. Jussim et al. first discuss early research on the self-fulfilling prophecy, and then provide a review and critical evaluation of research on the role of self-fulfilling prophecies in maintaining beliefs about stigmatized individuals in dyadic interaction. Although the processes underlying self-fulfilling prophecies are frequently initiated by the biased attitudes and stereotypes of perceivers, Jussim and his colleagues also note that targets' beliefs that another person stigmatizes them may also stimulate these processes. Like other chapters, this chapter emphasizes the importance of the interaction between targets and perceivers; however, Jussim and colleagues conclude by acknowledging that self-fulfilling prophecies may also occur at a sociological level, involving political and institutional policies. This again suggests the important role of collective representations in stigmatization.

The final chapter in this volume—Chapter 14, by Hebl and Kleck—explores the social consequences of a particular category of stigmas: physical limitations. The authors acknowledge that physical disabilities and their consequences are diverse, and thus that generalizations should be made cautiously. Nevertheless, Hebl and Kleck identify five fundamental issues for understanding the consequences of physical limitations. They first examine nonequitable and dysfunctional interaction outcomes that occur for physically disabled people. These range from direct and overt negative responses (e.g., jokes and rejection), to more indirect forms (e.g., avoidance) or more complex reactions (e.g., discrepant verbal and nonverbal responses), to unintentional forms (e.g., overly protective behaviors or unwanted and unnecessary assistance). The second dimension that Hebl and Kleck review involves both social and physical constraints on people with physical disabilities. In terms of social constraints, terms such as "the physically disabled" overemphasize the person's physical features, heighten awareness of difference, and threaten individual identity and "personhood." Physical constraints, such as restricted access (e.g., unavailability of elevators), can similarly increase the salience of a person's disability unnecessarily.

The other basic issues of physical disability that Hebl and Kleck discuss are dimensions of disability stigmas, attributions associated with these stigmas, and strategies for "unspoiling" interactions between physically disabled and nondisabled persons. In addition to the dimension of visibility controllability, which we have considered earlier in this chapter for stigmas more generally, Hebl and Kleck note that mobility impairment is an important additional dimension of stigmas associated with physical disability. The ways a person's physical disability is perceived along these dimensions, in turn, shape the types of attributions people make and influence their evaluations and expectations. The authors conclude their chapter by recognizing the role that a stigmatized person can play in reshaping these attributions, evaluations, and expectations. For example, individuals may try to downplay or hide their disability (i.e., try to "pass"). Alternatively, they may choose to openly acknowledge their stigma to others. The decision about which strategy to adopt, and the effectiveness of that strategy, are functions of the nature of the disability, the physical and social context, and the attitudes and expectations of the interactants. This chapter thus not only reflects the theme of the social interface in this section of the book. It also reinforces the volume's overall emphasis on the value of considering the perspectives of both the perceiver and the target; the relevance of both personal and collective identities; and the relations among cognitive, affective, and behavioral reactions in developing a comprehensive understanding of stigma and stigmatization.

ACKNOWLEDGMENTS

We express our appreciation to Bob Kleck for his helpful comments and guidance on earlier versions of this chapter, and to the editors for their support. Preparation of this chapter was supported by National Institute of Mental Health Grant No. MH 48721 to John F. Dovidio, and by National Institute of Mental Health Grant No. 1 R01 MH58869-01 to Jennifer Crocker.

REFERENCES

Adorno, T. W., Frenkel-Brunswik, E., Levinson, D. J., & Sanford, R. N. (1950). *The authoritarian personality.* New York: Harper.

Allport, G. (1979). *The nature of prejudice.* New York: Doubleday/Anchor. (Original work published 1954)

Archer, D. (1985). Social deviance. In G. Lindzey & E. Aronson (Eds.), *Handbook of social psychology* (3rd ed., Vol. 2, pp. 743–804). New York: Random House.

Ashmore, R. D. (1970). Prejudice: Causes and cures. In B. E. Collins (Ed.), *Social psychology: Social influence, attitude change, group processes, and prejudice* (pp. 245–339). Reading, MA: Addison-Wesley.

Brewer, M. B. (1988). A dual process model of impression formation. In T. S. Srull & R. S. Wyer (Eds.), *Advances in social cognition: Vol. 1. A dual process model of impression formation* (pp. 1–36). Hillsdale, NJ: Erlbaum.

Brewer, M. B., & Brown, R. J. (1998). Intergroup relations. In D. Gilbert, S. T. Fiske, & G. Lindzey (Eds.), *Handbook of social psychology* (4th ed., Vol. 2, pp. 554–594). Boston: McGraw-Hill.

Brigham, J. C. (1971). Ethnic stereotypes. *Psychological Bulletin, 76*, 15–38.

Cooley, C. H. (1956). *Human nature and the social order.* New York: Free Press. (Original work published 1902)

Crandall, C. S. (1994). Prejudice against fat people: Ideology and self-interest. *Journal of Personality and Social Psychology, 66*, 882–894.

Crocker, J. (1999). Social stigma and self-esteem: Situational construction of self-worth. *Journal of Experimental Social Psychology, 35*, 89–107.

Crocker, J., & Major, B. (1989). Social stigma and self-esteem: The self-protective properties of stigma. *Psychological Review, 96*, 608–630.

Crocker, J., & Major, B. (1994). Reactions to stigma: The moderating role of justifications. In M. P. Zanna & J. M. Olson (Eds.), *The Ontario Symposium: Vol. 7. The psychology of prejudice* (pp. 289–314). Hillsdale, NJ: Erlbaum.

Crocker, J., Major, B., & Steele, C. (1998). Social stigma. In D. T. Gilbert, S. T. Fiske, & G. Lindzey (Eds.), *Handbook of social psychology* (4th ed., Vol. 2, pp. 504–553). Boston: McGraw-Hill.

Crocker, J., & Quinn, D. M. (in press). Psychological consequences of devalued identities. In R. Brown & S. L. Gaertner (Eds.), *Blackwell handbook of social psychology, Vol. 4. Intergroup processes.* Cambridge, UK: Blackwell.

Crocker, J., Voelkl, K., Testa, M., & Major, B. (1991). Social stigma: The affective consequences of attributional ambiguity. *Journal of Personality and Social Psychology, 60*, 218–228.

Deaux, K., & Major, B. (1987). Putting gender into context: An integrative model of gender-related behavior. *Psychological Review, 94*, 369–389.

Deaux, K., Reid, A., Mizrahi, K., & Ethier, K. A. (1995). Parameters of social identity. *Journal of Personality and Social Psychology, 68*, 280–291.

Devine, P. G., & Vasquez, K. A. (1998). The rocky road to positive intergroup relations. In J. Eberhardt & S. T. Fiske (Eds.), *Confronting racism: The problem and the response* (pp. 234–262). Thousand Oaks, CA: Sage.

Douglas, M. (1966). *Purity and danger: An analysis of concepts of pollution and taboo.* New York: Praeger.

Dovidio, J. F., & Gaertner, S. L. (1998). On the nature of contemporary prejudice: The causes, consequences, and challenges of aversive racism. In J. Eberhardt & S. T. Fiske (Eds.), *Confronting racism: The problem and the response* (pp. 3–32). Thousand Oaks, CA: Sage.

Fields, B. J. (1990, May/June). Slavery, race, and ideology in the United States of America. *New Left Review, 181*, 95–118.

Fiske, S. T. (1982). Schema-triggered affect: Applications to social perception. In M. S. Clark & S. T. Fiske (Eds.), *The seventeenth annual Carnegie Symposium on Cognition* (pp. 55–78). Hillsdale, NJ: Erlbaum.

Fiske, S. T., & Neuberg, S. L. (1990). A continuum model of impression formation: From category based to individuating processes as a function of information, motivation, and attention. In M. P. Zanna (Ed.), *Advances in experimental social psychology* (Vol. 23, pp. 1–74). San Diego, CA: Academic Press.

Fiske, S. T., Neuberg, S. L., Beattie, A. E., & Milberg, S. J. (1987). Category-based and attribute-based reactions to others: Some informational conditions of stereotyping and individuating processes. *Journal of Experimental Social Psychology, 23,* 399–427.

Fiske, S. T., & Pavelchak, M. A. (1986). Category-based versus piecemeal-based affective responses: Developments in schema-triggered affect. In R. M. Sorrentino & E. T. Higgins (Eds.), *Handbook of motivation and cognition: Foundations of social behavior* (Vol. 1, pp. 167–203). New York: Guilford Press.

Fiske, S. T., & Taylor, S. E. (1991). *Social cognition.* New York: McGraw-Hill.

Frable, D. E. (1993). Dimension of marginality: Distinctions among those who are different. *Personality and Social Psychology Bulletin, 19,* 370–380.

Frable, D. E., Platt, L., & Hoey, S. (1998). Concealable stigmas and positive self-perceptions: Feeling better around similar others. *Journal of Personality and Social Psychology, 74,* 909–922.

Gaertner, S. L., & Dovidio, J. F. (1986). The aversive form of racism. In J. F. Dovidio & S. L. Gaertner (Eds.), *Prejudice, discrimination, and racism* (pp. 61–89). Orlando, FL: Academic Press.

Goffman, E. (1963). *Stigma: Notes on the management of spoiled identity.* Englewood Cliffs, NJ: Prentice-Hall.

Hamilton, D. L., & Sherman, S. J. (1996). Perceiving persons and groups. *Psychological Review, 103,* 336–355.

Harding, J., Proshansky, H., Kutner, B., & Chein, I. (1969). Prejudice and ethnic relations. In G. Lindzey & E. Aronson (Eds.), *Handbook of social psychology: Vol. 5. Applied social psychology* (2nd ed., pp. 1–76). Reading, MA: Addison-Wesley.

Hebb, D. O., & Thompson, R. (1968). The social significance of animal studies. In G. Lindzey & E. Aronson (Eds.), *Handbook of social psychology: Vol. 2. Research methods* (2nd ed., pp. 729–774). Reading, MA: Addison-Wesley.

Hebl, M. R., & Heatherton, T. F. (1998). The stigma of obesity in women: The difference is black and white. *Personality and Social Psychology Bulletin, 24,* 417–426.

Jones, E. E., Farina, A., Hastorf, A. H., Markus, H., Miller, D. T., & Scott, R. A. (1984). *Social stigma: The psychology of marked relationships.* New York: Freeman.

Jones, E. E., & Nisbett, R. E. (1971). *The actor and the observer: Divergent perceptions of the causes of behavior.* Morristown, NJ: General Learning Press.

Jones, J. M. (1986). Racism: A cultural analysis of the problem. In J. F. Dovidio & S. L. Gaertner (Eds.), *Prejudice, discrimination, and racism* (pp. 279–314). Orlando, FL: Academic Press.

Jost, J. T., & Banaji, M. R. (1994). The role of stereotyping in system-justification and the production of false consciousness. *British Journal of Social Psychology, 33*, 1–27.

Katz, I. (1981). *Stigma: A social-psychological perspective.* Hillsdale, NJ: Erlbaum.

Kleck, R. E., & Strenta, A. (1980). Perceptions of the impact of negatively valued physical characteristics on social interactions. *Journal of Personality and Social Psychology, 39*, 861–873.

Klinker, P. A., & Smith, R. M. (1999). *The unsteady march: The rise and decline of American commitments to racial equality.* New York: Free Press.

Kovel, J. (1970). *White racism: A psychohistory.* New York: Pantheon.

Lane, J. D., & Wegner, D. M. (1995). The cognitive consequences of secrecy. *Journal of Personality and Social Psychology, 69*, 1–17.

Lefebvre, A., & Munro, I. R. (1986). Psychological adjustment of patients with craniofacial deformities before and after surgery. In C. P. Herman, M. P. Zanna, & E. T. Higgins (Eds.), *The Ontario Symposium: Vol. 3. Physical appearance, stigma, and social behavior* (pp. 53–64). Hillsdale, NJ: Erlbaum.

Mackie, D. M., Hamilton, D. L., Susskind, J., & Rosselli, F. (1996). Social psychological foundations of stereotype formation. In N. Macrae, C. Stangor, & M. Hewstone (Eds.), *Stereotypes and stereotyping* (pp. 41–78). New York: Guilford Press.

Major, B., Barr, L., Zubek, J., & Babey, S. H. (1999). Gender and self-esteem: A meta-analysis. In W. B. Swan, J. H. Langlois, & L. A. Gilbert (Eds.), *Sexism and stereotypes in modern society: The gender science of Janet Taylor Spence* (pp. 223–254). Washington, DC: American Psychological Association.

Major, B., & Gramzow, R. H. (1999). Abortion as stigma: Cognitive and emotional implication of concealment. *Journal of Personality and Social Psychology, 77*, 735–745.

Miller, C. T., & Myers, A. M. (1998). Compensating for prejudice: How heavyweight people (and others) control outcomes despite prejudice. In J. K. Swim & C. Stangor (Eds.), *Prejudice: The target's perspective* (pp. 191–218). San Diego, CA: Academic Press.

Russell, K., Wilson, M., & Hall, R. (1992). *The color complex: The politics of skin color among African Americans.* New York: Harcourt Brace Jovanovich.

Siller, J., Ferguson, L. T., Vann, D. H., & Holland, B. (1968). Structure of attitudes toward the physically disabled: The disability factor scales—amputation, blindness, cosmetic conditions. *Proceedings of the 76th Annual Convention of the American Psychological Association, 3*, 651–652.

Snyder, M., Tanke, E. D., & Berscheid, E. (1977). Social perception and interpersonal behavior: On the self-fulfilling nature of social stereotypes. *Journal of Personality and Social Psychology, 35*, 656–666.

Solomon, S., Greenberg, J., & Pyszczynski, T. (1991). A terror management theory of social behavior: The psychological functions of self-esteem and cultural worldviews. In M. P. Zanna (Ed.), *Advances in experimental social psychology* (Vol. 24, pp. 93–159). San Diego, CA: Academic Press.

Steele, C. M. (1997). A threat in the air: How stereotypes shape intellectual identity and performance. *American Psychologist, 52*, 613–629.

Steele, C. M., & Aronson, J. (1995). Stereotype vulnerability and the intellectual test performance of African-Americans. *Journal of Personality and Social Psychology, 69*, 797–811.

Swann, W. B., Jr. (1987). Identity negotiation: Where two roads meet. *Journal of Personality and Social Psychology, 53*, 1038–1051.

Tajfel, H., & Turner, J. C. (1979). An integrative theory of intergroup conflict. In W. G. Austin & S. Worchel (Eds.), *The social psychology of intergroup relations* (pp. 33–48). Monterey, CA: Brooks/Cole.

Turner, J. C., Hogg, M. A., Oakes, P. J., Reicher, S. D., & Wetherell, M. S. (1987). *Rediscovering the social group: A self-categorization theory.* Oxford: Basil Blackwell.

Verkuyten, M., & Hagendoorn, L. (1998). Prejudice and self-categorization: The variable role of authoritarianism and in-group stereotypes. *Personality and Social Psychology Bulletin, 24*, 99–110.

Weiner, B. (1986). *An attributional theory of motivation and emotion.* New York: Springer-Verlag.

Weiner, B., Perry, R. P., & Magnusson, J. (1988). An attributional analysis of reactions to stigmas. *Journal of Personality and Social Psychology, 55*, 738–748.

Wills, T. A. (1981). Downward comparison principles in social psychology. *Psychological Bulletin, 90*, 245–271.

Wilson, E. O. (1975). *Sociobiology: The new synthesis.* Cambridge, MA: Belknap Press.

Zajonc, R. B. (1980). Feeling and thinking: Preferences need no inferences. *American Psychologist, 35*, 151–175.

I

THE PERCEIVER

2

Why People Stigmatize: Toward a Biocultural Framework

STEVEN L. NEUBERG
DYLAN M. SMITH
TERRILEE ASHER

With knives and branding irons, ancient Greeks would slice and burn criminals and traitors to denote their immorality or lack of fitness for regular society. Such a mark was called a "stigma," and an individual bearing a stigma was to be discredited, scorned, and avoided. We might consider this practice a behavioral manifestation of the more general process of psychological stigmatization—the process of cognitively marking an individual as possessing a negative characteristic so discrediting that it engulfs others' views of the individual. To stigmatize an individual is to *define* the individual in terms of this negative attribute, and then to devalue him or her in a manner "appropriate" to this label (e.g., Crocker, Major, & Steele, 1998; Goffman, 1963; Jones et al., 1984). Most researchers of stigma note that the process of stigmatization has a long history and is cross-culturally ubiquitous.

People may, of course, also mark others in favorable, nonstigmatizing ways. For instance, we frequently respond to an act of great courage by labeling the protagonist a "hero" and by marking that person with medals and awards, indicating that the individual is to be respected and adulated. Stigmatization thus represents one end of the continuum of the process of assigning positive or negative labels to those we come across, and then valuing or devaluing them as their labels warrant. We also note that responses to stigmatized individuals can vary in both their intensity and their quality, ranging from affective and behavioral dismissal (as might occur when we label someone "a person of little consequence") to hate and genocide (as might occur when we see members of other groups as threatening the safety and stability of our own group or society). Indeed, we may even feel ambivalence toward some of those we stigmatize—experiencing both sympathy and discomfort, for instance, when encountering facially disfigured individuals. More commonly, however, our reactions to those we stigmatize take the form of moderate dislike and avoidance. One feature of the framework to be presented below is that it suggests why the intensity and quality of reactions to various stigmatizing conditions differ as they do.

The predominant view of stigma researchers is that individual cultures and subcultures define which characteristics are stigmatizing and which are not (e.g., Archer, 1985; Crocker et al., 1998; Pfuhl & Henry, 1993). Advocates of this perspective may point to findings, for example, that being fat is more stigmatizing in some societies than in others (e.g., Crandall & Martinez, 1996). They further note that even within a single society, the identical person may be stigmatized in one social context but not in another—as when a body-pierced, spike-haired teenage boy is adored by his friends but derided by his parents' country club acquaintances. Moreover, they may cite instances in which stigmatization is clearly arbitrary and capricious. One can easily imagine, for example, a clique of grade-school children deciding to shun classmates who, say, wear shoes with laces. We agree that such cultural and subcultural variations in stigmatizing conditions are interesting and potentially important. However, such variations do not preclude the possibility that there exist equally fascinating, and perhaps more instructive, cross-cultural commonalities in stigmatizing conditions—commonalities inexplicable in terms of idiosyncratic and arbitrary decisions of individual groups and societies. Just as any full understanding of stigma needs to account for the ubiquity of the stigmatization process, and for the variations in stigma content, it must also account for the cross-cultural, historical, and cross-species commonalities in stigma content.

The task of this chapter is to explore why people stigmatize. In addressing this issue, we explicitly assume that stigmatizing others serves meaningful functions for those doing it. Certainly a functional approach to stigma is not novel (e.g., Snyder & Miene, 1994), and numerous benefits to the psychology of the individual stigmatizer have been proposed and empirically supported. For instance, people may stigmatize others partially to reduce the complexities of understanding them as multifaceted individuals (e.g., Allport, 1954; Hamilton, 1981; Fiske & Neuberg, 1990; Macrae, Milne, & Bodenhausen, 1994; Tajfel, 1969), to feel better about themselves (e.g., Ehrlich, 1973; Fein & Spencer, 1997; Wills, 1981), to feel better about their groups (e.g., Tajfel & Turner, 1986), to justify their preferential status in society (e.g., Jost & Banaji, 1994; Lerner, 1980; Major, 1994), or to validate an important world view (e.g., Greenberg et al., 1990) (for reviews of stigma functions, see Crocker et al., 1998; Jost & Banaji, 1994; Kenrick, Neuberg, & Cialdini, 1999, Ch. 11).

Our original intent was to focus this chapter on a review of such functions. As we considered these explanations more deeply, however, we found them to be less than completely satisfying (for a similar reaction, see Stangor & Crandall, Chapter 3, this volume). First, standing alone, these individual-level psychological explanations are often unable to predict which characteristics people use to stigmatize others. If you want to feel better about yourself, for instance, you could ostensibly denigrate *anyone*. Why, then, do members of North American society stigmatize ethnic minorities, people with AIDS, and child molesters, but not people with protruding belly buttons? Second, individual-level functional perspectives are generally unable to account for the many cross-cultural, historical, and even cross-species similarities in the contents of stigma. These perspectives cannot explain, for instance, why traitors have been routinely stigmatized across societies and across time, or why chimpanzees rebuff those individuals who violate the norm of reciprocity (e.g., de Waal, 1989) and attack members of their group who exhibit physical manifestations of communicable disease (e.g., Goodall, 1986). Third, such functional explanations say little about qualitative variations in *how* people treat stigmatized individuals—about why some such individuals are avoided; others are ridiculed; others are viewed with ambivalence; and yet others are quarantined, exiled, imprisoned, or executed. Finally, many such explanations ignore the interesting fact that stigmatization can be more than just a psychological process. It can also be a communicated, social process, as in the examples of the ancient Greek practice of physically branding criminals, the American Puritan use of the scarlet "A" to mark adulterers, or the Nazi demand that Jews wear yellow Stars of David to signify their religious status.

Because such issues frequently lie outside the theoretical machinery of individual-level functional explanations, we saw a need to look beyond the proximate psychology of the individual. In this chapter, then, we propose a broader, *biocultural* answer to the question "Why do people stigmatize?" We argue that the ubiquitous human practice of stigmatizing certain others is rooted primarily in the biologically based need to live in effective groups. Note that our biocultural approach does not, and is not intended to, render irrelevant functional approaches couched at the level of improving the proximate psychological welfare of the individual stigmatizer. Rather, we hope that the proposed framework provides a broader context in which these individual-level functions can be better understood.

Our primary theoretical proposition is that because group living is highly adaptive for human survival and gene transmission, people will stigmatize those individuals whose characteristics and actions are seen as threatening or hindering the effective functioning of their groups.[1] Fundamental to our position, then, is the necessary interaction of biological and cultural processes.

Our framework accounts for the ubiquity of the stigmatization process, and for the great similarity in stigma content, by positing that they emerge via processes of biological and social evolution from fundamental biological and group needs that exist (and have existed) across different cultures, time periods, and relevant social species. We also suggest that many observed societal variations in stigma content—variations that on their surface might seem incompatible with the present position—are actually predicted by this framework; we explore this possibility later.

Before continuing, we should make two comments. First, it is important to be explicit about our investigation strategy. Our overall aims are (1) to derive principles of stigmatization from what we know about the requirements of effective group functioning; (2) to generate concrete hypotheses from these principles—hypotheses about who will be targeted for stigmatization, who will be particularly motivated to stigmatize, what circumstances will facilitate stigmatization, and the form (i.e., the quality and intensity) this stigmatization will take; (3) to test these hypotheses against existing contemporary, historical, and cross-cultural data; (4) to gather new data to explore untested hypotheses; and (5) to assess the ability of this and alternative models to account for the data. This, of course, is a long-term strategy. Given the preliminary nature of this work, and the relative absence of analyzed empirical data testing our hypotheses, we focus in this chapter on steps 1 and 2. We request the reader's indulgence and acknowledge that assessing the ultimate viability of this framework will require us to go well beyond this chapter's presentation.

Second, we seek to avoid any misconceptions about our use of biological and evolutionary concepts. That the roots of stigma may lie in our evolutionary past in no way implies biological determinism; we firmly reject a deterministic view, as do most modern evolutionary theorists, for reasons explained by Kenrick (1994) and Buss (1999). Moreover, just because certain stigmas were adapted for the social and physical environments of our evolutionary past, this does not imply that they are adaptive today; they would only be adaptive to the extent that current environmental constraints are similar to past environmental constraints. Finally, just because some stigmas were (or even are) adaptive or "natural," this does not make them "good," "right," "morally justifiable," or anything of the sort; the morality of any particular stigma is independent of its existence (see Buss & Kenrick, 1998, on the "naturalistic fallacy").

HUMAN SOCIALITY AND STIGMA

Humans are, and have always been, social creatures (e.g., Coon, 1946; Mann, 1980). We do not review here the evolutionary history of *Homo sapiens*, but anthropological theorizing has it that changing environmental conditions (e.g., the receding of sub-Saharan African forests) and other factors (e.g., the shift toward increased meat eating and large-game hunting) gave significant advantages to individuals living in highly interdependent, cooperative groups (Leakey & Lewin, 1977). This human form of sociality—labeled "ultrasociality" by Campbell (1982) and "obligatory interdependence" by Brewer (in press)—generally facilitates individuals' abilities to eat well, build shelters, acquire knowledge, find mates, raise children, and protect themselves from rival species and bands of other humans. It makes sense, then, that individual humans are greatly committed to group living. This propensity for ultrasociality is further enhanced by the fact that throughout most of evolutionary history, we humans have lived in groups consisting primarily of kin. Interdependent group living, then, is more than just an investment in our own survival; it is also an investment, via inclusive fitness (Hamilton, 1964), in our genes that reside within fellow group members. Indeed, some researchers have posited that group living—characterized by prosocial tendencies such as sharing, cooperation, and mutual investment—is the primary human survival strategy: To the extent that the group operates effectively, its individual members benefit (Barchas, 1986; Brewer, 1997; Brewer & Caporael, 1990; Leakey, 1978). Moreover, the usefulness of the social group makes it an important selection environment, such that individuals who work well within the group structures should be more likely to transmit their genes into future generations. Over long periods of time, then, sociality could become a biologically based human characteristic (Campbell, 1983).

This is not to say, of course, that humans are fully prosocial in their aims and actions; far from it. Interestingly, a cooperative group context itself provides particularly rich opportunities for individuals to behave in selfishly exploitative ways. For instance, the prosocial propensity for sharing food gives a group's members greater access to nutrition than they would ever acquire as individuals. This sharing also provides a wonderful exploitation opportunity, however: An individual who eats the food gathered or killed by other group members, but fails to share his or her own food, is likely to survive longer and reproduce more successfully. The dual human propensities for prosociality and exploitation characterize group life, and are revealed nicely by research on helping and on behavior in social dilemma situations (Batson, 1998; Caporael, Dawes, Orbell, & van de Kragt, 1989; Pruitt, 1998; Schroeder, Penner, Dovidio, & Piliavin, 1995).

Exploitation within cooperative groups creates obvious problems. As individuals begin to exploit the efforts of others, those who continue to behave prosocially shoulder increasing amounts of the group burden, for decreasing gain. The rate of defection toward exploitation should thus increase, making it less likely that the group will hold together and eventually eliminating the group-living advantage for all members. Moreover, those continuing to cooperate will be less likely to survive (as their efforts begin to benefit others more than themselves) and less likely to transmit their genes into the future. Thus ultrasociality will be adaptive—and will persist—only to the extent that threats from within the group can be minimized. There must be mechanisms to identify individuals who threaten or hinder successful group functioning, to label them as such, to motivate group members to withhold group benefits from them, and to separate such individuals from the group if necessary.

We propose that stigmatization is such a mechanism; it represents one response to factors that threaten our ability to derive benefits from living in social groups. This view is consistent with Campbell's (1982) ideas about social control and mutual monitoring, and with Brewer's (1997) recent statement that "individuals will gain advantage if they selectively avoid, reject, or eliminate other individuals whose behaviors are disruptive to group organization" (p. 57). The present view also highlights, and brings to much greater prominence, the stigma dimension of "peril"—the extent to which an individual is viewed as threatening or dangerous—considered briefly by Jones and colleagues (1984).

What types of actions threaten groups, and thus require the kind of psychological and social restraint that stigmatization might provide? To derive those characteristics that people will see as stigmatizing, we need first to articulate those features of group structure that make groups effective, and therefore valuable to their members. Anthropologists suggest that both in the evolutionary past and currently, groups must successfully organize individual effort, share resources, create effective communication, protect individual members and gathered foods from predation and theft, and the like. Implicit in these features are requirements for establishing norms of reciprocity, truth telling, and trust; for creating a common group identity and stable bonds between members; for teaching needed competencies; and for establishing reliable mechanisms for group socialization. Such a list is no doubt incomplete, but it provides a useful starting point. In the remainder of the chapter, we illustrate the implications of these structural requirements for the stigmatization process with a few examples—focusing specifically on people's reactions to those who violate the norm of reciprocity, betray trust, disturb the group's socialization process, or threaten the group's survival from without.

STIGMATIZING NONRECIPROCATORS

The fundamental benefits of group living derive from the sharing of individual efforts, knowledge, and material resources. Tasks that an individual may be unable to accomplish alone may be facilitated by the shared, cooperative efforts of multiple individuals; problems that appear insoluble may yield to the shared knowledge and experience of multiple group members; a failure of one hunting party to "bring home the bacon" will be mitigated by the willingness of other parties to share their kill. However, the practice of sharing in these and related ways will only be beneficial to individual group members, and become a reliable part of the social system, if it is reciprocated—if the efforts, knowledge, or material resources of the givers are repaid by subsequently shared efforts, knowledge, or material resources of the recipients (Axelrod & Hamilton, 1981; Trivers, 1971). Not surprisingly, then, all human societies and many nonhuman group-living species have a norm of reciprocity (e.g., Becker, 1956; de Waal, 1996; Gouldner, 1960; Hobhouse, 1951; Thurnwald, 1916, 1932). Following the logic that people will stigmatize those seen as hindering the effective functioning of groups, we would hypothesize that individuals and subgroups perceived to be nonreciprocating in their actions will be stigmatized. We consider two such cases here: those who actively violate the norm of reciprocity via theft; and those who burden the group through no fault of their own, such as physically disabled individuals.

Thieves

There exist many forms of thievery. One may simply take some material object owned by another—a fishing rod, for instance. One may steal another's knowledge and services, as when people fail to pay their physicians, therapists, attorneys, accountants, or shamans. One may "free-ride" on the efforts of others, partaking of the fruits of other group members' efforts while contributing little effort of one's own. Such acts violate the social contract of reciprocity—whereby one is expected to pay for fishing rods and psychological services, and to contribute effort to joint projects—and the group and its individual members have an interest in reducing their frequency.

And so within-group thievery ought to be stigmatized. We have yet to do the archival search, but we suspect that a review of the laws of a wide range of cultures and subcultures, current and past, would reveal that within-group thievery is universally stigmatized. We would expect to find that the moral/religious books and socialization exercises of most cultures would discourage thievery. Even in groups such as criminal gangs that have pro-thievery norms, theft *within* the group should be proscribed. And members of working groups should stigmatize non-contributors.

Those who have accumulated resources and who have invested heavily in the group should be particularly likely to stigmatize thievery violations. For instance, individuals who actively and effortfully accumulate resources should be especially likely to stigmatize material thieves, and those who through similar efforts acquire knowledge (e.g., scientists) should be especially motivated to stigmatize knowledge thieves (e.g., plagiarists). We similarly suspect that people whose livelihoods depend on producing new music, software, and literature would be particularly harsh on thieves of intellectual property.

Stigmatization of within-group thievery should be particularly likely during times of economic stress, and in communities where that economic stress is greatest, because such circumstances make acquisition and replacement of material goods more difficult. Note that during these same times of scarcity, theft of resources from *other* groups may actually be encouraged—legends of Robin-Hood-like transfers of resources from "them" to "us" come easily to mind. Thus, consistent with the idea that the function of stigmatization is to facilitate group success, it should not be that people stigmatize those who steal per se, but rather stigmatize those whose thievery creates a burden within the group.

Thievery should evoke a range of negative stigmatization responses, even from those not directly victimized. The affect experienced should be straightforwardly negative: an anger at having the fundamental norm of reciprocity intentionally violated, and a contempt for those doing it. This anger and contempt should intensify with the magnitude of the offenses and their frequency—as the norm violation becomes greater, more clear in its meaning, and more indicative of a dispositional tendency on the part of the perpetrator to ignore the anti-theft norms of the group. Behaviorally, because most individuals are viewed as capable of adhering to the norm of reciprocity, initial violations may evoke attempts at further socialization. We see this in the ways that people deal with young children who get caught, sometimes quite literally, with their hands in the cookie jar. Subsequent violations, however, should be dealt with more punitively, eventually by separating the offender from the group and its resources. Prison sentences satisfy this aim and, as an added benefit, provide a socialization lesson to the broader community. In some cultures (e.g., the Taliban in present-day Afghanistan), theft may be punished through the amputation of the hands, which ostensibly makes stealing more difficult and reiterates symbolically the group's intolerance of theft.

Physically Disabled Individuals

Whereas some individuals, such as "free-riders" and material thieves, *choose* to violate the norm of reciprocity, others are *unable* to reciprocate the benefits they receive. Consider an ancestral group, for instance, where the primary male tasks were hunting, building shelters, and defending against predators. A male who was blind or had no use of his legs would have been of little use to this group; although he would have been able to consume the group resources of meat, housing, and protection, he would have been unable to reciprocate with any meat, housing, or protection of his own. In this sense, he was a burden. Given his inability to reciprocate investments made in him by the group, he would have hindered group effectiveness. And so our framework would predict that he would have been stigmatized. Much evidence reveals that the disabled are indeed stigmatized (see Jones et al., 1984, for a review).

Stigmatization of disabled individuals should be especially likely when material and behavioral resources are scarce; in these circumstances, unreciprocated investment becomes unaffordable, and people are likely to resent the great dependency of such individuals. Moreover, because disability can be defined in terms of one's inability to perform a task of value—in the group sense, as the inability to fill a needed performance niche—individuals disabled for one niche (e.g., hunting) should be particularly stigmatized in groups where no alternative niches exist. However, in groups where a disability (e.g., lower-body paralysis) allows an individual to contribute in alternative, valued ways (e.g., as a historian, teacher, or shaman), those having the disability should be stigmatized less.[2] Along these lines, as the tasks of greatest value shift from the physical to the cerebral, people with physical disabilities alone should become less burdensome and thus less stigmatized. And as niches for high-level cerebral activity become more central, those who are *mentally* less fit should become viewed as increasingly burdensome, and should thus become increasingly stigmatized.

In contrast to the manner in which thieves and other "active" nonreciprocators are stigmatized, disabled individuals and others unable to reciprocate should be viewed more ambivalently, with the natural desire to approach and invest in one's well-intentioned group members competing with the desire to avoid making costly, nonreciprocable investments. Indeed, people report ambivalent feelings toward persons with physical disabilities (e.g., Katz, 1981; Katz, Wackenhut, & Hass, 1986). Moreover, the behavioral manifestations of this stigmatization should primarily take the form of avoidance (rather than attack), as avoiding disabled persons will usually be sufficient for reducing the likelihood that one will invest in them. Some evidence suggests that avoidance is indeed a primary means of dealing with disabled individuals (e.g., Hardaway, 1991; Kleck, Ono, & Hastorf, 1966; Perlman & Routh, 1980; Snyder, Kleck, Strenta, & Mentzer, 1979; Stephens & Clark, 1987).

We have touched only briefly on perhaps the most important feature of group success—reciprocity—and its consequences for stigma. Nonetheless, it appears that our analysis possesses several strengths. It is able to organize under the same conceptual umbrella apparently disparate stigmatization phenomena (stigmatization of thieves and disabled persons). It provides a framework that explains why noncontributors of various sorts would be stigmatized across cultures, time, and relevant social species (because such behaviors fundamentally threaten the effective functioning of groups). It posits a priori why the affective and behavioral reactions to different types of noncontribution might differ (e.g., anger toward and punishment of thieves, ambivalence toward and avoidance of disabled persons). And it generates heretofore novel hypotheses (e.g., regarding people's reactions to intragroup versus extragroup thievery, concerning the moderating role of within-group economic resources).

STIGMATIZING THE TREACHEROUS

Traitors and cheaters directly threaten the ability to derive adaptive benefits from group living. For their own purposes, the treacherous exploit the social fabric that ties individuals together and, in so doing, make prosocial behavior injurious to those who perform it. That is, not only do they remove the adaptive advantages of cooperation and investment in the group, but they render such behavior directly *maladaptive*. When treacherous behavior goes unchecked, then, it breaks the bonds of trust so necessary for reciprocity, thereby threatening effective social relations and group functioning.

We would therefore expect those who cheat, betray, and lie to be powerfully stigmatized. This seems to be the case. In Norman Anderson's (1968) classic study of 555 traits and how people evaluate them, we see that 6 of the 10 least desirable traits directly imply violations of trust ("deceitful," "dishonorable," "untruthful," "dishonest," "phony," "liar").[3] Moreover, societies the world over have long stigmatized within-group lying and cheating, whether such behaviors occur in economic exchanges, Wild West poker games, or college admission exams. We also note the public scorn heaped upon those who betray others' confidences, as well as the ultimate severity with which traitors have long been treated. The 14th-century Florentine poet Dante Alighieri understood quite well the gravity of such offenses, reserving, in his *Inferno*, the deepest circle of hell for those who betray kin, country, hosts, guests, and benefactors (Pinsky, 1994).[4]

Cheaters

Cheating thrives on the prosocial trust of others. Con artists first create the impression of trustworthiness, placing their targets at ease before going in for the score. Child-molesting members of the clergy employ the trustworthiness afforded them by their position, and the natural naiveté of their victims, to practice their perversion. It is the presence of intragroup trust that makes group members susceptible to the manipulations of con artists, child molesters, and their ilk.

We humans trust others because to do otherwise makes social living difficult and ineffective. Without intragroup trust, dependable reciprocity cannot exist, making individuals reluctant to share efforts, material resources, and information. Without trust, people cannot rely on fellow group members to perform their assigned tasks, and so individuals must perform these tasks themselves. Without trust, group members must be constantly vigilant against exploitation—even more vigilant, perhaps, than they would be in solitary life, as group life maintains in immediate proximity individuals capable of exploiting. Because intragroup cheating renders insecure the premise of trust, it minimizes many of the great advantages of group life and threatens the stability and effectiveness of groups (Axelrod & Hamilton, 1981; Trivers, 1971; Williams, 1966). Our framework therefore predicts that cheaters would be heavily stigmatized. Indeed, not only are cheaters stigmatized, but recent research in cognitive psychology suggests that people may possess natural "cheater detectors" (Cosmides, 1989; Cosmides & Tooby, 1992; Gigerenzer & Hug, 1992; Mealey, Daood, & Krage, 1996).

Cheating should be particularly stigmatized by those who have gained their resources and status through legitimate means, and by those with the most to lose. In the world of scientific research, for instance, where truth telling is viewed as necessary for the field's advancement and where the discoveries (and therefore, successes) of individual scientists are usually built upon the (presumably truthful) discoveries of others, we see harsh stigmatization of those who falsify data (Hull, 1988). Cheating should also be highly stigmatized when cheaters have taken advantage of special positions of trust to practice their deception. Clergy who take sexual advantage of underage youth may be stigmatized to a greater degree than are individuals who perform the same act from a position of lesser "trust status" (Saenz & Neuberg, 1993). High-level corporate officers who embezzle from the company coffers should be stigmatized more harshly than should lower-level managers who do the same.

We predict that strong penalties for cheating will be found where group members are highly vulnerable to exploitation. For example, when people cheat those seen as unable to effectively defend themselves against it—when elderly persons are confronted by the complex and authority-tinged "bank examiner" scheme, when the emotionally and cognitively drained relatives of recently deceased individuals are set upon by unscrupulous funeral directors and insurance agents, or when children are manipulated and taken advantage of by adults—cheaters should be especially stigmatized. Cheaters should also be heavily penalized in circumstances where cheating is inherently difficult to detect, because in such cases the community has an especially large interest in deterring the behavior. For instance, in schools that do not proctor examinations (because they presume that students will adhere to a code of honor), apprehended cheaters and their accomplices should be punished more harshly (typically via expulsion) than in habitually vigilant schools where no such presumption of honor exists. When the costs of cheating are especially high—when an embezzler bankrupts a company, or when a shifty building contractor skims money by using inferior building materials—penalties for cheating should be commensurately high. And when the cheater is a previously trusted individual, with a presence in the public eye, he or she will be harshly stigmatized so as to remind the other group members of the importance of truth telling.

Like thieves, cheaters ought to evoke anger and contempt. Behaviorally, initial violations of trust may result in attempts to employ corrective socialization, particularly if the offender is a child. Repeat offenders, however, are likely to be viewed as dispositionally exploitative and thereby as presenting a continuing danger to the group, and so will be penalized more harshly. Because groups need their members to maintain their trust in one another, people are likely to publicly expose and label cheaters, to "spread the word" so that cheaters can be excluded from cooperative circumstances, and so that group members can be vigilant in that person's presence. Tarring and feathering a cheater, a punishment practiced in 18th-century America, would serve such a function. Avoidance and exclusion not only eliminate the cheater's access to exploitation opportunities and reduce his or her ability to enjoy group benefits, but also provide a message of deterrence to would-be cheaters. In smaller groups where social networks more effectively communicate information, public exposure and labeling may be sufficient to reduce the threat posed by cheaters. In larger, more anonymous groups, however, where one can be less confident that communication will effectively expose the perpetrator, imprisonment or banishment may be seen as necessary to reduce the threat.

Traitors

Cheating violates the presumption of trust because it involves lying—providing false information (lying by commission) or excluding relevant information (lying by omission). The act of betrayal often includes such forms of deception, but goes beyond them by additionally violating the implicit (and sometimes explicit) contract stating that special information or opportunity available to one *as a group member* will not be used to harm the group. The prototypical traitors, then, are the Benedict Arnolds, Ethel and Julius Rosenbergs, and Aldrich Ameses of the world, who take advantage of their positions to give security-threatening information to competing outgroups. The same contract exists within the context of interpersonal relationships, whereby the bond of that relationship implies that potentially sensitive information provided by one friend to another will not be made public. Betrayal, in this instance, is clearly exemplified by the actions of Linda Tripp, who betrayed confidences told to her by Monica Lewinsky about her sexual trysts with President Bill Clinton. Betrayal is costly. At minimum, reputations are damaged; at maximum, groups perish. For this reason, our framework holds that groups ought to have strong norms against betrayal. Consider, as a few instances, the "blue wall of silence" among police officers ("Code of Silence," 1999), the code of *omerta* among Mafiosi ("Mafia," 1999), or the norms against "whistle blowing" in corporate America (e.g., Miceli & Near, 1992) and "snitching" in prison (e.g., Akerstrom, 1986). And individuals who betray should be harshly stigmatized.

Betrayal should be particularly stigmatized by those who have invested trust in the betrayer. A group that has given a member special opportunities or access to information, or an individual who has confided to a friend a particularly sensitive piece of information, should be more likely to stigmatize the traitor than a group or an individual who has invested little trust in the traitor. Moreover, because betrayal is particularly threatening when the group or individual is already vulnerable, betrayal should be especially stigmatized when the group is in competition or conflict with the recipient of the "proprietary" information, or when the individual is already under scrutiny by scheming others. Traitorous behavior in times of war is commonly punished by death, and we suspect that Tripp would have been ostracized less had her betrayal of Lewinsky's secrets not made it to the ears of those seeking to remove Clinton from office.[5]

Traitors should elicit strong anger and contempt. Punishment for apprehended traitors should be quick and severe, commensurate with the level of threat they represent. As if Dante's ninth circle of hell were not enough, those who betray their friends, family, benefactors, and societies are punished with isolation at the least, and torture, exile, and death at the most severe. Traitors are rarely given a second chance; someone who has demonstrated the capacity for betrayal may be too dangerous to trust. Interestingly, money- or revenge-motivated traitors who successfully emigrate to the outgroup for whom they played turncoat often report great dissatisfaction with how they are treated by their new group, despite the valuable services they have rendered. As Benedict Arnold's treatment in England illustrates, they are rarely trusted in their new homes, and often feel isolated and rejected. Similarly, once one gains a reputation as an indiscreet and untrustworthy friend, friendships will probably be hard to come by. We suspect that even those individuals enthusiastic about Tripp's betrayal of Lewinsky would hesitate to entrust her with their own secrets. The harshness of the social and physical punishments for acts of betrayal seems quite functional, as behavior that is so injurious to the group and to the formation of interpersonal bonds needs to be strongly discouraged.

Like failures to reciprocate, then, acts of cheating and betrayal exploit the social cooperation and interpersonal investment required for successful group life. Stigmatization of treacherous persons is an attempt to deter those who threaten the group in this manner.

STIGMATIZING THOSE WHO COUNTER-SOCIALIZE

The amount of information needed to successfully manage the complex ultrasocial life of the human is imposing. Unfortunately, humans are not born knowing the rules of reciprocity or truth telling in all their textured sophistication. Nor do they come into this world preequipped with efficient strategies and techniques for large-game hunting, tuber gathering, medical healing, or home construction. To address such deficiencies, people put great effort toward educating their young—toward nurturing and developing their basic individual and social propensities into the competencies and values they will need to live effectively in social groups. We humans are taught by our elders how to acquire food, cook, build, and defend; we are socialized in the norms of reciprocity and truth telling, and in how and when these norms operate; and we discover through observation and direct lesson a grand range of subtle yet powerful strategies and tactics for effective social intercourse. It is clear that socialization mechanisms have been, and are, critical to the functioning of effective human groups (Levine & Moreland, 1994). Indeed, some evolutionary theorists hypothesize that the slow maturity process of humans is an adaptation to allow sufficient time for these socialization mechanisms to operate and have their intended impact (e.g., Geary, 1998).

If stigmatization is a response to those who threaten effective group functioning, people should stigmatize those who interfere with their preferred socialization lessons and processes—who publicly advocate or symbolize values incompatible with their own. Indeed, there is clear evidence that people tend to dislike individuals and groups who endorse (or appear to endorse) values different from their own (e.g., Biernat, Vescio, & Theno, 1996; Biernat, Vescio, Theno, & Crandall, 1996; Insko, Nacoste, & Moe, 1983; Katz & Hass, 1988; Kinder & Sears, 1981; Rokeach, 1972; Rosenbaum, 1986; Schwartz, Struch, & Bilsky, 1990). We would further suggest that such individuals or groups should become increasingly stigmatized as they are perceived to be effective threats to the preferred socialization messages. Thus individuals possessing fringe views in noncentral domains (e.g., tastes in music, haberdashery) should elicit little concern or hostility as long as they remain outside the socialization process. However, when these individuals challenge core values (related, for example, to sexual behavior, group safety, or authority structures), gather in groups, and gain access to powerful socialization positions (e.g., as educators or clergy) or media (e.g., print, television, radio, the Internet), they more effectively threaten desired socialization practices and, as a result, will become more greatly stigmatized.

As one illustration, a quick perusal of anti-Semitic World Wide Web sites reveals their tendency to list the Jewish-appearing surnames of the owners and high-level executives of major media and entertainment outlets, and to decry this powerful degrading influence on "American" life. Clearly there are other reasons why Jews are stigmatized, but we suspect that the threat they ostensibly pose to the mainstream Christian culture—because of their access to powerful socialization channels—plays an important role. The (albeit light) stigmatization of college pro-

fessors by politically and religiously conservative critics has a similar fla-
vor to it, as the purported academic "liberal elitism" ostensibly threatens, via classroom "indoctrination," the values held by our nation's best
and brightest young minds.

As a last example, consider that there have been large and meaningful increases in Americans' acceptance of homosexuals in the workplace
over the past 20 years. Nonetheless, Americans in 1996 were as relatively wary as they were in 1977 of having homosexuals employed as elementary school teachers or clergy, in contrast to their relative comfort
with having homosexuals employed as salespersons ("Americans
Growing More Tolerant of Gays," 1996). We suggest that the threat ostensibly posed by homosexuality to mainstream heterosexual values is
seen as all too real when potentially transmitted through professional socializers such as teachers and clergy. And so when individuals possessing
such deviating values occupy these positions, we would expect them to
be severely stigmatized. This should be especially the case when the deviating socializers have contact with those seen as highly susceptible to
such influences, such as children. This perhaps explains the Virginia
court verdicts in the case of *Bottoms v. Bottoms,* in which a grand-
mother gained legal custody of her 2-year-old grandson by convincing
judges that her daughter's homosexuality was an inappropriate and
harmful socialization environment for the child.

Stigmatization based on perceived socialization threat should be
particularly great among individuals highly invested in the values threatened, and among individuals with a vested interest in those potentially
influenced by the deviating values. For instance, teachers and clergy responsible for mainstream socialization, as well as the parents, grandparents, and other close relatives of children, should be especially likely to
stigmatize those who communicate deviating messages.

Finally, the affective responses to value deviates should range from
mild aversion (in the cases of apparently noninfluential value deviates)
to contempt, anger, and fear (in the cases of potentially influential deviates). Behaviorally, the responses should range from disinterest and dismissal in the former case to more extreme actions in the latter, where we
might expect attempts at conversion, ridicule, and verbal attack. If such
actions are insufficient to halt the perceived subversion of the socialization process, then separating the deviates from those potentially influenced may occur, as in the case of Sharon Bottoms and her son; such
separation could also include imprisonment, exile, or execution. Indeed,
judging from the Spanish Inquisition and from the Stalinist and Maoist
reeducation camps—as just a few of many examples—extreme behavioral reactions to value deviates may well be expected in cases where the
challenge to a group's core values is seen as potentially successful.

AN INTERIM SUMMARY

To this point, we have focused on threats from within the group—on how, when, and why people stigmatize fellow group members who create impediments to effective group functioning. We have illustrated our framework by showing how it applies to violations of the reciprocity norm, exploitation of trust, and interruptions of preferred socialization practices. By necessity, we have neglected other interesting cases that fit neatly within our framework. For example, because individuals need to remain physically healthy, group members with contagious diseases will be seen as a threat and will be stigmatized, via avoidance and quarantine (see Kurzban & Leary, 2000, for an argument along these lines). Because group life benefits from an understanding of and adherence to accepted rules and scripts for coordinated social action and interaction (e.g., Goffman, 1959), individuals seen as unpredictable (e.g., people labeled as having certain mental illnesses) are likely to be stigmatized (again, see Kurzban & Leary, 2000). Because groups need to get things done, individuals viewed as incompetent will be stigmatized. And because groups exist ultimately to enhance the reproductive fitness of their members, individuals seen as threatening effective reproduction (e.g., those possessing congenital physical deformities, rapists) should be stigmatized. Of course, existing research indicates that carriers of infectious diseases (Stangor & Crandall, Chapter 3, this volume), those with mental illness diagnoses such as schizophrenia (e.g., Linsky, 1970; Morrison, 1980; Rabkin, 1974), people who fail at group tasks (e.g., Rosenfield, Stephan, & Lucker, 1981; Worchel, Andreolli, & Folger, 1977), and those possessing what Goffman (1963) referred to as congenital "abominations of the body" (see Jones et al., 1984) are indeed stigmatized. We suspect that a more thorough treatment of the kind we are advocating in this chapter will lend greater texture to our understanding of why, when, by whom, and in what ways such individuals are treated as they are.

We would be remiss, however, if we failed to discuss briefly one last application of our framework—an application that differs from the others in that the threat to the group comes not from within, but from without (from other groups). We turn to that now.

STIGMATIZING THREATS FROM THE OUTSIDE

Stigmatizing members of other groups appears to be a cross-cultural feature of human life, and some theorists argue that this tendency has its roots in human evolutionary history (Brewer, in press; Eibl-Eibesfeldt, 1989; Fishbein, 1996; Fox, 1992; Schaller, 1999; van der Dennen &

Falger, 1990). For reasons briefly discussed earlier, it has been highly advantageous for humans to live in groups. It should be no surprise, then, that people value the groups to which they belong. Valuing one's own group relative to other groups increases the likelihood that one's efforts and resources will go toward those who are already committed to reciprocate, and not toward those (i.e., members of other groups) with whom one has no established reciprocity-based bonds or trust. Indeed, members of all cultures appear to display a strong ingroup preference—a preference so strong that mere surface indications of common group membership are often sufficient to lead people to benefit strangers (e.g., Brewer, 1979; Mullen, Brown, & Smith, 1992; Tajfel, 1982).

The existence of ingroup *preference*, however, does not alone explain why people *stigmatize* members of other groups. Why don't people just ignore other groups and leave them alone? Part of the answer to this question may lie in the previously discussed aversions people have toward those whose values appear different from theirs. We suspect that the larger part of the answer, however, may lie in two factors. First, because people have no established reciprocity-based bonds with members of outgroups, they are likely to mistrust them (Brewer, in press). Indeed, data ranging from the stereotypes held by East Africans (Brewer & Campbell, 1976) to the perceptions of American students about to play the Prisoner's Dilemma game in the experimental laboratory (Insko, Schopler, Hoyle, Dardis, & Graetz, 1990) suggest that people tend to mistrust members of other groups. Second, members of other groups may pose very real threats to one's own group's well-being. Valuable resources are often limited; within any physical territory, for example, there will exist only so many sources of potable water, nutritious foods, weather-resistant places to live, and the like. If multiple groups live within this territory, and if the territory is not particularly rich in its resources, then the different groups will have to compete to maintain their well-being (e.g., Keeley, 1996).[6] This is the view espoused by realistic group conflict theory: Intergroup conflict, and the outgroup stigmatization that usually accompanies it, emerge when groups see themselves as competing for the same resources (e.g., Bonacich, 1972; Campbell, 1965; Sherif, Harvey, White, Hood, & Sherif, 1961/1988). Just as people stigmatize those ingroup members they see as hindering the ability of the group to operate effectively, they also stigmatize those outgroups they see as hindering the ability of the group to operate effectively.

All this is not to say that groups always stigmatize one another. Rather, the critical issue is whether groups view themselves as competing for a common pot of important resources. When resources are plentiful, or when it is clear that intergroup cooperation enables groups to do well, intergroup stigmatization is less likely. When resources become more scarce, however—when economic times are tough and jobs are difficult to come by, for instance, or when natural disaster or environmental destruction leave a territory poor in natural resources—intergroup competition heats up and stigmatization should follow. Analyses of economic conditions and intergroup conflict are consistent with this (e.g., Hepworth & West, 1988; Hovland & Sears, 1940; Olzak, 1992), and results from the classic Robbers Cave field study by Sherif and his colleagues (1961/1988) demonstrate this experimentally. More recently, Pettigrew and Meertens (1995) have presented survey data from Europe showing that people direct their hostilities toward those groups they view as competition.

Outgroup threat should evoke fear and unambiguous dislike—fear, because threats to resources are potentially deadly; and unambiguous dislike, because members of other groups elicit none of the positive feelings that naturally exist toward ingroup members with whom one has reciprocity-based bonds. Behavioral responses toward stigmatized outgroups should be defensive if one's existing resources are sufficient to sustain the group in the desired manner, and more aggressive if the other group needs to be displaced from resources or kept from moving toward them. When people perceive that outgroups threaten important resources, arms buildups, mass killings, and genocide become increasingly possible.

PERCEIVING GROUPS, PERCEIVING THREAT, PERCEIVING CHOICE

We have posited that people stigmatize those seen as threatening the successful functioning of their groups. People are flexible in the ways they conceive of their multiple group memberships, however, viewing themselves as members of group A at one moment and as members of groups B, C, or D at another (e.g., Brewer, 1991). This flexibility has important implications for our framework. For instance, a supermarket employee who identifies with his or her employer is likely to stigmatize a coworker who pilfers a steak at the end of the shift. In contrast, an employee who identifies with the other workers, and who sees management and the corporation as the outgroup, may applaud this theft. The theft is a violation of ingroup reciprocity for the first employee, but not for the second. As a second example, to the extent that "we" view immigrants as "them," we are likely to stigmatize immigrants *just for being here*, as we fear that they will usurp resources meant for us. However, if we view these very same immigrants as, say, "new members of our society," we are likely to stigmatize them only if they violate reciprocity, trust, or other within-group practices. As a last example, we might note that Jews and Moslems tend to be stigmatized in predominantly Christian societies, Christians and Jews in Moslem societies, and Moslems and Christians in Jewish societies. Many social constructivists would point to these variations as evidence for the arbitrariness of stigma. After all, sometimes thieves are stigmatized, sometimes not; sometimes immigrants are stigmatized, sometimes not; sometimes Moslems are stigmatized, sometimes not. We disagree with this interpretation, however, as such variations in stigma are far from arbitrary. Rather, they all emerge from the same fundamental principle: People stigmatize those who threaten the success of their *own* groups. The variation exists in how people draw the ingroup–outgroup boundary, not in the reasoning that determines who gets stigmatized. Stable throughout apparently unrelated stigmas, then, are the principles governing what actions constitute threats to one's group and how such threats should be addressed. Thus we concur with those who emphasize that where one places the boundary of "we" has great implications for social relations (e.g., Brewer, 1991; Cialdini, Brown, Lewis, Luce, & Neuberg, 1997; Gaertner, Dovidio, Anastasio, Bachman, & Rust, 1993; Turner, Hogg, Oakes, Reicher, & Wetherell, 1987).

Our framework further implies that the manner in which one defines the threat posed by an individual determines whether (or how) that individual will be stigmatized. Consider the following example: A mother who is receiving welfare and who is perceived as unintentionally violating the norm of reciprocity, because of an inability to contribute, will be viewed ambivalently. If, however, she is seen as able but unwilling to contribute, she will evoke anger and contempt. And if she is joined by many able "welfare moms" who claim entitlement to their benefits, she may be seen as threatening the society's desired socialization practice, evoking even more extreme stigmatization. As the number and intensity of threats posed by individuals or groups increase, then, they will be stigmatized in commensurate ways. Similarly, as the actual or perceived threat is reduced, traditionally stigmatized individuals or groups should find others reacting to them in less damaging ways.

An understanding of this relationship between threat and stigmatization has proven useful to those interested in marginalizing individuals or groups. By escalating the rhetoric of threat, one can justify increasingly hostile and punitive actions toward the stigmatized. As one example, we may consider the systematic Nazi labeling of Jews—as sneaky, insincere, exploitative, oppressing, satanic, and polluting the genetic purity of the Aryan race—and the ability of this rhetoric to facilitate the escalation of stigmatizing actions against them (Bar-Tal, 1990). We see our framework, then, as having interesting ramifications for the rhetoric of social communication and for large-scale movements of social devaluation, hate, and hostility.

Finally, much research reveals that people are particularly harsh in their reactions to those seen as *choosing* the behaviors that create their stigma (e.g., Crandall & Moriarty, 1995; Weiner, Perry, & Magnusson, 1988; see Jones et al., 1984, for a review). Adult thievery and betrayal are usually chosen behaviors—they rarely occur by accident—and readily elicit negative responses from other group members. People who believe that welfare recipients are lazy are more likely to stigmatize them than are those who believe them to have been unfairly victimized by poor educational opportunities. And so on.

We explain such findings in terms of the additional threat to the social group implied by choice: According to attribution theory (e.g., Jones & Davis, 1965), individuals who choose to be burdens or to disturb socialization, for instance, represent a great threat because such choices imply dispositional tendencies to act similarly in the future. Just as we might surmise that a woman receiving welfare because of an unexpected job layoff will be motivated to remove herself from the public dole, we might surmise that a woman who chooses welfare because she is uninterested in working will be similarly uninterested in reducing her burden on the group in the future. Thus, just as discourse can alter the fate of the potentially stigmatized by altering how the public views their group memberships and the severity of threat they impose, it can do the same by altering perceptions of whether they have chosen their behaviors and circumstances.

FINAL COMMENTS

We have presented a preliminary view of our developing framework. It differs from some other functional perspectives in that it focuses not on proximal psychological benefits to be gained by stigmatizing others (e.g., elevated self-esteem), but rather on the biologically based social foundations from which stigmatization emerges. For humans to gain advantages from ultrasociality, their groups require certain structural, task, and normative features. In this manner, our views are explicitly biocultural; biology heavily influences culture. Our perspective is also biocultural in the sense that it proposes *interacting* influences of biological predispositions and cultural forces. Whereas we posit that the process of stigmatizing certain categories of people (e.g., nonreciprocators, traitors) is biologically based, the ways in which many of these categories manifest themselves may be context-specific and culturally determined: Although humans have evolved to stigmatize certain types of people, which individuals fall into these types is determined at least partially by culture.[7] We thus encourage interested readers to attend to the chapters in this volume that explore how social and cognitive processes maintain and exaggerate the importance of the categories of stigmas discussed here (Stangor & Crandall, Chapter 3, and Biernat & Dovidio, Chapter 4). We see the views presented here as quite compatible with cultural and cognitive mechanisms of stigma development and influence; we believe our framework sets a foundation of stigma content upon which these other mechanisms operate.

Some researchers and theoreticians still believe that evolutionary reasoning implies biological determinism and the stasis of existing conditions. It does not. Indeed, our framework has direct and clear implications for reducing stigmatization: Eliminate the threat (or perception of threat) posed by individuals or groups, and they should become decreasingly stigmatized. The history of 19th- and 20th-century America demonstrates that new immigrant groups can become decreasingly stigmatized as they are seen to be adopting "American" values and contributing to the common good. Observers of the Takamiut Eskimos note that elderly women can stave off abandonment during the resource-depleted times of late winter by becoming midwives (Graburn, 1969). A study from the experimental laboratory suggests that people become less likely to stigmatize physically disabled individuals after considering that such individuals might perform difficult tasks despite their disabilities (Langer, Bashner, & Chanowitz, 1985); indeed, we suspect that physically disabled people will be stigmatized less as enhanced technologies better enable them to assume important responsibilities for their groups. And research in Thailand reveals that as cures for the visible symptoms of leprosy improve, lepers gain greater social acceptance (Navon, 1996). By reducing the perceived and actual threats to group functioning created by marked individuals and groups, we should be able to reduce the extent to which they are stigmatized.

We have yet to expose the biocultural framework to sufficient empirical test, although we are encouraged by our early explorations of existing data. We are especially excited, however, by its potential for parsimoniously organizing a wide range of interesting and important social phenomena. It is one of few perspectives to make explicit predictions about the likely contents of stigma, and it appears unique in providing a common foundation for explaining the devaluation of people whose "infractions" range widely—from free-riding on group projects to being gay, from betraying a friend to having a facial disfigurement, from being a stranger to being blind. Moreover, unlike other perspectives, our framework generates explicit predictions about which behaviors and characteristics are most likely to be stigmatized cross-culturally, historically, and across relevant species. The functional basis of the framework also enables explicit predictions about how individuals are likely to be stigmatized: Instead of speaking vaguely of "liking" and "disliking," it posits affective states ranging from anger to disgust, from fear to ambivalence; instead of speaking vaguely of "social distance," it posits behavioral reactions ranging from avoidance to shunning, from indoctrination to quarantine, from imprisonment to genocide. Furthermore, the framework has the potential to bring together the phenomena of stigmatization, in which people are devalued and discredited, with the phenomena of hero making, in which people are highly valued and revered.

More broadly, we note that our developing framework can inform our understanding of social cognition and self-presentation. Researchers in the fields of social cognition have focused primarily on process—on *how* people pay attention, interpret, remember, analyze, and judge. Little attention has been paid to the *contents* of people's thoughts.[8] A framework such as this one can begin to remedy this inattention, as it addresses content explicitly: As group-living creatures, people need to pay attention to information relevant to reciprocity, to ponder whether others are telling them the truth, to remember well those individuals who have lied to them, and so forth. The actions that threaten group living should be those to which people attune themselves. Moreover, because people's success in social life is predominantly determined by how others view them, they should be especially cognizant of whether others see them as reciprocal in their efforts and actions, as worthy of trust, and so forth. Just as our framework has straightforward implications for what people think about, it also has straightforward implications for the manner in which people want to present themselves to others.

In closing, we believe that the biocultural perspective shows promise for explicating the issue of why people stigmatize, whom they stigmatize, when they stigmatize, and how they stigmatize. We continue to develop the general framework, and have begun to gather archival and new data bearing on the fitness of the model.

ACKNOWLEDGMENT

We thank Doug Kenrick, Mark Schaller, Jon Maner, and Jennifer Jordan for their very helpful comments on this chapter, and the University of Maryland social psychology group for their feedback on an early presentation of these ideas.

NOTES

1. Of course, the obverse of this proposition is that people will value those individuals seen as benefiting the group, and will revere those whom they view as benefiting the group in particularly effective ways. We are currently developing these ideas further. In this chapter, however, we focus on the concepts of group threat and hindrance and on their implications for stigmatization.

2. One might think of elderly people in similar terms. As physical skills diminish through aging, elderly individuals potentially become a greater burden in those societies where physical labor is critically important, and so they may be exiled or killed. This is particularly the case when the groups are nomadic, as in the Krangmalit and Takamiut Eskimos of Arctic North America (de Coccola & King, 1986; Graburn, 1969), the Mataco of the Bolivian Gran Chaco (Alvarsson, 1988), and the Murngin of Australia (Warner, 1937). Interestingly, infanticide is often similar to geronticide in its function in such nomadic groups—as a response to having too many very young children, who require scarce nutritional resources and human transportation but who are unable to contribute themselves (e.g., Alvarsson, 1988; Condon, 1987; de Coccola & King, 1986). When societies value the wisdom of the past, however, and possess an important niche for a historian/teacher, elderly individuals remain potentially able to contribute as long as their memories remain accessible. In such societies, then, elders should be revered and not stigmatized. In contrast, in societies where the future is extolled relative to the past—for instance, where wisdom is seen as coming from rapidly developing technological and informational innovation—there is a smaller niche for the historian, and thus elderly individuals should be stigmatized more as burdens.

3. In symmetrical fashion, five of the six most highly rated traits in Anderson's (1968) study were "sincere," "honest," "loyal," "truthful," and "trustworthy."

4. We also note that a fundamental feature of outgroup stereotypes is that such groups are seen as untrustworthy (Brewer & Campbell, 1976).

5. An alternative form of betrayal—cowardice displayed by those responsible for the group's safety and welfare—may also be dealt with harshly in times of great threat. A soldier who flees in the face of attack violates the trust placed in him or her and places the group in harm's way. It is thus unsurprising that desertion while one's nation is at war is often a capital offense. By assuming certain critical protection-related roles in a group (e.g., warriors, firefighters), individuals commit to summoning the physical and moral courage needed to perform their tasks, even when doing so may leave them personally vulnerable. Cowardly behavior violates this critical social contract, and is therefore stigmatized.

6. The value of land as the repository of needed resources helps explain why intergroup hatreds are so often based on territorial disputes. The importance of land goes beyond its value for providing natural resources, however. Land is also a keeper of social resources—of group history, in the form of monuments, shrines, and sites of important events. And so we see that Serbs and Albanians fight to the death over Kosovo, that Jews and Moslems fight over Jerusalem, and so on.

7. We thank Jon Maner for stimulating in us greater thought on this issue.
8. The senior author must plead guilty to this crime, with the others.

REFERENCES

Akerstrom, M. (1986). Outcasts in prison: The case of informers and sex offenders. *Deviant Behavior, 7,* 1–12.

Allport, G. W. (1954). *The nature of prejudice.* Reading, MA: Addison-Wesley.

Alvarsson, J.-A. (1988). *The Mataco of the Gran Chaco: An ethnographic account of change and continuity in Mataco socio-economic organization.* Uppsala, Sweden: Academiae Upsaliensis.

Americans growing more tolerant of gays. In *The Gallup Organization* [Online]. Available: http://www.gallup.com/poll/news/961214.html [1996, November]

Anderson, N. H. (1968). Likableness ratings of 555 personality trait words. *Journal of Personality and Social Psychology, 9,* 272–279.

Archer, D. (1985). Social deviance. In G. Lindzey & E. Aronson (Eds.), *Handbook of social psychology: Vol. 2. Special fields and applications* (3rd ed., pp. 743–804). New York: Random House.

Axelrod, R., & Hamilton, W. D. (1981). The evolution of cooperation. *Science, 211,* 1390–1396.

Barchas, P. (1986). A sociophysiological orientation to small groups. In E. Lawler (Ed.), *Advances in group processes* (Vol. 3, pp. 209–246). Greenwich, CT: JAI Press.

Bar-Tal, D. (1990). *Group beliefs: A conception for analyzing group structure, processes, and behavior.* New York: Springer-Verlag.

Batson, C. D. (1998). Altruism and prosocial behavior. In D. T. Gilbert, S. T. Fiske, & G. Lindzey (Eds.), *Handbook of social psychology* (4th ed., Vol. 2, pp. 282–316). Boston: McGraw-Hill.

Becker, H. (1956). *Man in reciprocity.* New York: Praeger.

Biernat, M., Vescio, T. K., & Theno, S. A. (1996). Violating American values: A "value congruence" approach to understanding outgroup attitudes. *Journal of Experimental Social Psychology, 32,* 387–410.

Biernat, M., Vescio, T. K., Theno, S. A., & Crandall, C. S. (1996). Values and prejudice: Toward understanding the impact of American values on outgroup attitudes. In C. Seligman, J. M. Olson, & M. P. Zanna (Eds.), *The Ontario Symposium: Vol. 8. The psychology of values* (pp. 153–189). Mahwah, NJ: Erlbaum.

Bonacich, E. (1972). A theory of ethnic antagonism: The split labor market. *American Sociological Review, 37,* 547–559.

Brewer, M. B. (1979). In-group bias in the minimal intergroup situation: A cognitive-motivational analysis. *Psychological Bulletin, 86,* 307–324.

Brewer, M. B. (1991). The social self: On being the same and different at the same time. *Personality and Social Psychology Bulletin, 17,* 475–482.

Brewer, M. B. (1997). On the social origins of human nature. In C. McGarty & S. A. Haslam (Eds.), *The message of social psychology: Perspectives on mind in society* (pp. 54–62). Cambridge, MA: Blackwell.

Brewer, M. B. (in press). Ingroup identification and intergroup conflict: When does ingroup love become outgroup hate? In R. Ashmore, L. Jussim, & D. Wilder (Eds.), *Social identity, intergroup conflict, and conflict reduction*. New York: Oxford University Press.

Brewer, M. B., & Campbell, D. T. (1976). *Ethnocentrism and intergroup attitudes: East African evidence*. Beverly Hills, CA: Sage.

Brewer, M. B., & Caporael, L. R. (1990). Selfish genes versus selfish people: Sociobiology as origin myth. *Motivation and Emotion, 14,* 237–242.

Buss, D. M. (1999). *Evolutionary social psychology: The new science of the mind*. Needham Heights, MA: Allyn & Bacon.

Buss, D. M., & Kenrick, D. T. (1998). Evolutionary social psychology. In D. T. Gilbert, S. T. Fiske, & G. Lindzey (Eds.), *Handbook of social psychology* (4th ed., Vol. 2, pp. 982–1026). Boston: McGraw-Hill.

Campbell, D. T. (1965). Ethnocentric and other altruistic motives. In D. LeVine (Ed.), *Nebraska Symposium on Motivation* (Vol. 13, pp. 283–311). Lincoln, NE: University of Nebraska Press.

Campbell, D. T. (1982). Legal and primary-group social controls. *Journal of Social and Biological Structures, 5,* 431–438.

Campbell, D. T. (1983). Two distinct routes beyond kin selection to ultrasociality: Implications for the humanities and social sciences. In D. Bridgeman (Ed.), *The nature of prosocial development: Theories and strategies* (pp. 11–41). New York: Academic Press.

Caporael, L. R., Dawes, R. M., Orbell, J. M., & van de Kragt, A. J. C. (1989). Selfishness examined: Cooperation in the absence of egoistic incentives. *Behavioral and Brain Sciences, 12,* 683–739.

Cialdini, R. B., Brown, S. L., Lewis, B. P., Luce, C., & Neuberg, S. L. (1997). Reinterpreting the empathy–altruism relationship: When one into one equals oneness. *Journal of Personality and Social Psychology, 73,* 481–494.

Code of silence. In *Human Rights Watch* [Online]. Available: http://www.hrw.orh/reports98/police/uspo27.htm [1999, October 11]

Condon, R. G. (1987). *Inuit youth: Growth and change in the Canadian Arctic*. New Brunswick, NJ: Rutgers University Press.

Coon, C. S. (1946). The universality of natural groupings in human societies. *Journal of Educational Sociology, 20,* 163–168.

Cosmides, L. (1989). The logic of social exchange: Has natural selection shaped how humans reason? Studies with the Wason selection task. *Cognition, 31,* 187–276.

Cosmides, L., & Tooby, J. (1992). Cognitive adaptations for social exchange. In J. Barkow, L. Cosmides, & J. Tooby (Eds.), *The adapted mind: Evolutionary psychology and the generation of culture* (pp. 163–228). New York: Oxford University Press.

Crandall, C. S., & Martinez, R. (1996). Culture, ideology, and antifat attitudes. *Personality and Social Psychology Bulletin, 22,* 1165–1176.

Crandall, C. S., & Moriarty, D. (1995). Physical illness stigma and social rejection. *British Journal of Social Psychology, 34,* 67–83.

Crocker, J., Major, B., & Steele, C. (1998). Social stigma. In D. T. Gilbert, S. T. Fiske, & G. Lindzey (Eds.), *Handbook of social psychology* (4th ed., Vol. 2, pp. 504–553). Boston: McGraw-Hill.

de Coccola, R., & King, P. (1986). *The incredible Eskimo: Life among the barren land Eskimos.* Surrey, British Columbia, Canada: Hancock House.

de Waal, F. (1989). Food sharing and reciprocal obligations among chimpanzees. *Journal of Human Evolution, 18,* 433–459.

de Waal, F. (1996). *Good natured: The origins of right and wrong in humans and other animals.* Cambridge, MA: Harvard University Press.

Ehrlich, H. J. (1973). *The social psychology of prejudice.* New York: Wiley.

Eibl-Eibesfeldt, I. (1989). *Human ethology.* New York: Aldine de Gruyter.

Fein, S., & Spencer, S. J. (1997). Prejudice as self-image maintenance: Affirming the self through derogating others. *Journal of Personality and Social Psychology, 73,* 31–44.

Fishbein, H. D. (1996). *Peer prejudice and discrimination: Evolutionary, cultural, and developmental dynamics.* Boulder, CO: Westview Press.

Fiske, S. T., & Neuberg, S. L. (1990). A continuum of impression formation, from category-based to individuating processes: Influences of information and motivation on attention and interpretation. In M. P. Zanna (Ed.), *Advances in experimental social psychology* (Vol. 23, pp. 1–74). San Diego, CA: Academic Press.

Fox, R. (1992). Prejudice and the unfinished mind: A new look at an old failing. *Psychological Inquiry, 3,* 137–152.

Gaertner, S. L., Dovidio, J. F., Anastasio, P. A., Bachman, B. A., & Rust, M. C. (1993). The common ingroup identity model: Recategorization and the reduction of intergroup bias. In W. Stroebe & M. Hewstone (Eds.), *European review of social psychology* (Vol. 4, pp. 1–26). Chichester, England: Wiley.

Geary, D. C. (1998). *Male, female: The evolution of human sex differences.* Washington, DC: American Psychological Association.

Gigerenzer, G., & Hug, K. (1992). Domain-specific reasoning: Social contracts, cheating, and perspective change. *Cognition, 43,* 127–171.

Goffman, E. (1959). *The presentation of self in everyday life.* Garden City, NJ: Doubleday.

Goffman, E. (1963). *Stigma: Notes on the management of spoiled identity.* Englewood Cliffs, NJ: Prentice-Hall.

Goodall, J. (1986). Social rejection, exclusion, and shunning among the Gombe chimpanzees. *Ethology and Sociobiology, 7,* 227–236.

Gouldner, A. W. (1960). The norm of reciprocity: A preliminary statement. *American Sociological Review, 25,* 161–178.

Graburn, N. H. H. (1969). *Eskimos without igloos: Social and economic development in Sugluk.* Boston: Little, Brown.

Greenberg, J., Pyszczynski, T., Solomon, S., Rosenblatt, A., Veeder, M., Kirkland, S., & Lyon, D. (1990). Evidence for terror management theory: II. The effects of mortality salience on reactions to those who threaten or bolster the cultural worldview. *Journal of Personality and Social Psychology, 58,* 308–318.

Hamilton, D. L. (Ed.). (1981). *Cognitive processes in stereotyping and intergroup behavior.* Hillsdale, NJ: Erlbaum.

Hamilton, W. D. (1964). The genetic evolution of social behavior: I & II. *Journal of Theoretical Biology, 7,* 1–32.

Hardaway, B. (1991). Imposed inequality and miscommunication between physically impaired and physically nonimpaired interactants in American society. *Howard Journal of Communications, 3,* 139–148.

Hepworth, J. T., & West, S. G. (1988). Lynching and the economy: A time-series reanalysis of Hovland and Sears (1940). *Journal of Personality and Social Psychology, 55,* 239–247.

Hobhouse, L. T. (1951). *Morals in evolution: A study in comparative ethics.* London: Chapman & Hall.

Hovland, C. J., & Sears, R. R. (1940). Minor studies in aggression: VI. Correlations of lynchings with economic indices. *Journal of Psychology, 9,* 301–310.

Hull, D. L. (1988). *Science as a process.* Chicago: University of Chicago Press.

Insko, C. A., Nacoste, R., & Moe, J. L. (1983). Belief congruence and racial discrimination: Review of the evidence and critical evaluation. *European Journal of Social Psychology, 13,* 153–174.

Insko, C. A., Schopler, J., Hoyle, R., Dardis, G., & Graetz, K. (1990). Individual–group discontinuity as a function of fear and greed. *Journal of Personality and Social Psychology, 58,* 68–79.

Jones, E. E., & Davis, K. E. (1965). From acts to dispositions: The attribution process in person perception. In L. Berkowitz (Ed.), *Advances in experimental social psychology* (Vol. 2, pp. 220–266). New York: Academic Press.

Jones, E. E., Farina, A., Hastorf, A. H., Markus, H., Miller, D. T., & Scott, R. A. (1984). *Social stigma: The psychology of marked relationships.* New York: Freeman.

Jost, J. T., & Banaji, M. R. (1994). The role of stereotyping in system-justification and the production of false consciousness. *British Journal of Social Psychology, 33,* 1–27.

Katz, I. (1981). *Stigma: A social psychological analysis.* Hillsdale, NJ: Erlbaum.

Katz, I., & Hass, R. G. (1988). Racial ambivalence and American value conflict: Correlational and priming studies of dual cognitive structures. *Journal of Personality and Social Psychology, 55,* 893–905.

Katz, I., Wackenhut, J., & Hass, R. G. (1986). Racial ambivalence, value duality, and behavior. In J. F. Dovidio & S. L. Gaertner (Eds.), *Prejudice, discrimination, and racism* (pp. 35–59). Orlando, FL: Academic Press.

Keeley, L. H. (1996). *War before civilization.* New York: Oxford University Press.

Kenrick, D. T. (1994). Evolutionary social psychology: From sexual selection to social cognition. In M. P. Zanna (Ed.), *Advances in experimental social psychology* (Vol. 26, pp. 75–122). San Diego, CA: Academic Press.

Kenrick, D. T., Neuberg, S. L., & Cialdini, R. B. (1999). *Social psychology: Unraveling the mystery.* Boston: Allyn & Bacon.

Kinder, D. R., & Sears, D. O. (1981). Prejudice and politics: Symbolic racism versus racial threats to the good life. *Journal of Personality and Social Psychology, 40,* 414–431.

Kleck, R. E., Ono, H., & Hastorf, A. H. (1966). The effects of physical deviance upon face-to-face interaction. *Human Relations, 19,* 425–436.

Kurzban, R., & Leary, M. R. (2000). *Evolutionary origins of stigmatization: The functions of social exclusion.* Manuscript submitted for publication.

Langer, E. J., Bashner, R. S., & Chanowitz, B. (1985). Decreasing prejudice by increasing discrimination. *Journal of Personality and Social Psychology, 49,* 113–120.

Leakey, R. E. (1978). *People of the lake: Mankind and its beginnings.* New York: Avon.

Leakey, R. E., & Lewin, R. (1977). *Origins: What new discoveries reveal about the emergence of our species and its possible future.* New York: Dutton.

Lerner, M. J. (1980). *The belief in a just world: A fundamental delusion.* New York: Plenum Press.

Levine, J. M., & Moreland, R. L. (1994). Group socialization: Theory and research. In W. Stroebe & M. Hewstone (Eds.), *European review of social psychology* (Vol. 5, pp. 305–336). Chichester, England: Wiley.

Linsky, A. S. (1970). Who shall be excluded: The influence of personal attributes in community reaction to the mentally ill. *Social Psychiatry, 5,* 166–171.

Macrae, C. N., Milne, A. B., & Bodenhausen, G. V. (1994). Stereotypes as energy-saving devices: A peek inside the cognitive toolbox. *Journal of Personality and Social Psychology, 66,* 37–47.

Mafia. In *Encyclopaedia Britannica online* [Online]. Available: http://www.eb.com:180/bol/topic?eu=51169&sctn=1 [1999, September 20].

Major, B. (1994). From social inequality to personal entitlement: The role of social comparisons, legitimacy appraisals, and group membership. In M. P. Zanna (Ed.), *Advances in experimental social psychology* (Vol. 26, pp. 293–348). San Diego, CA: Academic Press.

Mann, L. (1980). Cross-cultural studies of small groups. In H. C. Triandis & R. W. Brislin (Eds.), *Handbook of cross-cultural psychology: Vol. 5. Social psychology* (pp. 155–209). Boston: Allyn & Bacon.

Mealey, L., Daood, C., & Krage, M. (1996). Enhanced memory for faces of cheaters. *Ethology and Sociobiology, 17,* 119–128.

Miceli, M. P., & Near, J. P. (1992). *Blowing the whistle: The organizational and legal implications for companies and employees.* New York: Lexington Books.

Morrison, J. K. (1980). The public's current beliefs about mental illness: Serious obstacle to effective community psychology. *American Journal of Community Psychology, 8,* 697–707.

Mullen, B., Brown, R., & Smith, C. (1992). Ingroup bias as a function of salience, relevance, and status: An integration. *European Journal of Social Psychology, 22,* 103–122.

Navon, L. (1996). Cultural notions versus social actions: The case of the socio-cultural history of leprosy in Thailand. *Social Analysis, 40,* 95–119.

Olzak, S. (1992). *The dynamics of ethnic competition and conflict.* Stanford, CA: Stanford University Press.

Perlman, J. L., & Routh, D. K. (1980). Stigmatizing effects of a child's wheelchair in successive and simultaneous interactions. *Journal of Pediatric Psychology, 5,* 43–55.

Pettigrew, T. F., & Meertens, R. W. (1995). Subtle and blatant prejudice in western Europe. *European Journal of Social Psychology, 25,* 57–75.

Pfuhl, E. H., & Henry, S. (1993). *The deviance process* (3rd ed.). New York: Aldine de Gruyter.

Pinsky, R. (1994). *The Inferno of Dante: A new verse translation*. New York: Farrar, Straus & Giroux.

Pruitt, D. G. (1998). Social conflict. In D. T. Gilbert, S. T. Fiske, & G. Lindzey (Eds.), *Handbook of social psychology* (4th ed., Vol. 2, pp. 470–503). Boston: McGraw-Hill.

Rabkin, J. (1974). Public attitudes toward mental illness: A review of the literature. *Schizophrenia Bulletin, 10*, 9–33.

Rokeach, M. (1972). *Beliefs, attitudes, and values*. San Francisco: Jossey-Bass.

Rosenbaum, M. E. (1986). The repulsion hypothesis: On the nondevelopment of relationships. *Journal of Personality and Social Psychology, 61*, 1156–1166.

Rosenfield, D., Stephan, W. G., & Lucker, G. W. (1981). Attraction to competent and incompetent members of cooperative and competitive groups. *Journal of Applied Social Psychology, 11*, 416–433.

Saenz, D. S., & Neuberg, S. L. (1993). *When good folks do bad things: Evaluation extremity due to expectancy violation*. Unpublished manuscript, Arizona State University.

Schaller, M. (1999). *Intergroup vigilance theory: An evolutionary theory of intergroup cognition*. Manuscript submitted for publication.

Schroeder, D. A., Penner, L. A., Dovidio, J. F., & Piliavin, J. A. (1995). *The psychology of helping and altruism*. New York: McGraw-Hill.

Schwartz, S. H., Struch, N., & Bilsky, W. (1990). Values and intergroup social motives: A study of Israeli and German students. *Social Psychology Quarterly, 53*, 185–198.

Sherif, M., Harvey, O. J., White, B. J., Hood, W. R., & Sherif, C. W. (1988). *The Robbers Cave experiment: Intergroup conflict and cooperation*. Middletown, CT: Wesleyan University Press. (Original work published 1961)

Snyder, M. L., & Miene, P. (1994). On the function of stereotypes and prejudices. In M. P. Zanna & J. M. Olson (Eds.), *The Ontario Symposium: Vol. 7. The psychology of prejudice* (pp. 33–54). Hillsdale, NJ: Erlbaum.

Snyder, M. L., Kleck, R. E., Strenta, A., & Mentzer, S. J. (1979). Avoidance of the handicapped: An attributional ambiguity analysis. *Journal of Personality and Social Psychology, 37*, 2297–2306.

Stephens, K. K., & Clark, D. W. (1987). A pilot study on the effect of visible physical stigma on personal space. *Journal of Applied Rehabilitation Counseling, 18*, 52–54.

Tajfel, H. (1969). Cognitive aspects of prejudice. *Journal of Social Issues, 25*, 79–97.

Tajfel, H. (1982). Social psychology of intergroup relations. *Annual Review of Psychology, 33*, 1–39.

Tajfel, H., & Turner, J. C. (1986). The social identity theory of intergroup behavior. In S. Worchel & W. Austin (Eds.), *Psychology of intergroup relations* (2nd ed., pp. 7–24). Chicago: Nelson-Hall.

Thurnwald, R. (1916). Banaro society: Social organization and kinship system of a tribe in the interior of New Guinea. *Memoirs of the American Anthropological Association, 3*(4).

Thurnwald, R. (1932). *Economics in primitive communities*. London: Oxford University Press.

Trivers, R. L. (1971). The evolution of reciprocal altruism. *Quarterly Review of Biology, 46*, 35–57.

Turner, J. C., Hogg, M. A., Oakes, P. J., Reicher, S. D., & Wetherell, M. S. (1987). *Rediscovering the social group: A self-categorization theory.* Oxford: Blackwell.

van der Dennen, J., & Falger, V. (Eds.). (1990). *Sociobiology and conflict: Evolutionary perspectives on competition, cooperation, violence, and warfare.* London: Chapman & Hall.

Warner, L. (1937). *A black civilization: A social study of an Australian tribe.* New York: Harper.

Weiner, B., Perry, R. P., & Magnusson, J. (1988). An attributional analysis of reactions to stigma. *Journal of Personality and Social Psychology, 55*, 738–748.

Williams, G. C. (1966). *Adaptation and natural selection.* Princeton, NJ: Princeton University Press.

Wills, T. A. (1981). Downward comparison principles in social psychology. *Psychological Bulletin, 90*, 245–271.

Worchel, S., Andreolli, V. A., & Folger, R. (1977). Intergroup cooperation and intergroup attraction: The effects of previous attraction and outcome of combined effort. *Journal of Experimental Social Psychology, 13*, 131–140.

3

Threat and the Social Construction of Stigma

CHARLES STANGOR
CHRISTIAN S. CRANDALL

One of the main goals of this book is to clarify our thinking about stigma, and our goal in this chapter is to consider one of the fundamental questions about stigma: Where does stigma come from? That is, what is stigmatizing, and why? Although fundamental, this topic has rarely been addressed within the social psychology literature. Indeed, three of the fundamental volumes about stigma (Goffman, 1963; Katz, 1981; Wright, 1960) do not address it at all, although a fourth (Jones et al., 1984) does, at least to some extent. Because this topic has not heretofore been considered in much detail, our analysis remains at least partially tentative; we have little direct empirical evidence for our claims. Still, by extrapolating from the stereotyping and prejudice literatures, and building on the stigma literature that does exist, we can develop a basic theory of the origins of stigma.

Our chapter focuses on three issues. We first consider why some attributes appear to be universally stigmatizing, and yet for others there is wide variation across cultures, as well as over time within cultures. Second, we review and then apply several theoretical approaches, derived from the literature on prejudice and stereotyping, to the development of stigmatized social categories. Finally, we present a theory of stigma development: We propose that stigma develops out of an initial, universally held motivation to avoid danger, followed by (often exaggerated) perception of characteristics that promote threat, and accompanied by a social sharing of these perceptions with others. These three processes are sufficient to provide a general account of the perceptions of stigma. Moreover, we emphasize a fundamental conclusion—namely, that stigmas exist primarily in the minds of stigmatizers and stigmatized individuals as cultural social constructions, rather than as universally stigmatized physical features.

That the origins of stigma are poorly understood is not surprising, given that we also know little about where the related concepts of social stereotypes and group prejudice come from. In fact, Schneider (1996) recently lamented the paucity of data concerning stereotype development. Nevertheless, because we know of few data and are aware of little prior speculation about the origins of stigma (but see Schaller, 1999; Neuberg, Smith, & Asher, Chapter 2, this volume), we draw at least to some extent in this review from the (also limited) literature on stereotyping and prejudice. Since prejudice is based, at least to some extent, on perceptions of *deviance* (Katz & Hass, 1988), such an approach does not seem unreasonable. In fact, we follow the example of Goffman (1963), who included the "tribal" stigmas of race, nationality, and religion in his seminal book on stigma. Like stigmas, stereotypes come from (among other things) the perception of group boundaries, the sense of "us" versus "them," perceptual distinctiveness, and so on (see Biernat & Dovidio, Chapter 4, this volume). Thus the same forces that lead to social categorization and beliefs about group members may also lead to perceptions of value and devaluation, interruption in normal social flow, and the discrediting that characterizes stigmatization.

WHAT NEEDS EXPLAINING?

According to Goffman (1963), "stigma" refers to a mark or sign of some sort that is seen as disqualifying individuals from the full social acceptance of a society; it also refers to the beliefs about individuals with such a mark. As he put it, "Society establishes the means of categorizing persons and the complement of attributes felt to be ordinary and natural for members of each of these categories" (p. 2). One task of a theory regarding the origins of stigma is to explain how a given society or culture comes to share its beliefs about stigmatization. For a characteristic to be a stigma, it must be shared among the members of a given group. You may prefer long blonde hair and detest short dark hair, whereas I may have the opposite inclinations. But these personal evaluative beliefs do not constitute stigma: Stigmas must be shared to be so considered, such that they "spoil" interactions not only at an individual level, but also at a group level.

Nevertheless, the question of "among whom" the sharing must take place is complex. The negotiation of shared reality may take place at the very broadest social contexts (such as within historical eras), within the briefest of dyadic social interactions, or at any level in between. Shared realities, including the definition of stigmas and the stereotypic attributes and social roles that accompany them, are constantly negotiated by large and small social groups. Furthermore, "local" social negotiations always take place in reference to a larger social context. And so whenever a group defines an attribute as a stigma, or whenever it defines a typically stigmatizing attribute (such as race, gender, or physical disability) as nonstigmatizing, the attributes are never stigmatizing per se, but are rather defined by the relation of the group's and its members' beliefs with beliefs held in the larger social world. Indeed, people often seek out groups in which their stigma "disappears," such as among like-minded or similarly stigmatized others, or groups in which a stigma (such as body piercing) is shared and thus enhanced. In such cases the negotiated shared reality in the group is one of acceptance and fraternity, which diminishes or enhances the stigma's power.

Despite this constant negotiation, relative stability is usually achieved; this smooths over social interactions, making them reliable, meaningful, and predictable. Conflict often appears when realities are not shared. For example, a stigma-defined group may have quite conflictual relations with outgroup members who do not share their stigma-diminishing reality.

The second task for a theory of stigma origins is accounting for both cross-cultural similarity and cross-cultural variability in perceptions of stigma (Archer, 1985). Evidence that some characteristics—such as facial distortions, mental illness, and homosexuality—are stigmatized across many cultures suggests that there is a common underlying component to stigma. As other examples, it has been argued both that dark skin is universally more stigmatized than light skin, and that height is a universally positively valued feature (Chaiken, 1986; Collins & Zebrowitz, 1995; Roberts & Herman, 1986; Wilson, 1968). Another powerful and probably universal stigma is facial disfigurement. A grossly distorted face is very disturbing to viewers, and this profound reaction appears in newborns and across cultures (Johnson, Dziurawiec, Ellis, & Morton, 1991). Facial perception appears to have a specific locus in the brain (Trehub, 1997), suggesting that a distorted face may be a "hard-wired" stigma (Johnson et al., 1991).

Despite these cross-cultural commonalities in stigma perceptions, there is nevertheless substantial evidence that stigmas are locally and culturally constructed. What is stigmatizing varies both across and within cultures, as well as across time within a culture. In short, as Weiner (1993) puts it, what is "sin" for one culture at one time is "sickness" in another culture or another time. For example, the extent to which homosexuality is seen as stigmatizing turns to a great degree on whether it is viewed as a "lifestyle choice" (as in much of the United States) or as an issue based on religion, morals, and "cleanliness" (as in Venezuela) (D'Anello & Crandall, 2000). Similarly, fatness is seen as more stigmatizing in the United States more than in Mexico (Crandall & Martinez, 1996); and age is seen as evidencing sickness and weakness in the United States, but signifies moral wisdom and status in Japan (O'Leary, 1993). Sexual behaviors, such as divorce and polygamy, also vary substantially in the extent to which they are culturally accepted or stigmatized. And we find similar differences across subcultures with a broader culture. For instance, some social groups in the United States value body piercing, tattoos, and scarification with knives, whereas others value modesty, sensible shoes, and natural hair colors. Each group, of course, views the other's valued marks of identity as stigmas.

Under certain circumstances, characteristics that appear to be universally stigmatizing are in fact determined by the local "culture." For instance, although a distorted face is sometimes referred to as a "universal" stigma, there are a variety of social interactions in which a deformed face might not be stigmatizing. A facially distorted person may interact smoothly with a blind person who may not be aware of the other's stigma—or, if aware of it, nevertheless lacks the automatic and visceral response that characterizes the sight of disfigurement. Sighted people often interact with others without seeing them; telephone conversations may be unaffected by disfigurement, rendering the attribute nonstigmatizing. An expanding area of social interaction that avoids face-to-face interaction is the Internet. Growing numbers of relationships have begun through chat rooms, e-mail, Usenet newsgroups, mailing lists, and electronic personal ads. These relationships can be intimate, long-lasting, satisfying, and entirely independent of visual interaction. Thus what appears to be a universal and hard-wired stigmatization reaction may play no role in some social situations. On the other hand, the local culture may not be able to destigmatize an attribute entirely. For instance, even in a setting in which all group members have distorted facial features, the stigma may still persist—especially if there are inborn "expectations" about what defines a "normal" face (Zebrowitz, 1997).

What is perceived as stigma also changes relatively quickly over time within a single culture. It has been observed that stereotypes about competing nations change quickly as a function of international relationships, such as wars. Perceptions of appropriate body weight, and corresponding stigmas for those who violate these norms—as well as even whether weight is a relevant variable—have changed over the centuries. Attitudes toward homosexuality, mental illness, divorce, and ethnicity also evolve over time. Italian immigrants, once vilified and characterized as intellectually inferior to other ethnic groups, are now esteemed members of U.S. society. Blacks, once held as slaves, now have (ostensibly) equal status with Whites. The American Psychiatric Association's *Diagnostic and Statistical Manual of Mental Disorders*—the bible of the definitions of mental disorders—has shown changes in the definition of what is a mental illness in virtually every diagnostic category.

To consider one example, although homosexuality is stigmatizing in many cultures, historically it was not so reliably rejected (Katz, 1984). Although homosexuality is commonly stigmatizing in the United States, it is far more accepted now than in early American days. Early Puritan colonies had the death penalty for both adultery and sodomy (homosexual acts), and executed men for both; however, a conviction of sodomy was more likely to lead to execution, and adultery was more likely to lead to a severe lashing (Katz, 1996). In some societies, the "natural" and "normal" (and therefore unstigmatizing) progression of sexual development begins with a homosexual stage for all males, prior to their ascending into "adult" heterosexuality (Mead, 1949). Although the Catholic Church now squarely stigmatizes homosexuality as a matter of moral principle, there is evidence that it sanctioned homosexual marriages during the Middle Ages (Boswell, 1995).

EXISTING APPROACHES

We need fresh insights into the development of stigma because existing models from the stigma literature, as well as those from the closely related work on stereotyping, prejudice, and discrimination, have not provided complete theories to account for the development of social stigma. However, theories of stereotype development may provide clues to the etiology of stigma, and thus a foundation for the development of new approaches. Theories of the development of stereotypes and prejudice fall into three general categories—"functional" theories, "perceptual" theories, and "consensus" theories—each of which appears to be relevant to a full understanding of stigma. Yet, although each theory accounts for some aspects of group perceptions, no theory seems by itself to provide a full answer to our fundamental question of why some groups are stigmatized and not others. Nevertheless, we can learn something important about the potential determinants of stigma from each.

Functional Theories

Functional theories assume that individuals perceive members of their own and other groups, and create associated stereotypes and prejudices about these groups, in such a way as to provide personal benefits (Snyder & Miene, 1994). For instance, it is frequently argued that stereotypes provide initial and potentially valid information about others, and that they thus simplify social perception (Allport, 1954; Esses, Haddock, & Zanna, 1992; Ford & Stangor, 1992; Macrae, Milne, & Bodenhausen, 1994; Macrae, Stangor, & Milne, 1994; Stangor & Ford, 1992; Turner, 1987). Another set of such functional theories assumes that stereotyping and prejudice, and particularly comparisons between ingroups and outgroups, enhance self-esteem or social identity for the individual perceiver, as a result of downward comparison with relatively devalued outgroups (Brewer, 1979; Fein & Spencer, 1997; Lemyre & Smith, 1985; Rubin & Hewstone, 1998; Wills, 1981).

Although functional approaches based on cognitive economy or self-enhancement can account for category use, they cannot well account for the initial creation of social stigma. Once a category and its associated stereotypes exist, it can be used to simplify social perception. But the theory of cognitive economy is not particularly specific about which categories (as long as they differentiate individuals) will initially become the foundation of social perception. Similarly, according to social identity formulations, perceiving one's ingroups as better than outgroups is important for identity enhancement, but it does not say much about which groups should be used for this function.

However, still another potential function—the protection of the self from threat or harm—provides a rather straightforward explanation for the development of stigma, and thus may be more relevant to understanding its origins. Avoiding dangerous and threatening situations, and thus assuring survival through an accurate perception of potential of threat, should be an important perceptual function for all organisms, including humans. Indeed, it is a fundamental assumption of many theories of emotion that displays of threat will be more easily detected and more quickly responded to than other equivalently extreme negative and positive emotional displays (Hansen & Hansen, 1988), precisely because of their adaptive significance. Perceiving the physical features of others may allow the quick and accurate detection of threat, and thus groups may initially become stigmatized to the extent that they are perceived as threatening (Zebrowitz, 1996). Indeed, as reviewed by Dovidio, Major, and Crocker in Chapter 1 of this volume, Jones et al. (1984) saw "peril" as an important determinant of stigma, and our analysis expands upon this idea. Because perception of threat appears to be a likely foundation for the development of stigma, we consider it in more detail later in this chapter.

In sum, the important, and necessary, contribution of a functional approach to a model of stigma development is the specification of an initial function or motivation—an impetus for stigma. In this sense, stigmas may be assumed to have their origins because they provide appropriate meaning about the environment, because they provide support for the individual perceiver's self-concept, and (perhaps particularly) because they provide cues about the potential of danger for the perceiver.

Perceptual Theories

There are various perceptual theories of stereotyping, each based on the assumption that the initial categorization of individuals into groups and the resulting group stereotypes are the results of direct observation of the social environment. These approaches share the underlying assumption that social perception will be biased, such that group perceptions as well as stereotypes about groups will be both distorted and amplified. Perceptual theories can themselves be divided into two types: "belief creation" theories and "accentuation" theories.

Belief Creation Theories

Two perceptual approaches—illusory correlation (Hamilton, 1981) and the ecological theory of social perception (Gibson, 1979; Zebrowitz, 1996)—may provide insights into the initial development of social stigma. According to the illusory-correlation approach, negative traits will be ascribed to minority groups as a result of inaccurate perceptions of the relationships between group characteristics and group size. Thus, because they are both less frequent, minority groups and negative behaviors will be particularly distinctive and thus will become (erroneously) associated. Although designed to account for the development of social stereotypes, illusory-correlation theory also appears able to account for stigma development in its expectation that unusual or infrequent characteristics will be stigmatized. Although the theory does not make clear which unusual stigmas will be important, this theory is informative because it suggests that since stigmas are unusual, they will also be associated with negative beliefs.

The ecological approach to social perception also provides a mechanism for stigma development by proposing that the characteristics of a person—for instance, facial appearances, body movements, and voice qualities—provide useful, and potentially accurate, information about the individual's personality. These physical features are proposed to reveal a person's "affordances"—the behavioral opportunities that the person provides. For instance, individuals with "baby faces" are perceived as naive, dependent, and attractive, and criminals are also perceived to have distinct facial features. Moreover, there is evidence that these perceptions have some basis in fact (Zebrowitz, 1996). Thus the ecological approach assumes an initial "kernel of truth" to a stigma, which is then accentuated and overgeneralized through perceptual accentuations. Similarly, faces that are symmetrical are argued to denote physical health and the lack of genetic defects—characteristics important in sexual partners (Gangestad & Thornhill, 1998).

Accentuation Theories

The assumption underlying theories of perceptual accentuation is that perceived differences in group behaviors or characteristics (actual or misperceived) are exaggerated through cognitive biases. Thus these theories (Ford & Stangor, 1992; Turner, 1987) do not account for the initial development of stigma, but rather explain how existing (actual) group differences are perceptually exaggerated because individuals seek for meaning in these differences. According to the accentuation approach, ingroup favoritism occurs because individuals exaggerate the extent of differences between ingroup and outgroup members, and stereotypes are exaggerated because of biased information search (Trope & Thompson, 1997), biased memory (Fyock & Stangor, 1994), and biased attributions (Hewstone, 1988) about social groups.

   Thus, as a set of theories, the perceptual models each predict that individuals, on an individual basis, seek meaning by observing their social environments, determining consistencies in behavior across individuals who share common categories, and subsequently exaggerating the consistencies as a result of cognitive biases. These theories seem to be applicable to stigma development, because they provide a foundation for the exaggerated characteristics of group beliefs.

Consensus Theories

Functional theories provide an initial impetus for stigmas, and perceptual theories provide a means by which they are subsequently accentuated. But neither of these approaches provides a full explanation for how each or most members of a given society end up finding the same dimensions meaningful. However, still another set of theories about stereotyping, based on social exchange and communication, is designed to do so (Harasty, 1997; Hardin & Higgins, 1996; Haslam et al., 1998; Levine & Moreland, 1991; Levine, Resnick, & Higgins, 1993; Ruscher,

Hammer, & Hammer, 1996; Schaller & Conway, 1999, in press; Schaller & Latané, 1996). These models, which are currently receiving much research attention, are particularly capable of accounting for agreement within the members of a culture on beliefs about stigma because they assume that stereotypes (like all beliefs) are transferred throughout the society through communication, and that individuals by and large tailor their opinions to conform to the opinions of others.

In an influential study concerning the importance of social norms in prejudice, Pettigrew (1959) studied anti-Black and pro-apartheid beliefs of White South Africans. He found that these beliefs were not so much predicted by individual personality constructs such as authoritarianism, but rather were predicted most reliably from two sources: cultural norms about the acceptability of prejudice toward Blacks, and individual conformity to the norms. Pettigrew found that the social norms about racial differences in status and privilege in South African society permeated all levels of society. To the extent that individuals conformed to these social norms, they endorsed racialist beliefs and policies. Thus he concluded that stigmatization was a problem not so much of the individual perceiver as of the social context. That is, a stigmatized target person is not really stigmatized at an individual level (i.e., by other individuals), but rather by the society that creates, condones, and maintains such attitudes and behavior. And an individual stigmatizer is only, by and large, repeating his or her society's norms about appropriate behavior.

According to the consensus approach, shared beliefs about social stigma—although they may initially be developed and amplified through interactions with *outgroup* members—are further accentuated and socially consensualized through communication and other contact with *ingroup* members. In this sense, beliefs about the appropriate reactions to an individual with mental illness, the morality of divorce, or the appropriateness of excluding gays from elementary school teaching positions are not determined only by an individual's interactions with members of those groups, but also by the individual's perceptions of the culturally normative beliefs about them.

In one experiment that demonstrated the importance of social norms as determinants of stigma (Crandall, Eshleman, & O'Brien, 2000), 120 undergraduates were asked to sort a list of 105 social groups into one of three categories: "OK to feel negatively toward this group," "Maybe OK to feel negatively toward this group," and "Not OK to feel negatively toward this group." The groups were based on a long list of groups of people (generated by University of Kansas undergraduates) that or who could plausibly be targets of prejudice. The list included the usual ethnic, racial, and religious groups, but also rapists, physically disabled persons, child molesters, politicians, stars of pornographic films, accountants, gay soldiers, students at Kansas State University, college teachers with poor English skills, and so on. From these data, Crandall and colleagues were able to create an ordering of the groups in terms of a "normatively acceptable to express prejudice toward" dimension.

Another 120 undergraduates were asked to fill out "feeling thermometers" on the same 105 groups. These thermometers represent a relatively straightforward affective measure of prejudice or stigmatization. Crandall, Eshleman, and O'Brien (2000) collapsed the data into mean ratings, so that each group had a mean rating of "OK to express prejudice" from the first sample, and a mean rating of prejudice from the second sample. With the 105 groups as a unit of analysis, the correlation between the normative acceptability of expressing prejudice and the actual expression of prejudice was .97! These data suggest that the willingness to express rejection and negative affect toward group members is almost completely a function of the perceived normative acceptability of that prejudice. If holding negative attitudes is perceived as socially appropriate, then it is condoned. In this sense, individual differences in prejudice are more likely to indicate differences in conformity to perceived group norms than personal motivations for cognitive parsimony or self-esteem.

Social beliefs, including those about stigmas, are transmitted within the members of a society in both an active and a passive sense. In some cases an individual may relatively passively assimilate the beliefs that are culturally available through exposure to those messages. The mass media, particularly television, depict interactions between stigmatized and nonstigmatized individuals in stereotyped ways. Stigma are also particularly common sources of humor, and thus they are highly likely to be consensually transmitted (LaFrance & Woodzicka, 1998).

Stigma may also be shared actively, through communication. Indeed, Schaller and Conway (in press) recently investigated the extent to which the traits that were perceived as true of social groups remained stable over time by analyzing the agreement in stereotype ascription across three stereotyping studies over several decades (Gilbert, 1951; Karlins, Coffman, & Walters, 1969; Katz & Braly, 1933). Schaller and Conway also had undergraduates rate the extent to which there was a tendency to communicate the trait ("Suppose you met a person who had this trait, and now you're talking to others about this person; how likely it is that you'll tell these others that this person has this trait?"). Schaller and Conway found that the extent to which a trait remained part of a cultural stereotype over time (as assessed by a lack of change across the three studies) was strongly related to the rated likelihood of communicating the trait.

Also supporting the importance of consensus, Stasser and his colleagues have shown that information that is common to group members prior to a discussion is much more likely to be openly discussed than information that some members have prior to the discussion but other members do not (see Stasser, 1992). Thus initial consensus tends to create even more consensus (Allen & Levine, 1968; Miller & Prentice, 1996). Interestingly, Latané's model of dynamic social influence (Schaller & Latané, 1996) explicitly predicts that although consensus will develop within a group that communicates, pockets of disagreement will always remain. Consensus is never perfect.

Beliefs about stigmas may also become consensual within a society because individuals are motivated to share their beliefs with others. Indeed, a fundamental assumption of many social-psychological approaches is that individuals are motivated to be part of groups, and that sharing beliefs allows them to be accepted (Baumeister & Leary, 1995). Sharing beliefs provides positive affect, as well as a sense of security and epistemological validity. Stangor, Sechrist, and Jost (in press) tested the hypothesis that individuals' beliefs about the stereotypes of other social groups would be a direct function of the individuals' perceptions of the stereotypes of other members of their own social groups (Haslam et al., 1996; Wittenbrink & Henly, 1996). It was found both that individuals overestimate the negative stereotypes held by other members of their groups, and that stereotypes can be significantly changed by altering people's perceptions of the stereotypes held by others.

Creating consensus can also occur as a result of negotiation between the stigmatizer and the stigmatized (Goffman, 1963; Pfuhl & Henry, 1993). Typically, both the stigmatized and the nonstigmatized agree that the mark or attribute that serves as a stigma is in fact a potential disqualifier or "interaction interrupter." Thus stigma and the stigmatization process are socially constructed, even in a small, local social group of two. The two parties may also agree that the attribute does not serve as a stigma, either because they both carry the mark, or because they deem it nondisqualifying, or because they are unaware of the stigma. However, the negotiation of stigma does not always go smoothly. In the early days of the U.S. civil rights movement, Black students sitting at lunch counters presented themselves in a situation where White employees and business owners perceived the customers' race as a disqualifying attribute, but the Blacks did not. Conflict ensued.

In sum, consensus theories suggest that there will be general, but not perfect, agreement among the members of a society because they share communications with each other, and this results in shared group representations. And this approach provides mechanisms for this sharing. Not only are stereotypes of, attitudes toward, and proscriptive responses to stigmatized persons created through social learning and social interaction; even the initial determination of what is stigmatized is also socially constructed.

A THEORY OF STIGMA ETIOLOGY

Our reading of the relatively limited literature concerning the development of stigma, as well as of the theoretical approaches to understanding the etiology of stereotypes within social psychology, suggests that an adequate theory of the development of social stigma will involve consideration of three major components: function, perception, and social sharing. Thus knowledge about social stigma will be initially acquired because it serves a basic function for the individual or the society; will be learned, and potentially distorted, through direct experience with the social environment and subsequent perceptual distortion; and will be consolidated culturally through communications expressed to and by relevant others. This model is presented in Figure 3.1.

Stigma requires, first, an initial functional impetus. Although there are many potential functions, we believe that the goal of avoiding threat to the self is the most likely candidate (see also Neuberg et al., Chapter 2, this volume). Furthermore, this initial function is then accentuated through perception and subsequently consolidated at a social level through social sharing of information. The result is a sharing of stigma, such that stigmatization becomes part of the society that creates, condones, and maintains such attitudes and behavior (Jones, 1997).

Our theory has the advantage of providing an explanation for the sharing of at least some stigmas cross-culturally (the common goal of

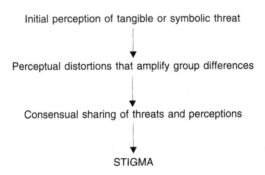

FIGURE 3.1. The role of threat, perceptual distortions, and societal sharing in the development of stigma.

protecting against threat), and yet it is also consistent with variation across cultures due to differential perception and sharing. Different societies have different tastes in food (Americans love hamburgers, whereas inhabitants of India would be disgusted by them), but nevertheless food (whatever its form) satisfies an underlying need (that of providing nourishment) for all individuals (Asch, 1952).

Stigma as Threat

Because the perception of threat provides such an important component of our analysis, it is worth considering in more detail. It is our general expectation that a characteristic becomes stigmatizing when it is perceived, at either an individual or a social level, to pose a threat to the vitality of the individual or the culture. In this section we consider some of the many potential threats that may be conveyed through stigma. Our review considers threats that are tangible, such as contagious diseases and their markers, as well as threats that are symbolic in nature, such as threats to belief in a just world. Tangible threats are "instrumental"— that is, they threaten a material or concrete good, such as health, safety, wealth, or social position (Schaller, 1999). Symbolic threats, on the other hand, threaten beliefs, values, ideology, and an understanding of how the social, political, and/or spiritual worlds work. Both kinds of threats are unwelcome; both are anxiety- or fear-provoking; and both can produce and increase stigmatization. Furthermore, many stigmas (e.g., AIDS, radical political beliefs, and schizophrenia) appear to be the result of both tangible and symbolic threats, and it is not unlikely that threats that were originally tangible are later generalized to become symbolic (Schaller, 1999).

Intergroup Conflict

According to realistic group conflict theory (Sherif & Sherif, 1953), social categories or characteristics may demonstrate threat when they are associated with intergroup conflict. Groups that threaten other groups' livelihood are likely to be stigmatized. For instance, attitudes within a country toward individuals from friendly countries will generally be positive, whereas attitudes toward warring nations will be negative (Brewer & Campbell, 1976). But similar outcomes can occur within groups. In a classic study, Hovland and Sears (1940; see also Hepworth & West, 1988) found that the number of lynchings (of Blacks by Whites) in the South varied with the price of cotton; as cotton prices fell, lynchings increased. Such a correlation can be accounted for in terms of realistic group conflict theory (Sherif & Sherif, 1953). When economic times are hard, competition for scarce resources produces intergroup conflict. Furthermore, individuals who steal, cheat, lie, or betray the group (or who are members of social groups that are believed to do so) are stigmatized (Neuberg et al., Chapter 2, this volume).

According to our approach, perceived threat from outgroup members may provide an initial impetus for stigmatization. When individuals initially perceive that their individual livelihood is threatened, they then exaggerate these perceptions (blaming all Blacks for the problem, for instance) and share the beliefs with each other. In the end, perceptions or behaviors (such as the lynchings) are social phenomena, occurring when members of a group collectively decide that they are threatened, and convince each other that the stigmatized individuals (in this case, the Blacks) are an appropriate target. Thus in the end a lynch mob reflects not only individual fears of deprivation, but also the norms of the society (Cantril, 1941). The perceptions of wartime enemies represent a similar phenomenon.

Health Threats

Just as threats may endanger one's financial well-being, they may also directly endanger one's physical health (Jones et al., 1984). Crandall and Moriarty (1995) tested the hypothesis that stigmatization is associated with perceived threats to health by studying individual reactions to 66 different illnesses, representing a wide range of possible physical illnesses and disease states (e.g., tuberculosis, venereal disease, diabetes, cancer, Hodgkin's disease, renal disease, rabbit fever, plantar warts, etc.). Participants read a realistic case report of a person who presented to a physician with the classic symptoms of one of the illnesses. The case report listed the typical course of disease and outlined treatment options. The disease outcomes for both treated and untreated individuals were described, although in the case report the patient always received the recommended treatment.

After reading about the illness, participants rated it on a variety of dimensions, including how severe, contagious, controllable, and sexually transmitted it was. In addition the participants filled out a social distance scale, indicating the degree of stigmatization of the diseased person. Crandall and Moriarty (1995) collapsed the data across raters, treating the disease as the unit of analysis, and predicted social distance from the illness ratings. Each of the predictor variables significantly predicted social distance (all r's > .30). Taken together, these data suggest that stigma may come from two independent causes: the extent to which a stigma is severe, contagious, and sexually transmitted; and the extent to which it is perceived to be under personal control. Furthermore, responsibility was found to be highly correlated with the contagiousness of the illness and with whether it was sexually transmitted. In a series of regressions, it was shown that personal responsibility explained the same variance as contagiousness and sexual transmission. This suggests that in some cases, personal responsibility may serve as a signal or proxy for instrumental threat, particularly in the case of disease and illness.

This study is one of the few that has attempted to delineate the underlying structure of what leads to stigmatization in the form of social rejection. The two factors that emerged (how dangerous the stigma was believed to be and whether the person was seen as responsible for it) can be used to characterize almost any stigma, and the higher a stigma is on either dimension, the more severe the stigmatization reaction is likely to be; the most disruptive stigmas will be seen both as severe and as the results of individual responsibility (Weiner, Perry, & Magnusson, 1988).

A similar argument has been developed for the cross-cultural analysis of anti-fat prejudice (Crandall, 1994; Crandall & Martinez, 1996) and for prejudice and stigma in general (Crandall, Eshleman, & O'Brien, 2000). Crandall et al. (2000) have shown that variables representing the extent to which a stigma is (1) negative, culturally devalued, disruptive, or severe and (2) under individual control accurately predict anti-fat prejudice in six nations, although the element of individual control is more important in individualist cultures than in collectivist cultures.

Although disease states that people are held responsible for lead to greater stigmatization than do disease states that are uncontrollable, the controllability of the stigma appears to be an essential component of stigmatization in Western cultures (Weiner et al., 1988) but not in more collectivist cultures (Crandall et al., 2000). In non-Western cultures, purity seems to take the role of controllability, and purity is often the standard that can lead to the rejection of outsiders (e.g., the perception of some ethnic groups as "dirty" because of strange foods and smells, nonnormative clothing and bathing practices, etc.; Schweder, Much, Mahapatra, & Park, 1997). As with many threats, then, the tangible threat of disease appears to be blended into the perception of symbolic threats, such as the lack of restraint and control (in Western cultures) and violation of religious codes (in non-Western cultures).

In sum, health states are stigmatizing to the extent that they are severe and thus disruptive of normal social relations. Although this is likely to be a general rule cross-culturally, and thus one that can help explain communalities in stigmas, there will also be cultural differences. The notion of "disruptive" will depend upon the locally constructed consensus on what is disruptive. As an example, the deformed facial features and blindness that come from onchocerciasis ("river blindness") on the upper Nile River are only modestly stigmatizing among subsistence farmers and fishing people of this region, where it is relatively common; however, these features would be highly stigmatizing in the United States.

Physical Features That Denote Threat

Some faces are inherently more threatening than others, and this perception may be a source of stigma. For example, people with "baby faces" (large eyes, small concave nose, light coloring, large forehead, and small chin) are perceived as less threatening and are liked more than people with more mature faces are (Borkenau & Liebler, 1992; Kenny, Horner, Kashy, & Chu, 1992). Criminals have more unattractive, angular faces, and a wide variety of mental and physical illnesses can reduce facial attractiveness (Zebrowitz, 1997). One notable exception to this pattern is Down's syndrome, which creates a face that is babyish and distinctly nonthreatening, but is still stigmatized.

One outcome of unusual or distorted physical features (Goffman's "abominations of the body") is a direct, visceral physiological arousal, experienced by an individual as aversion or disgust when in direct contact with a stigmatized person. Severe facial deformities tend to produce this type of affective reaction. Such stigmas may increase perceptions of mortality salience (Solomon, Greenberg, & Pyszczynski, 1991), such that they produce a subjective rather than an objective concern with death. Although it may be true that stigmas based on physical deformities do not involve misperceptions or social sharing of negative views to the same extent that other ("tribal") stigmas do (see Biernat & Dovidio, Chapter 4, this volume), the negative affective reactions that they promote are nevertheless generally consensual (Kleck, Ono, & Hastorf, 1966; Kleck & Strenta, 1980) and thus likely to be damaging to the stigmatized individuals.

Belief in a Just World

When individuals or groups are disadvantaged in some way, they may ironically become even more stigmatized by more fortunate individuals or groups in order to justify the former's negative outcomes (Lerner, 1980). In this way, for example, AIDS becomes perceived as a punishment for homosexual behavior, and poverty becomes viewed as a punishment for laziness or lack of intelligence (Furnham & Gunter, 1984; Robinson & Bell, 1978). Lerner (1980) argues that people are highly motivated to believe in a world that is just and fair, and that they will defend such a view against counterexamples. Threats to belief in a just world may lead to a defensive assertion of belief in justice. Indeed, in a series of studies, people who read about a positively described young boy who was said to have contracted HIV through a blood transfusion subsequently reported higher levels of belief in a just world, when compared to a control group (Crandall, Britt, & Glor, 1999). Paradoxically, then, when someone's stigmatized state appears to be unfairly earned, an observer may respond in a dissonance-like fashion with a number of justice- and fairness-related cognitions, which in turn may serve to justify and enhance the stigmatization.

Moral Threats

Threats to a way of life or a society can also come in the form of the perceived potential for "moral undermining" of the society. Indeed, it is not unreasonable for the members of a society to develop a shared ideology that creates and supports an important value hierarchy, and to search for and condemn violations of this moral order. Perception of shared common values is a necessary component of a successful society. Groups that do not have a collective sense of the "group beliefs" (Bar-Tal, 1990) that define their very essence are not likely to prosper.

Societies naturally differ in terms of which beliefs are central. For instance, in the United States the underlying value system is based upon principles of individualism, with an emphasis on personal freedom, self-reliance, and achievement. Thus it would be expected that individuals who are perceived to violate these basic principles will be perceived as threatening, and thus will be stigmatized. One such group is Black Americans, and several current theories of racial prejudice are based on the belief that Blacks do not live up to traditional American values (Katz & Hass, 1988; Kinder & Sears, 1981). Surveys show that White Americans tend to see Blacks as lazy and lacking in ambition (Schuman, Steeh, Bobo, & Krysan, 1997). Thus Blacks may be stigmatized at least in part because they are perceived to violate basic cultural values (Biernat, Vescio, Theno, & Crandall, 1996), and the same is also true of homosexuals (Biernat, Vescio, & Theno, 1996).

Some of this can be motivated by psychological balance (Heider, 1958). We humans believe that people who are like us are good people with good values, whereas people with different values from us are perceived as "other" and thus are seen more negatively. In general, we believe that people who are in different groups have different values than we do (Wilder, 1985). Rokeach (1960) showed that rejection of a person based on the perception of a different value system is more powerful than rejection based on race. This may result in part from the tendency to see people with the same values as good people (Heider, 1958, 1988).

In addition, we tend to attribute moral goodness and value similarity to people to whom we are similar (Byrne, 1971).

Homosexuality is often construed as a moral threat. One of us lives in a small town that is constantly picketed by a very active and committed anti-homosexual group, whose signs and placards vividly illustrate their stigmatization of homosexuals by claim of moral impurity. One typical sign, often carried by preteen children, involves a silhouette of two people engaging in anal sex, with the caption "AIDS = Anally Injected Death Sentence"; another common sign reads "God Hates Fags." The equation of homosexuality with "unclean" sex, disease, and death on the one hand, and with value violation on the other, forms the tacit argument that homosexuals should be stigmatized because of their impurity and value violations.

Interim Summary

The perception of a person as "threatening," broadly defined, can lead to stigmatization. Perceived threat can be the result of either of two basic kinds of threat—one tangible and realistic, the other intangible and symbolic. Some stigmatization comes from realistic threat: Outgroup members may threaten to reduce access to some finite resource, such as in war, competition for scarce jobs, or the potential for disease transmission. The other major source of stigmatization is more symbolic; in this case, the threat is to one's moral and political world view. This type of stigmatization comes from violations of values, such as religious beliefs or the value of hard work and "fair play." In most cases—such as threats to "purity" values, which can appear in the form of unusual body odors, sexual practices outside the norm, piercing/marking/scarring of the body, the eating of "unclean" foods, touching "unclean" parts of the body, and so on—the two types of threats are intertwined.

Other Possibilities and Limitations

Our analysis to this point has suggested that the most likely candidate for the initial motivation to construct stigma is potential threat, and that subsequent cognitive and social processes amplify these beliefs and "consensualize" them. We have no direct evidence to support this theory, although we also know of no data that directly contradicts it. However, we should consider some other possibilities, as well as some potential alternatives.

One difficulty in assuming that the initial foundations of stigma relate to threat is that these cues may occasionally be contradictory. For instance, some homosexuals may also have baby faces. Similarly, some stigmatized targets, such as people with physical disabilities or elderly individuals, tend to be quite low in physical threat and quite supportive of traditional cultural values (Lambert & Chasteen, 1997). However, although some groups may pose little or no tangible threat, stigmatization may occur when *any* potential threat is perceived. Thus, even when threats are contradictory, the mere presence of any one significant perceived threat is likely to lead to stigmatization.

Other theories of stigma have pointed to deviance, unusualness, or the violation of social norms as the source of stigmatization (Pfuhl & Henry, 1993). This is certainly a reasonable idea, and it is certain that many stigmatized attributes are deviant. But being deviant is just as likely to be positive as it is to be negative, and many normative abnormalities (e.g., red hair, violet eyes) are not usually stigmatized. We suggest that only those "deviances" that pose a threat to safety, self-interest, or the social order will lead to stigmatization.

Another potential function of stigma is the detection of weakness. If we humans see others as weak, this may allow us to take advantage of them. This translates stigma theory into a theory of power and advantage, where stigma is conceived as an opportunity for social control (Schur, 1980). However, assuming that the initial function of stigma is to detect threat has the advantage of explaining why most stigmas are negative, whereas assuming that this function is the detection of weakness does not.

Yet another possibility (and one that social psychologists may not wish to take seriously) is an anarchic theory of stigmatization. Perhaps there is no particular motivation whatsoever for stigmatization; perhaps the characteristics that become stigmatizing are essentially determined by the outcome of random events. For example, in the United States, the common "dumb Swede" jokes from the 1950s were transformed into "dumb Polish" jokes and then "dumb blonde" jokes over time, although it is difficult to point to immigration, mass media effects, or events in world history that could account for such a change. Some change in stigmas is likely to be chaotic and essentially unpredictable.

CONCLUSIONS

Our approach in this chapter has been to consider the concept of stigma from a quasi-sociological perspective. We have argued that those interested in stigma must ask this important question: Where does stigma come from? We have taken a page from the stereotyping literature and suggested that stigma has its basis first in threat, be it symbolic or tangible. The merest glimmer of threat from some group may be exaggerated, distorted, and enhanced. This threat ultimately leads to a negotiation of shared understanding, and this negotiation takes place at many levels: face to face, in friendship groups, within social organizations, regionally, and across cultures. These processes lead to full-blown stigmatization.

As a result, we believe that individual approaches are not sufficient to answer this question, because they cannot explain many phenomena related to stigma—including change across cultures and time, the waxing and waning of the potency of some stigmas, and subgroup variations in stigmas. This is not to argue that individual approaches are not important. We need to understand why some people use stigmas when responding to others, while others are more able to get beyond them. Furthermore, there are individual differences in resistance to change; some people rapidly destigmatize "marked" individuals after brief periods of interaction with them, whereas others cling to their rejection of these individuals.

Ultimately, however, a theory of stigma creation must focus on both individuals and the context in which we find them. The process of stigma is particularly interesting because it illuminates the liminal space that social psychology occupies, between the individual and the collective. As our model in Figure 3.1 suggests, the process of stigmatization is an intricate dance between individual perceptions and beliefs, and group sharing of these same cognitions. Stigmatization can be a result of threat, but it requires social communication and sharing on the one hand, and individual distortions and enhancements on the other.

ACKNOWLEDGMENTS

This research was supported in part by Grant No. 9729739 from the National Science Foundation. We thank Mark Schaller for his insightful and helpful comments.

REFERENCES

Allen, V. L., & Levine, J. M. (1968). Social support, dissent and conformity. *Sociometry, 31*, 138–149.

Allport, G. W. (1954). *The nature of prejudice*. Reading, MA: Addison-Wesley.

Archer, D. (1985). Social deviance. In G. Lindzey & E. Aronson (Eds.), *Handbook of social psychology: Vol. 2. Special fields and applications* (3rd ed., pp. 743–804). New York: Random House.

Asch, S. E. (1952). *Social psychology*. Englewood Cliffs: Prentice-Hall.

Bar-Tal, D. (1990). *Group beliefs*. New York: Springer-Verlag.

Baumeister, R., & Leary, M. (1995). The need to belong: Desire for interpersonal attachments as a fundamental human motivation. *Psychological Bulletin, 117,* 497–529.

Biernat, M., Vescio, T. K., & Theno, S. A. (1996). Violating American values: A "value congruence" approach to understanding outgroup attitudes. *Journal of Experimental Social Psychology, 32,* 387–410.

Biernat, M., Vescio, T. K., Theno, S. A., & Crandall, C. S. (1996). Values and prejudice: Toward understanding the impact of American values on outgroup attitudes. In C. Seligman, J. M. Olson, & M. P. Zanna (Eds.), *The Ontario Symposium: Vol. 8. The psychology of values* (pp. 153–189). Hillsdale, NJ: Erlbaum.

Borkenau, P., & Liebler, A. (1992). Trait inferences: Sources of validity at zero acquaintance. *Journal of Personality and Social Psychology, 62,* 645–657.

Boswell, J. (1995). *Same-sex unions in pre-modern Europe.* New York: Vintage.

Brewer, M. B. (1979). In-group bias in the minimal intergroup situation: A cognitive–motivational analysis. *Psychological Bulletin, 86,* 307–324.

Brewer, M. B., & Campbell, D. T. (1976). *Ethnocentrism and intergroup attitudes: East African evidence.* Beverly Hills, CA: Sage.

Byrne, D. (1971). *The attraction paradigm.* New York: Academic Press.

Cantril, H. (1941). *The psychology of social movements.* London: Chapman & Hall.

Chaiken, S. (1986). Physical appearance and social influence. In C. Herman, M. P. Zanna, & E. Higgins (Eds.), *The Ontario Symposium: Vol. 3. Physical appearance, stigma, and social behavior* (pp. 143–177). Hillsdale, NJ: Erlbaum.

Collins, M., & Zebrowitz, L. (1995). The contributions of appearance to occupational outcomes in civilian and military settings. *Journal of Applied Social Psychology, 25,* 129–163.

Crandall, C. S. (1994). Prejudice against fat people: Ideology and self-interest. *Journal of Personality and Social Psychology, 66,* 882–894.

Crandall, C. S., Britt, T. W., & Glor, J. (1999). *When ideology is challenged: Pediatric AIDS and the belief in the just world.* Manuscript submitted for publication.

Crandall, C. S., Eshleman, A., & O'Brien, L. (2000). *Social norms and the expression of prejudice.* Unpublished manuscript.

Crandall, C. S., & Martinez, R. (1996). Culture, ideology, and antifat attitudes. *Personality and Social Psychology Bulletin, 22,* 1165–1176.

Crandall, C. S., & Moriarty, D. (1995). Physical illness stigma and social rejection. *British Journal of Social Psychology,, 34,* 67–83.

Crandall, C. S., D'Anello, S., Sakalli, N., Lazarus, E., Nejtardt, G. W., & Feather, N. T. (in press). An attribution-value model of prejudice: Anti-fat attitudes in six nations. *Personality and Social Psychology Bulletin.*

D'Anello, S., & Crandall, C. S. (2000). *Prejudice against fat people and homosexuals in Venezuela and the USA: Attributions and values.* Unpublished manuscript, University of the Andes, Merida, Venezuela.

Esses, V. M., Haddock, G., & Zanna, M. P. (1993). Values, stereotypes and emotions as determinants of intergroup attitudes. In D. Mackie & D. Hamilton

(Eds.), *Affect, cognition and stereotyping: Interactive processes in group perception* (pp. 137–166). New York: Academic Press.

Fein, S., & Spencer, S. J. (1997). Prejudice as self-image maintenance: Affirming the self through derogating others. *Journal of Personality and Social Psychology, 73,* 31–44.

Ford, T. E., & Stangor, C. (1992). The role of diagnosticity in stereotype formation: Perceiving group means and variances. *Journal of Personality and Social Psychology, 63,* 356–367.

Furnham, A., & Gunter, B. (1984). Just world beliefs and attitudes towards the poor. *British Journal of Social Psychology, 23,* 265–269.

Fyock, J., & Stangor, C. (1994). The role of memory biases in stereotype maintenance. *British Journal of Social Psychology, 33,* 331–343.

Gangestad, S., & Thornhill, R. (1998). Human sexual selection and developmental stability. In J. Simpson & D. Kenrick (Eds.), *Evolutionary social psychology* (pp. 169–196). Mahwah, NJ: Erlbaum.

Gibson, J. (1979). *The ecological approach to visual perception.* Boston: Houghton Mifflin.

Gilbert, G. M. (1951). Stereotype persistence and change among college students. *Journal of Abnormal and Social Psychology, 46,* 245–254.

Goffman, E. (1963). *Stigma: Notes on the management of spoiled identity.* Englewood Cliffs, NJ: Prentice-Hall.

Hamilton, D. L. (1981). Illusory correlation as a basis for stereotyping. In D. L. Hamilton (Ed.), *Cognitive processes in stereotyping and intergroup behavior* (pp. 115–144). Hillsdale, NJ: Erlbaum.

Hansen, C. H., & Hansen, R. D. (1988). Finding the face in the crowd: An anger superiority effect. *Journal of Personality and Social Psychology, 54,* 917–924.

Harasty, A. S. (1997). The interpersonal nature of social stereotypes: Differential discussion patterns about in-groups and out-groups. *Personality and Social Psychology Bulletin, 23,* 270–284.

Hardin, C., & Higgins, E. T. (1996). Shared reality: How social verification makes the subjective objective. In R. M. Sorrentino & E. T. Higgins (Eds.), *Handbook of motivation and cognition: Vol. 3. The interpersonal context* (pp. 28–84). New York: Guilford Press.

Haslam, S. A., Oakes, P. J., McGarty, C., Turner, J. C., Reynolds, K. J., & Eggins, R. A. (1996). Stereotyping and social influence: The mediation of stereotype applicability and sharedness by the views of ingroup and outgroup members. *British Journal of Social Psychology, 35,* 369–397.

Haslam, S., Turner, J., Oakes, P., Reynolds, K., Eggins, R., Nolan, M., & Tweedie, J. (1998). When do stereotypes become really consensual?: Investigating the group-based dynamics of the consensualization process. *European Journal of Social Psychology, 28,* 755–776.

Heider, F. (1958). *The psychology of interpersonal relations.* Hillsdale, NJ: Erlbaum.

Heider, F. (1988). *The notebooks of Fritz Heider: Vol. 4. Balance theory* (M. Benesh-Weiner, Ed.). Munich: Psycologie Verlags Union.

Hepworth, J. T., & West, S. G. (1988). Lynchings and the economy: A time-series reanalysis of Hovland and Sears (1940). *Journal of Personality and Social Psychology, 55,* 239–247.

Hovland, C. I., & Sears, R. R. (1940). Minor studies of aggression: VI. Correlation of lynchings with economic indices. *Journal of Psychology, 9,* 301–310.

Johnson, M. H., Dziurawiec, S., Ellis, H., & Morton, J. (1991). Newborns' preferential tracking of face-like stimuli and its subsequent decline. *Cognition, 40,* 1–19.

Jones, E. E., Farina, A., Hastorf, A., Markus, H., Miller, D., & Scott, R. (1984). *Social stigma: The psychology of marked relationships.* New York: Freeman.

Jones, J. M. (1997). *Prejudice and racism.* New York: McGraw-Hill.

Karlins, M., Coffman, T., & Walters, G. (1969). On the fading of social stereotypes: Studies in three generations of college students. *Journal of Personality and Social Psychology, 13,* 1–16.

Katz, D., & Braly, K. W. (1933). Racial stereotypes of one hundred college students. *Journal of Abnormal and Social Psychology, 28,* 280–290.

Katz, I. (1981). *Stigma: A social psychological analysis.* Hillsdale, NJ: Erlbaum.

Katz, I., & Hass, R. G. (1988). Racial ambivalence and American value conflict: Correlational and priming studies of dual cognitive structures. *Journal of Personality and Social Psychology, 55,* 893–905.

Katz, J. (1984). *Gay American history.* New York: Avon.

Katz, J. (1996). *The invention of heterosexuality.* New York: Dutton.

Kenny, D. A., Horner, C., Kashy, D. A., & Chu, L. C. (1992). Consensus at zero acquaintance: Replication, behavioral cues, and stability. *Journal of Personality and Social Psychology, 62,* 88–97.

Kinder, D. R., & Sears, D. O. (1981). Prejudice and politics: Symbolic racism versus racial threats to the "good life." *Journal of Personality and Social Psychology, 40,* 414–431.

Kleck, R., Ono, H., & Hastorf, A. H. (1966). The effects of physical deviance upon face-to-face interactions. *Human Relations, 19,* 425–436.

Kleck, R., & Strenta, A. (1980). Perceptions of the impact of negatively-valued physical characteristics on social interaction. *Journal of Personality and Social Psychology, 39,* 861–873.

LaFrance, M., & Woodzicka, J. (1998). No laughing matter: Women's verbal and nonverbal reactions to sexist humor. In J. K. Swim & C. Stangor (Eds.), *Prejudice: The target's perspective* (pp. 62–80). San Diego, CA: Academic Press.

Lambert, A., & Chasteen, A. (1997). Perceptions of disadvantage versus conventionality: Political values and attitudes toward the elderly versus Blacks. *Personality and Social Psychology Bulletin, 23,* 469–481.

Lemyre, L., & Smith, P. M. (1985). Intergroup discrimination and self-esteem in the minimal group paradigm. *Journal of Personality and Social Psychology, 49,* 660–670.

Lerner, M. J. (1980). *The belief in a just world: A fundamental delusion.* New York: Plenum Press.

Levine, J. M., & Moreland, R. (1991). Culture and socialization in work groups. In L. B. Resnick, J. M. Levine, & S. D. Teasley (Eds.), *Perspectives on socially shared cognition* (pp. 257–279). Washington, DC: American Psychological Association.

Levine, J. M., Resnick, L. B., & Higgins, E. T. (1993). Social foundations of cognition. *Annual Review of Psychology, 44*, 585–612.

Macrae, C. N., Milne, A. B., & Bodenhausen, G. V. (1994). Stereotypes as energy-saving devices: A peek inside the cognitive toolbox. *Journal of Personality and Social Psychology, 66*, 37–47.

Macrae, C. N., Stangor, C., & Milne, A. B. (1994). Activating social stereotypes: A functional analysis. *Journal of Experimental Social Psychology, 30*, 370–389.

Mead, M. (1949). *Male and female: A study of the sexes in a changing world.* New York: Morrow.

Miller, D. T., & Prentice, D. A. (1996). The construction of social norms and standards. In E. T. Higgins & A. W. Kruglanski (Eds.), *Social psychology: Handbook of basic principles* (pp. 799–829). New York: Guilford Press.

O'Leary, J. S. (1993). A new look at Japan's honorable elders. *Journal of Aging Studies, 7*, 1–24.

Pettigrew, T. F. (1959). Regional differences in anti-Negro prejudice. *Journal of Abnormal and Social Psychology, 59*, 28–36.

Pfuhl, E. H., & Henry, S. (1993). *The deviance process* (3rd ed.). New York: Aldine de Gruyter.

Roberts, J., & Herman, C. (1986). The psychology of height: An empirical review. In C. Herman, M. P. Zanna, & E. T. Higgins (Eds.), *The Ontario symposium: Vol. 3. Physical appearance, stigma, and social behavior* (pp. 113–140). Hillsdale, NJ: Erlbaum.

Robinson, R. V., & Bell, W. (1978). Equality, success, and social justice in England and the United States. *American Sociological Review, 43*, 125–143.

Rokeach, M. (1960). *The open and closed mind.* New York: Basic Books.

Rubin, M., & Hewstone, M. (1998). Social identity theory's self-esteem hypothesis: A review and some suggestions for clarification. *Personality and Social Psychology Review, 2*, 40–62.

Ruscher, J. B., Hammer, E. Y., & Hammer, E. D. (1996). Forming shared impressions through conversation: An adaptation of the continuum model. *Personality and Social Psychology Bulletin, 22*, 705–720.

Schaller, M. (1999). *Intergroup vigilance theory: An evolutionary theory of intergroup cognition.* Manuscript submitted for publication.

Schaller, M., & Conway, G. (1999). Influence of impression-management goals on the emerging content of group stereotypes: Support for a social-evolutionary perspective. *Personality and Social Psychology Bulletin, 25*, 819–833.

Schaller, M., & Conway, L. (in press). From cognition to culture: The origins of stereotypes that really matter. In G. Moscowitz (Ed.), *Cognitive social psychology on the tenure and future of social cognition.* Mahwah, NJ: Erlbaum.

Schaller, M., & Latané, B. (1996). Dynamic social impact and the evolution of social representations: A natural history of stereotypes. *Journal of Communication, 46*, 64–77.

Schneider, D. (1996). Modern stereotype research: Unfinished business. In C. N. Macrae, C. Stangor, & M. Hewstone (Eds.), *Stereotypes and stereotyping* (pp. 419–453). New York: Guilford Press.

Schuman, H. S., Steeh, C., Bobo, L., & Krysan, M. (1997). *Racial attitudes in America: Trends and interpretations*. Cambridge, MA: Harvard University Press.

Schur, E. M. (1980). *The politics of deviance: Stigma contests and the use of power*. Englewood Cliffs, NJ: Prentice-Hall.

Schweder, R., Much, N., Mahapatra, M., & Park, L. (1997). The "big three" of morality (autonomy, community, divinity) and the "big three" explanations of suffering. In A. Brandt & P. Rozin (Eds.), *Morality and health* (pp. 119–169). New York: Routledge.

Sherif, M., & Sherif, C. W. (1953). *Groups in harmony and tension*. New York: Harper & Row.

Snyder, M., & Miene, P. (1994). On the function of stereotypes and prejudice. In M. P. Zanna & J. Olson (Eds.), *The Ontario Symposium: Vol. 7. The psychology of prejudice* (pp. 33–54). Hillsdale, NJ: Erlbaum.

Solomon, S., Greenberg, J., & Pyszczynski, T. (1991). A terror management theory of social behavior: The psychological functions of self-esteem and cultural worldviews. In M. P. Zanna (Ed.), *Advances in experimental social psychology* (Vol. 24, pp. 93–159). San Diego, CA: Academic Press.

Stangor, C., & Ford, T. E. (1992). Accuracy and expectancy-confirming processing orientations and the development of stereotypes and prejudice. *European Review of Social Psychology, 3*, 57–89.

Stangor, C., Sechrist, G., & Jost, J. (in press). Changing racial beliefs by providing consensus information. *Personality and Social Psychology Bulletin*.

Stasser, G. (1992). Pooling of unshared information during group discussions. In S. Worchel, W. Wood, & J. Simpson (Eds.), *Group processes and productivity* (pp. 48–67). Newbury Park, CA: Sage.

Trehub, A. (1997). Sparse coding of faces in a neuronal model: Interpreting cell population response in object. In J. W. Donahoe & V. P. Dorsel (Eds.), *Neural-network models of cognition: Biobehavioral foundations* (pp. 189–202). Amsterdam: Elsevier/North-Holland.

Trope, Y., & Thompson, E. (1997). Looking for truth in all the wrong places?: Asymmetric search of individuating information about stereotyped group members. *Journal of Personality and Social Psychology, 73*, 229–241.

Turner, J. C. (1987). *Rediscovering the social group: A self-categorization theory*. Oxford: Blackwell.

Weiner, B. (1993). On sin versus sickness: A theory of perceived responsibility and social motivation. *American Psychologist, 48*, 957–965.

Weiner, B., Perry, R., & Magnusson, J. (1988). An attributional analysis of reactions to stigmas. *Journal of Personality and Social Psychology, 55*, 738–748.

Wills, T. A. (1981). Downward social comparison principles in social psychology. *Psychological Bulletin, 90*, 245–271.

Wilson, P. (1968). The perceptual distortion of height as a function of ascribed academic status. *Journal of Social Psychology, 74*, 97–102.

Wittenbrink, B., & Henly, J. R. (1996). Creating social reality: Informational social influence and the content of stereotypic beliefs. *Personality and Social Psychology Bulletin, 22*, 598–610.

Wright, B. (1960). *Physical disability: A psychological approach*. New York: Harper & Row.

Zebrowitz, L. A. (1996). Physical appearance as a basis of stereotyping. In C. N. Macrae, C. Stangor, & M. Hewstone (Eds.), *Stereotypes and stereotyping* (pp. 79–120). New York: Guilford Press.

Zebrowitz, L. A. (1997). *Reading faces: Window to the soul?* Boulder, CO: Westview Press.

4

Stigma and Stereotypes

MONICA BIERNAT
JOHN F. DOVIDIO

"Stigma" has traditionally been defined as a sign or a mark that designates the bearer as defective and therefore as meriting less valued treatment than "normal" people (Goffman, 1963). As Goffman (1963) suggested in his classic volume on the subject, different varieties of stigma or stigmatizing conditions can be distinguished. He focused on three types: (1) "tribal identities" (e.g., race, sex, religion, or nation), (2) "blemishes of individual character" (e.g., mental disorders, addictions, unemployment), and (3) "abominations of the body" (e.g., physical deformities). According to Crocker, Major, and Steele (1998), "stigmatized individuals possess (or are believed to possess) some attribute, or characteristic, that conveys a social identity that is devalued in some particular social context" (p. 505). Thus the major negative impact of stigmatization normally resides not in the physical consequences of the mark, but rather in its psychological and social consequences. The psychological and social consequences of stigma involve the responses both of the perceivers and of stigmatized people themselves.

The process of generalizing from an observable physical characteristic to a set of assumed traits is an essential aspect of the more general process of "stereotyping." Stereotypes have historically been viewed as unjustified because they reflect faulty thought processes or overgeneralization, factual incorrectness, inordinate rigidity, an inappropriate pattern of attribution, or a rationalization for a prejudiced attitude or discriminatory behavior (Brigham, 1971). However, even though they are inaccurate to varying degrees, stereotypes also serve fundamental functions for perceivers, such as providing explanations for others' behavior, supporting the perceiver's motivations (Kunda & Sinclair, 1999; Sinclair & Kunda, 1999), satisfying needs for cognitive closure (Jost, Kruglanski, & Simon, 1999), and enhancing personal and collective self-esteem (Stangor & Schaller, 1996). Many classic discussions of stigmatization propose not only that stigmatization involves social stereotyping in forms reflecting both these "unjust" and functional qualities, but also that it involves the internalization of these stereotypes by those who are stigmatized (Allport, 1954; Fanon, 1952/1967; Sartre, 1946/1965). This chapter examines stereotypes and stereotyping, and assesses their relevance to understanding stigma and stigmatization. We focus primarily on the response of perceivers to stigmatized persons; the four chapters in Part II of this volume consider issues relating to how people respond to being stigmatized.

Within the framework of the three dimensions of stigmatization introduced by Dovidio, Major, and Crocker in Chapter 1, stereotypes and stereotyping are mainly relevant to "collective" stigmas (or, in Goffman's terms, "tribal" stigmas) from the perspective of the "perceiver" (i.e., a person who evaluates the stigmatized), with a primary emphasis on "cognitive" processes. A "stereotype" has traditionally referred to the content of an assumed set of characteristics associated with a particular social group or type of person. Stereotypes are involved in stigmatization to the extent that the response of perceivers is not simply a negative one (i.e., dislike of "devalued identity"), but also that a specific set of characteristics is assumed to exist among people sharing the same stigma (i.e., the stigma evokes a *social* identity).

Because of the common mechanism of group-based inferences, stereotyping and tribal stigmas are closely related. Indeed, tribal stigmas have been of most interest to stereotyping researchers, as the large literatures on racism and sexism can attest. There is a simple explanation for the this interest: Tribal or group-based stigmas have consensually held, culturally transmitted stereotypes associated with them. White Americans endorse stereotypes about Black Americans that include traits such as "lazy," "athletic," and "streetwise" (see Devine & Elliot, 1995; Dovidio, Brigham, Johnson, & Gaertner, 1996; Wittenbrink, Judd, & Park, 1997), and gender stereotypes have been fairly steady in content for generations (Lueptow, Garovich, & Lueptow, 1995; Williams & Best, 1982).

Stereotyping is also involved in stigmas based on blemishes of individual character, although to a lesser extent. For example, people with mental disorders, although not typically perceived as an organized group, are assumed to possess common negative characteristics (Corrigan, 1998). People perceive those seeking psychological counseling as generally defensive, awkward, insecure, sad, cold, and unsociable (Sibicky & Dovidio, 1986). Fear of being perceived negatively by others leads many people who need psychological assistance not to seek it (Wills, 1983).

In contrast, abominations of the body (e.g., facial disfigurement, blindness, infertility), perhaps because they are more idiosyncratic and relatively rare, are less associated with a coherent set of presumed characteristics other than their defining qualities. Thus perceivers share beliefs that facially disfigured individuals are unattractive, that blind persons cannot see, and that infertile people cannot have children, but perceivers typically do not respond with broad-based inferences about these groups in general. Beliefs about these defining attributes certainly carry a negative evaluative tone, and someone with such a stigma is generally viewed as "the type of person that is devalued" (Crocker et al., 1998, p. 505). "Normals" may also assume that individuals with such stigmas are unhappy, and associated attributes of unhappiness may be inferred. Visible physical stigmas in particular may also provide information that "facilitates adaptive action" (e.g., "avoid those with communicable diseases"), and in that sense, beliefs about these stigmas exist (Zebrowitz, 1996). Nonetheless, explicit, specific, consensually held stereotypes of these more individually based stigmas are rarer than are stereotypes for Goffman's (1963) other two classifications of stigmas.

To summarize thus far, although stereotyping and stigmatization are closely related terms, they are not identical. Stigmatization can sometimes occur in the absence of consensual stereotypes; at other times—perhaps more often—its effects are closely affiliated with those of stereotyping. Jones and colleagues (1984), for example, write: "We assume that there is always a strong tendency for stigmatizing reactions to move in the direction of stereotypes that rationalize or explain the negative affect that is involved. This is true whether we are talking about the stereotypes associated with racial prejudice or serving to rationalize one's avoidance of the physically handicapped" (p. 10). The development of cultural stereotypes, however, also involves social influences and consensus (see also Jones et al., 1984; Schaller & Conway, 1999). Thus we propose that cultural stereotypes develop more readily for socially identifiable groups (groups with tribal stigmas, or people who share common blemishes of character)—to explain and justify negative attitudes, discrimination, and control and/or exploitation through institutional policies—than for people with more idiosyncratic "marks" (such as disfigurements) that produce more immediate and easily explained affective reactions. In the next section we consider factors that influence the relationship between stigmatization and stereotyping.

WHAT MAKES A STIGMA A STEREOTYPE?

Researchers have identified a range of cognitive and motivational factors that contribute to the development of stereotypes (see Mackie, Hamilton, Susskind, & Rosselli, 1996). Many of these general processes readily apply to stigmatization. For example, when a stigma involves a distinguishing physical or social feature, the feature can serve as a cue for social categorization. Once others are categorized into social groups, members of the group are seen as similar to one another and to a group prototype (Hogg & Hains, 1996), and differences between that group and other groups become exaggerated (Tajfel, 1969). Social categorization involves both information reduction and elaboration: Some information is lost about specific individuals, but the category allows for the assumption (perhaps often erroneous) that each member possesses a range of qualities characteristic of the group (Mackie et al., 1996; Spears & Haslam, 1997). Furthermore, social categorization subsequently affects how information is processed, stored, and retrieved (Linville, Salovey, & Fischer, 1986; Park & Rothbart, 1982; von Hippel, Sekaquaptewa, & Vargas, 1995) and how behavior is interpreted and explained (Hewstone, 1990; Maass & Arcuri, 1996; Pettigrew, 1979). These effects are especially strong when the target person has a distinguishing characteristic that makes him or her more salient (Taylor, 1981)—a process of obvious relevance to people with visible stigmas.

Motivationally, stereotypes and stereotyping may help perceivers achieve a flattering self-image (Dunning, 1999) and attain a sense of positive group distinctiveness that enhances self-esteem (Tajfel & Turner, 1979). Recent research also suggests that when individuals experience self-esteem threat, stereotypes are readily activated, and negativity toward stereotyped targets increases as a means of restoring the threatened self-image (Fein & Spencer, 1997; Spencer, Fein, Wolfe, Fong, & Dunn, 1998). Stereotypes may also originate from motivations, not necessarily conscious, to maintain the status quo that provides advantages to one's own group. Perceiving members of other groups not only as inferior but as possessing specific characteristics (e.g., "unintelligent but athletic") can justify their unequal treatment, which, in turn, leads to disparate outcomes (Jost & Banaji, 1994; Pettigrew, 1981; Yzerbyt, Rocher, & Schadron, 1997; see also Major, 1994). Then, because people are also motivated to see the world as fair and just (Lerner, 1980), they tend to explain the different statuses of groups in terms of differences in their characteristics, a process that reinforces stereotypes. Thus, from this motivational perspective, negative stereotyping is a self-perpetuating phenomenon. Moreover, Schaller and Conway (1999) argue that goals and motives further shape which aspects of cultural stereotypes are attended to and eventually learned. Those aspects that enhance one's collective self-esteem and that improve one's physical as well as psychological well-being are those most likely to be accepted and internalized or applied to outgroups.

Beyond what is shared with other forms of social categorization, what is it about stigmas that particularly contributes to the development of stereotypes about the individuals who have them? One is the "groupiness" factor. To the extent that a stigma is based on membership in a definable group, stereotypes are likely to develop and persevere. This is presumably the case because categories (even diffuse ones such as gender or race) can imply a substantial amount of other information about a person. By categorizing others, we humans "go beyond" given information and view objects with "more elaborated, connotative meaning" (Bruner, 1957, p. 148); categorization generates expectations about individual group members (Medin, 1988; see Oakes, Haslam, & Turner, 1994).

This may be particularly true of categories that are viewed in "essentialistic" terms. Essentialism is apparent when "perceivers appraise category membership of targets as reflecting their true identity, their real nature. Associated is a strong feeling of unalterability: Membership to an essentially defined social category can hardly be modified" (Yzerbyt et al., 1997, pp. 36–37). Racial and gender groups tend to be viewed in this way (Martin & Parker, 1995), and such "essential" categories have high "inductive potential"—that is, they allow for inferences about a wide range of attributes (Rothbart & Taylor, 1992). McGill (1998), for instance, found that people more readily accept natural categories (e.g., race) as causal explanations for an individual's behavior without probing deeply for alternative explanations than they do for arbitrary or "nonessential" categories (e.g., people grouped by preferences). Thus stigmas based on group-level attributes may trigger stereotyping to the extent that the categories are perceived to mark "natural kinds."

In a related vein, Hamilton and Sherman (1996) have emphasized that some groups are more "groupy," or higher in "entitativity," than others (see Brewer & Harasty, 1996; Campbell, 1958). Antecedents of perceived entitativity include organization and structure (e.g., differentiation of roles and functions; power and status differentials), high levels of interaction among group members, and shared goals. Interestingly, the groups with "tribal" stigmas are *not* the most entitative of groups (Hamilton, 1998); the size of the group "Black Americans" alone may prohibit a clear sense of group organization and interaction (e.g., compare "Blacks" to groups such as "fraternity" or "rock band"). Nonetheless, an entitative group will probably trigger stereotyping to the extent that entitativity is based on perceived similarity among members (Brewer & Harasty, 1996; Brewer, Weber, & Carini, 1995; Hamilton & Sherman, 1996). Similarity implies homogeneity, and low perceived within-group variability is one of the hallmark features of stereotypes (Park & Hastie, 1987; Park & Judd, 1990; Tajfel, 1969). In short, the tendency for stigmas that carry group-level associations to elicit stereotypes and stereotyping is probably based in part on the entitativity or within-group similarity that the group conveys. Whether entitativity is linked to perceptions of essence is unclear; these two features may independently create a climate conducive to the development of stereotypes.

Another factor that may affect whether a stigma becomes associated with a well-formed stereotype is the extent to which the stigmatizing attribute is confounded with "role division," or segregation at the societal level. Eagly's (1987) social role theory makes such an argument in the domain of gender stereotypes. Eagly suggests that beliefs about gender are shaped by the observation of women and men in different roles in daily life: Because women are often seen in domestic roles and men in the labor force, stereotypes that fit these roles have developed (e.g., women are nurturing and communal, whereas men are agentic; Eagly & Steffen, 1984; Yount, 1986). More generally, if members of a stigmatized group are disproportionately found in particular roles in society, we might expect that stereotypes will develop *and* that the content of the stereotypes will be tied to those roles. That Black and Hispanic Americans are more likely than White Americans to be found in low-paying jobs may therefore contribute to racial stereotypes regarding intelligence; that elderly people tend to be retired from paid employment may facilitate stereotypes about failing cognitive abilities. But when individuals with a particular stigma can be found in a wide variety of roles and across many contexts (as is true of many visible and concealable stigmas), the ground for stereotype development is less solid.

Zebrowitz (1996; see also Zebrowitz & Montepare, Chapter 12, this volume) has also proposed that physical characteristics of an individual or a group of individuals can influence not only whether stereotypes will be formed (e.g., through distinctiveness), but what the nature of those stereotypes will be. Drawing on Gibson's (1979) ecological theory of social perception, Zebrowitz suggests that "perceptible stimulus qualities provided in a person's movements, vocal qualities, and facial appearance provide socially useful information" (1996, p. 81), and that people are highly attuned to this information. As a consequence, people tend to make systematic, although often overgeneralized, judgments of others' characters. For instance, individuals with facial physiognomies that are more neotenous are perceived to have more "babyish" or childlike characteristics, such as being naive, dependent, submissive, and affectionate. Because women tend to have more neotenous features (e.g., large eyes, full lips) than men, women as a group are more likely to be stereotyped along these lines than are men. Facial appearance may also suggest health or illness and produce corresponding impressions (Zebrowitz, 1996). Perhaps because abominations of the body suggest ill health to perceivers, they produce virtually universally negative reactions and attributions.

In addition to groupiness, role division, and shared physical characteristics, stigmas may generate stereotypes if certain kinds of *attributions* for the stigmatizing condition are made. Wright (1983) noted that people often ask physically disabled individuals, "How did this happen?" This explicit search for cause also occurs for the less visible stigmas— "Why was she raped?" "What led him to drug use?"—and the perceived answer in each case may determine beliefs about the person, affective reactions, and behavior toward the individual. This is a central tenet of Weiner's (1986, 1993; Weiner, Perry, & Magnusson, 1988) model of attribution-based affect and behavior.

The inference that a stigmatized individual is responsible for his or her condition leads to a predictable pattern of affective response and intended behavior: Responsibility attributions lead to anger toward and punishment of the stigmatized individual; an attributed lack of responsibility prompts sympathy and helpful support. Weiner (1993) suggests that sometimes "the stigma itself implies a cause" (p. 959), as when AIDS is associated with homosexual activity or obesity with overeating—supposedly controllable events that imply personal responsibility (see also Crandall, 1994). Although stereotypes are not an explicit part of Weiner's model, we suggest that when stigmas are regularly attributed to internal, controllable causes, negative stereotypes (in addition to negative affect) are increasingly likely to develop. By this reasoning, a culture is more likely to develop stereotypes about people with obesity or alcoholism than about children with birth defects and people with Alzheimer's disease. Of course, this logic cannot account for stereotypes about racial, gender, and age groups: Ascribed group membership, by definition, is not controllable. Nonetheless, for less collectivistic stigmas, responsibility attributions may influence whether a stigma becomes associated with a stereotype.[1]

In summary, the nature of the stigma, the entitativity of the individuals who share the stigmatizing characteristic, the shared physical characteristics involved, and the degree to which people are seen as responsible for their stigma all help to shape whether a stigma will become associated with stereotypes. Stereotypes and stereotyping, in turn, can reciprocally contribute to stigmatization—a topic we examine in the next section.

WHAT IS THE ROLE OF STEREOTYPING IN STIGMATIZATION?

This section begins by considering what stereotypes are and what processes they involve. We then explore general consequences of stereotyping, focusing on their implications for cognition, affect, and behavior.

Stereotypes and Stereotyping

Stereotypes have traditionally been considered to be *descriptions* of groups, though faulty, incomplete, and overly rigid, that extend to group members. More recent approaches, in line with the cognitive orientation that has characterized research on stereotyping during the past two decades, have stressed the information-processing and schematic characteristics of stereotypes while deemphasizing any necessary objectionable aspects. For example, Hamilton and Trolier (1986) defined stereotypes simply as "cognitive categories that are used by the social perceiver in processing information about people" (p. 128; see also Fiske, 1998; Hilton & von Hippel, 1996). Similarly, stereotyping is defined as "the use of stereotypic knowledge in forming an impression of an individual" (Brewer, 1996, p. 254).

Despite considerable debate about the specific structure and organization of stereotypic representations (see Stangor & Schaller, 1996), there is widespread consensus that stereotypes are cognitive schemas (Hamilton & Sherman, 1994). People within a culture consensually ascribe certain traits to social groups (e.g., Karlins, Coffman, & Walters, 1969) and perceive that these groups possess distinctive characteristics (McCauley & Stitt, 1978). These group schemas, which may be spontaneously accessible, influence how information is encoded, stored, and retrieved: "Once cued, schemas affect how quickly we perceive, what we notice, how we interpret what we notice, and what we perceive as similar and different" (Fiske & Taylor, 1991, p. 122). In general, the activation of stereotypes produces an information-processing advantage for stereotypical traits (Macrae, Stangor, & Milne, 1994). In short, stereotypes may represent the cognitive component within the tripartite view of intergroup attitudes (cognition, affect, conation; Harding, Proshansky, Kutner, & Chein, 1969).

However, stereotypes may involve affective reactions as well as cognitive representations. That is, when stereotypes are activated, both cognitive and affective information becomes accessible (Fiske, 1982; Fiske, Neuberg, Beattie, & Milberg, 1987; Fiske & Pavelchak, 1986). Affective responses involve a "range of preferences, evaluations, moods, and emotions" (Fiske & Taylor, 1991, p. 410). Information about groups, like information about persons (Wyer & Gordon, 1984), may be represented twice in memory: independently in a trait–behavior cluster (based on its descriptive implications), and in an evaluation-based representation (based on its affective implications) (Dovidio & Gaertner, 1993; Stephan & Stephan, 1993).

Consequences of Stereotypes and Stereotyping

Much empirical research suggests that stereotypes and stereotyping have important consequences for attitudes and behaviors toward social groups. Stereotypes influence how people think about others (information processing), how they feel about them (attitudes and prejudice), and how they act and react to others (discrimination and self-fulfilling prophecies).

Information Processing

Once established, stereotypes operate as cognitive structures that influence how information about others is encoded, stored, and retrieved (von Hippel et al., 1995). These stereotyping processes operate in unconscious and unintentional ways, as well as consciously (Greenwald & Banaji, 1995). Repetition during socialization or personal experience may make some social stereotypes so overlearned that they will automatically become activated when people are presented with a representative or symbol of that group (Devine, 1989; cf. Lepore & Brown, 1997).

When stereotypes are activated, individual group members are judged in terms of group-based expectations or standards. The most common form of this tendency is an assimilative one: Perceptions of group members are drawn toward relevant stereotypes. Thus individual men may be judged as more aggressive or better at leadership roles than individual women. This assimilative pattern typically emerges in situations where little information besides category membership is known about a target, or when available information is ambiguous (see Kunda & Thagard, 1996, and von Hippel et al., 1995, for reviews).

In contrast, group stereotypes may also serve as standards of comparison, thereby producing contrast effects in judgment. For example, female attorneys may be judged as more competent than male attorneys (Abramson, Goldberg, Greenberg, & Abramson, 1977), and women may be judged as more financially successful than men (Biernat, Manis, & Nelson, 1991), presumably because of lower standards for women relative to men on the dimensions of job competence and financial success (see Biernat & Kobrynowicz, 1997). Contrastive patterns tend to emerge more frequently when target behavior is inconsistent with group stereotypes—that is, when expectancies are violated (Bettencourt, Dill,

Greathouse, Charlton, & Mulholland, 1997; Jussim, Coleman, & Lerch, 1987). However, these contrast effects tend to be restricted to certain kinds of judgments, such as subjective or global evaluations. Other measures of perceivers' impressions of individual group members (e.g., objective indicators and behavioral choices) continue to show a confirmatory influence of group stereotypes (Biernat et al., 1991; Glick, Zion, & Nelson, 1988; Kunda & Thagard, 1996).

In their role as interpretive frameworks, group stereotypes may also affect the meaning or construal of other information one might learn about a member of a social category. "Aggressiveness" may be construed as "arguing and complaining" if the target is a lawyer, but as "punching and yelling insults" if the target is a construction worker (Kunda, Sinclair, & Griffin, 1997); similarly, the behavior of "rushing to the department store checkout counter" is likely to be remembered as "gingerly dodging" if the actor is a nurse, but as "hurriedly pushing" if he is a bar bouncer (Dunning & Sherman, 1997; see also Kunda & Sherman-Williams, 1993; Kobrynowicz & Biernat, 1997). These influences on construal of information indicate a subtle manner in which stereotypes may color impressions of individual group members.

Finally, people tend not only to interpret the behaviors of others in ways consistent with group stereotypes, but also to show a bias in the way that information is subsequently recalled. In general, stereotype-consistent information has a recall advantage: People have better memory for information that is consistent rather than inconsistent with a preexisting stereotype (Bodenhausen, 1988; Cohen, 1981; Fyock & Stangor, 1994; Hastie & Kumar, 1979; Rothbart, Evans, & Fulero, 1979). Nevertheless, some memory indicators (e.g., recognition sensitivity) show an advantage to expectancy-inconsistent information (Stangor & McMillan, 1992), and some research suggests that inconsistent information gains a memory advantage when the stereotype is well established (presumably because the inconsistency is particularly striking in these cases; Borgida & DeBono, 1989; Srull, Lichtenstein, & Rothbart, 1985; Wyer & Martin, 1986). Processing goals may also moderate these effects. Specifically, when people are directed to form accurate or complete impressions of individuals, their "inconsistency resolution" motivation is high; therefore, stereotype-incongruent material may be better recalled (Fiske, 1989). However, perceivers who are motivated to maintain a simple, coherent impression may "ignore, filter, or distort" inconsistent information (Stangor & McMillan, 1992, p. 57).

In sum, people develop expectations about others substantially on the basis of their group membership and the associated stereotypes, although this effect may be undermined by providing information about the unique characteristics of a person (Fiske, 1998; Kunda & Thagard,

1996) or as a function of the perceiver's motivations and goals (Fiske, 1989; Kunda & Sinclair, 1999). Stereotypes are particularly likely to influence expectations, inferences, and impressions when people are not motivated to attend to individuating information, or when they are limited in their capacity to process information due to other demands on their attention and thoughts. Because stereotypes shape interpretations, influence how information is recalled, and guide expectations and inferences in systematic ways, they tend to be self-perpetuating (see also Trope & Thompson, 1997). These fundamental effects of stereotypes and stereotyping suggest more pervasive effects of stereotyping—for example, in creating and supporting prejudice.

Prejudice

Traditional and contemporary views of stereotyping suggest a positive relationship between stereotypes and prejudice. Although relatively little research has explicitly examined the association between these two constructs (Stangor, Sullivan, & Ford, 1991), a recent meta-analysis documented that a modest positive relationship between stereotypes and prejudice does exist (r = +.25; Dovidio et al., 1996). The precise nature of this relationship is less clear. On the one hand, stereotypes may form the cognitive basis for (i.e., lead to) prejudice (e.g., Harding et al., 1969; Jones, 1986). Brigham (1971) reasoned that "in order to feel negatively toward a group, one must be able to perceive the different individuals of the given ethnic group as having certain constant characteristics, as being similar to other individuals in the same group, and as being different from individuals not of that ethnic group" (p. 26). On the other hand, several researchers have proposed that stereotypes perform a function for prejudiced people by allowing them to rationalize their hostility and negative feelings toward particular groups (e.g., Simpson & Yinger, 1965). In this view, prejudice may lead to stereotypes. Still another possibility is that stereotypes and prejudice are related indirectly, via their connection to other constructs. For example, individual differences on dimensions such as authoritarianism may affect both stereotyping and prejudice (Haddock, Zanna, & Esses, 1993; Saenger & Flowerman, 1954).

Whatever the nature of the stereotypes–prejudice relationship, it may prove to be even stronger to the extent that researchers adopt a broader conceptualization of prejudice. Smith (1993) suggested that prejudice, rather than being viewed simply as a negative attitude, can be thought of in terms of a broad range of social emotions. In this "prejudice-as-emotions" conceptualization, a wide variety of situationally specific emotions can be triggered by a group or individual, depending on the appraisals one makes in those particular contexts. For example, if people appraise an individual as violating ingroup norms, they may experience disgust, which in turn may prompt avoidance. Such a reaction may be typical for stigmas such as homosexuality, which seem to be tied to the perceived violation of ingroup norms and values (Haddock et al., 1993; Herek, 1991). If people appraise an individual as making unfair demands, however, they may experience anger, which may lead them to move against or to closely monitor the individual's actions. This reaction may be typical for the tribal stigmas, particularly when members of the stigmatized group take collective action to improve their lot. In fact, one item of the Modern Racism Scale (McConahay, 1986) reflects this type of appraisal: "Blacks are getting too demanding in their push for equal rights." In general, to the extent that the specific contents of stereotypes guide appraisals of group members, different affective responses may result, only some of which may be captured under the rubric of traditional measures of prejudice. With more precise characterization and operationalization of prejudice, stronger links between stereotypes and prejudice may be established.

Discrimination and Other Effects on the Stigmatized

If stereotypes are cognitive structures that, like other schemas, influence how people perceive, process, store, and retrieve information and how they feel about other groups, then stereotypes are likely to affect behaviors that are based on these biased processes. Although relatively few studies have addressed this issue, Dovidio and colleagues' (1996) meta-analysis indicated only a modest relationship between stereotypes and direct manifestations of discriminatory behavior ($r = .16$). It appears, however, that the association between stereotypes and discrimination may be subtle, complex, or indirect (e.g., moderated by situational factors). For example, stereotypes may be more directly associated with subsequent behavior when stereotypic attributes (e.g., "violent") are directly relevant to the nature of the behavior to be elicited (e.g., juridic decisions) or support the perceiver's general motivational orientation to the other person (Sinclair & Kunda, 1999).

Stereotypes may exert a weak influence on overt discrimination in part because discrimination violates prevailing norms of fairness and egalitarianism (Dovidio & Gaertner, 1986). Perceivers may be inclined to inhibit stereotype-based responding at various points in the behavioral sequence (Bodenhausen & Macrae, 1998), and therefore the effects of stereotypes may appear in relatively subtle or covert ways (see Crosby, Bromley, & Saxe, 1980). Furthermore, stereotypes may trigger self-fulfilling prophecies in social interaction, in which the stereotypes of the perceiver influence the interaction in ways that conform to stereotypical expectations (Jussim, 1991; Snyder, 1981; Word, Zanna, & Cooper, 1974). And under conditions that make stereotypes salient (e.g., aptitude testing, solo/token status), the performance of members of the stereotyped group may be adversely affected (Cohen & Swim, 1995; Spencer, Steele, & Quinn, 1999; Steele & Aronson, 1995).

Under some conditions, however, awareness of stereotypes can be self-protective. Crocker and Major (1989; see also Major & Crocker, 1993) have argued that the causes of outcomes for stigmatized individuals are likely to be attributionally ambiguous. For example, negative outcomes can be attributed to one's poor performance, lack of effort, or lack of ability; alternatively, they can be attributed to prejudice and discrimination. If the negative outcomes can be attributed to others' prejudice, then this attributional ambiguity may protect one's self-esteem and general well-being, perhaps via increases in group identification (Branscombe, Schmitt, & Harvey, 1999). However, individuals and members of different groups may differ in the extent to which they expect to be stereotyped by others (Pinel, 1999), and making attributions to prejudice may come with the cost of perceived loss of control over one's outcomes (Ruggiero & Taylor, 1997).

In short, considerable research documents a range of negative consequences of stereotypes and stereotyping. The impact may not always be especially strong or direct, but it is systematic and pervasive. Stereotypes affect the ways people think about outgroup members, their attitudes toward them, and their behavior with them during interactions. Awareness of stereotypes can interfere with the performance of members of stereotyped groups and may produce attributional ambiguity in response to both negative and positive outcomes.

STEREOTYPING AND STIGMATIZATION: SOME EXAMPLES

In the preceding section we have reviewed how stereotypes influence information processing, attitudes and feelings, and action toward stigmatized group members, as well as the feelings and beliefs the stigmatized have about themselves. In this section we illustrate the role of stereotyping in examples of the three bases of stigmas described by Goffman (1963): "tribal identities," "blemishes of individual character," and "abominations of the body."

"Tribal Stigma": Racism

The racism of White Americans toward Black Americans has been a defining feature in the history of the United States. It is also a classic example of the processes involved in tribal stigmas. Most fundamentally, it involves the social categorization of people into ingroups and outgroups on the basis of readily available physical characteristics. These characteristics may provide immediate cues of "entitativity" (see Brewer & Harasty, 1996; Campbell, 1958) and may activate related knowledge structures. In this way, the categorization of people into ingroup and outgroup, "we" and "they," is associated not only with general differences in overall evaluation (i.e., preference for the ingroup), but also with specific beliefs about outgroup members—stereotypic traits regarding Blacks, such as "violent," "athletic," "musical," and "lazy" (Devine & Elliot, 1995; Dovidio & Gaertner, 1991). Prejudice and personal endorsement of stereotypes are positively related (Dovidio et al., 1996).

Although the development of racial stereotypes is typically assumed to be a consequence of social categorization that precedes discriminatory behavior, the particular content of stereotypes may be reciprocally shaped by the nature of discriminatory actions. Explicitly race-based policies tend to be associated with the development of ideologies that justify them. During the early history of the United States, for example, White Americans developed ideologies about race that helped them to rationalize laws permitting them to carry out two important types of economic exploitation: slavery and the takeover of lands from Native Americans (Klinker & Smith, 1999). Thus racial stereotypes are tied to a particular ideology that justifies discrimination and exploitation (Fields, 1990). Moreover, because of repeated exposure to racial stereotypes through common socialization experiences, White Americans generally develop a knowledge of cultural stereotypes of Blacks that is activated spontaneously by the direct or symbolic presence of a member of that group (Devine, 1989), though this effect seems to occur more strongly among Whites who are highly prejudiced (Kawakami, Dion, & Dovidio, 1998; Lepore & Brown, 1997).

More generally, exposure to Black targets increases the accessibility of stereotypic and negative thoughts (Dovidio, Evans, & Tyler, 1986), often automatically (Fazio, Jackson, Dunton, & Williams, 1995; Wittenbrink et al., 1997). These associations may then influence how new information is interpreted. For example, both White children and adults tend to interpret ambiguously aggressive behaviors as more threatening and violent when they are performed by a Black person than by a White person (Duncan, 1976; Sagar & Schofield, 1980). These interpretations and attributions can then lead to different outcomes and actions, such as longer prison sentences and greater likelihood of receiving the death penalty in murder cases for Blacks than for Whites (see Dovidio & Gaertner, 1998). They can also promote the development of institutional racism, which involves the differential impact of policies, practices, and laws on members of racial groups and on the groups as a whole (e.g., differential mandatory penalties for trafficking in crack and powdered cocaine). Institutional racism is typically not recognized as being racially unfair, because it is embedded in laws (which are normally assumed to be right and moral), is ritualized, and is accompanied by racial ideologies and stereotypes that justify it. Nevertheless, it systematically reinforces disparities in resources between the groups.

Besides their expression in overt discrimination, racial stereotypes and prejudiced feelings can shape interpersonal interactions in subtle but significant ways. These can produce self-fulfilling prophecies. For example, Word and colleagues (1974) found that White interviewers behaved in a more cold and distant manner *nonverbally* (e.g., in eye contact, interpersonal distance, awkwardness of speech) toward Black interviewees than toward White interviewees. Such effects seem to occur without Whites' even being aware of them (e.g., Weitz, 1972). Regardless of their self-reported (and presumably conscious) racial attitudes, individual differences in automatically and unconsciously activated attitudes predict how friendly White individuals' behavior will be overall (Fazio et al., 1995) and nonverbally (Dovidio, Kawakami, Johnson, Johnson, & Howard, 1997) toward a Black person. Also consistent with the operation of self-fulfilling prophecies was a second study by Word and colleagues (1974): White interviewees who interacted with interviewers displaying the nonverbal style that characterized interactions with Blacks, relative to the style that characterized interactions with Whites, performed significantly more poorly in the situation as assessed by independent observers.

Finally, racial identities develop and diverge as a function of one's group's experiences and of how one interprets, internalizes, and adjusts to those experiences. The racial identity and culture of Black Americans have been hypothesized to reflect an evolutionary component, which developed from the cultural foundation of an African past, and a reactionary component, which is an adaptation to the historical and contemporary challenges of minority status in the United States (see also Helms, 1995). Because of the pervasiveness of racism, Black Americans may implicitly internalize racial stereotypes—perhaps by disidentifying with a stereotyped domain (e.g., academics; Steele, 1992), or by performing poorly under conditions of "stereotype threat" (e.g., on achievement tests)—even when the stereotypes are not personally endorsed (Steele, 1998).

This brief analysis illustrates the central role of stereotypes in the stigmatization of Black Americans. Exposure to Blacks generally and often automatically activates racial stereotypes among Whites. The particular nature of these stereotypes is used to justify individual treatment and institutional policies that produce disparate outcomes. These effects may occur subtly and indirectly in individual interactions, and the pervasiveness of the effects can also influence the individual reactions of Blacks and the development of personal and social identities. Thus, at least for some types of tribal stigmas, stereotyping and stigmatization are intimately intertwined.

"Blemishes of Character": Mental Illness

The processes of categorization, stereotyping, discrimination, and self-fulfilling prophecy can also apply to stigmas based on blemishes of individual character. The case of people with psychological problems provides one such example. Because the dynamics are fundamentally similar to those illustrated for race, our review of these processes is relatively brief.

Responses to persons with mental illnesses include recognition of difference associated with devaluation, existence of stereotypes, biased evaluations and attributions, and self-fulfilling consequences. Within the United States, mentally ill and formerly mentally ill individuals have traditionally been degraded and rejected; they have experienced prejudice similar to that experienced by racial and ethnic minorities (Calicchia, 1981; Farina, 1998; Farina, Gliha, Boudreau, Allen, & Sherman, 1971; Katz, 1981; Link, Struening, Rahav, & Phelan, 1997; cf. Hayward & Bright, 1997). Moreover, these negative attitudes extend to others who are associated with them (McGuire & Borowy, 1979; Mehta & Farina, 1988)—a "courtesy stigma" (Goffman, 1963; see also "stigma by association" in attitudes toward homosexuals; Neuberg, Smith, Hoffman, & Russell, 1994). In part to avoid being stigmatized themselves, people frequently attempt to conceal the mental illness of their family members (Phelan, Bromet, & Link, 1998).

Besides being associated with generally negative attitudes, persons with mental illnesses are represented in specific, stereotypic ways (see Scheff, 1966). They are described as "sick," "dangerous," "worthless," "cold," "unpredictable," and "insincere" (Crumpton, Weinstein, Acker, & Annis, 1967); they are characterized in the mass media in negative and violent ways (Fisher, 1982). Like racial stereotypes, stereotypes of people with psychological problems can be activated spontaneously by the presence (real or symbolic) of a representative of that category (Sibicky & Dovidio, 1985). Moreover, stereotypic perceptions persist even if the behavior of the particular person does not justify such negative attributions (e.g., Farina, Felner, & Boudreau, 1973). Mental illness, at least in some forms, is a potentially concealable stigma. Because of concerns about attitudes and stereotypes about people with psychological problems, a significant proportion of people in need of psychological assistance will choose not to seek it (Wills, 1983)—or, if they do, will pay for it themselves rather than use their insurance benefits (Sobel, 1981). One can also imagine that fear of confirming negative stereotypes may plague mentally ill individuals, in the same manner that Blacks and women are vulnerable to stereotype threat in performance domains (Steele, 1998).

Beliefs about people with mental illnesses can also produce a self-fulfilling prophecy. Sibicky and Dovidio (1986) found that college students expected partners who they believed to be seeking psychological counseling (but who actually were naive peers) to be cold, unsociable, incompetent, and defensive. Because of these expectations, the students then behaved in a relatively distant, closed, insecure, incompetent way. In turn, and consistent with a self-fulfilling prophecy, independent raters found that students believed to be experiencing psychological problems behaved in more defensive, insecure, cold, unsociable, and incompetent ways, compared to students who were not believed to be seeking counseling.

Visible (i.e., unconcealable) stigmas related to blemishes of individual character, such as the stigma of overweight,[2] show similar patterns of responses: social categorization, devaluation, stereotypes, biased evaluations and attributions, and self-fulfilling prophecies (Crandall & Biernat, 1990; Crandall, 1994; Crandall & Martinez, 1996; DeJong & Kleck, 1986; Miller & Myers, 1998; Stunkard & Sobal, 1995; Yuker & Allison, 1994). However, depending on the nature of the stigmatizing mark, some *concealable* blemishes of individual character may be more closely related to social categorization and stereotyping than others. For example, "criminals" may be more likely than "liars" to be seen as a social category because of their common treatment, common fate, and potential threat (elements of entitativity). Thus criminals may elicit more consensual stereotyping, whereas liars may prompt more individualistic attributions and responses. The former reflects on social identity, the latter on personal identity. Differences in level of categorization may also be revealed in the descriptions that people apply to others (e.g., "He is a criminal" vs. "He is a person who committed a crime"). Stereotyping is a more prominent factor for blemishes of individual character ascribed to social identity than to personal identity. The distinction between social category responses and individually oriented reactions is more fully illustrated in stigmas based on abominations of the body.

"Body Abominations": Disability and Disfigurement

Like other forms of stigma, stereotypes are associated with what Goffman (1963) terms "abominations of the body" that are both more and less visible (e.g., physical disabilities and illnesses such as cancer; Rounds & Zevon, 1993; see also Crandall & Moriarty, 1995). However, whereas stereotypes associated with tribal stigmas and blemishes of individual character are well documented, sufficiently strong to produce automatic activation, and consensually held, stereotypes for abominations of the body are rarer, weaker, and more variable across individuals (as opposed to cultural and consensual). Some reasons for this have been outlined earlier in this chapter (e.g., lesser entitativity, segregation into particular social roles, attributions of responsibility). In addition, there may be a broader range of differences within a category (e.g., physical disabilities involving paralysis or loss of limbs; facial disfigurement from burns, accidents, or birth defects), and this may reduce the likelihood of forming prototypic, category-based representations relative to more individualized impressions (Fiske & Neuberg, 1990). Furthermore, many of these types of marks are relatively rare, thus limiting the experience necessary to develop elaborate stereotypes (Jones et al., 1984). Finally, individuals with these types of stigmas may be less likely to function collectively for political action that could pose the social or economic threat productive of general ideologies to justify resistance and discrimination. Consistent with each of these reasons, among the marks for this type of stigmatization that are most strongly associated with stereotypes are beliefs about deaf and hearing-impaired individuals—for whom the mark is specifically defined, with whom contact is more common, and who are politically organized in visible ways.

Whereas the functions of stigmatization based on tribal identities or blemishes of individual character may be largely social and collective, involving needs for positive social identity, system justification, or social control over a category of people (see Crocker et al., 1998), the functions of stigmatization based on body abominations may be more individualistic. Individualistic functions may involve self-enhancement through downward comparison with less fortunate others (Wills, 1981).[3] Alternatively, self-protective motivations may be involved. To the extent that physical cues are signs of ill health or questionable genetic fitness (Zebrowitz, 1996), rejection of people with abominations of the body—particularly in intimate relationships—may be functional for ensuring the perpetuation of one's genes in future generations. In addition, Crocker and colleagues (1998) propose that one "function that social stigma may serve for the individual is that of providing a world view and meaning system that buffers one against existential anxiety" (p. 510). Individuals with body abominations are likely to be perceived as different or deviant; they "make salient the lack of social consensus for our views and thus threaten our confidence in the absolute validity of our world views" (Solomon, Greenberg, & Pyszczynski, 1991, p. 125).

Abominations of the body may be particularly threatening forms of deviance because they increase the salience of a perceiver's own mortality. According to terror management theory (Solomon et al., 1991), increasing awareness of one's mortality creates anxiety and a motivation to reinforce the validity of one's world view, often leading to the rejection and derogation of those perceived to be different. Thus, the trepidation experienced during interactions with people with these types of marks may reflect not only the general anxiety response that occurs during interactions with others who are different (Stephan & Stephan, 1985), but also the reaction to a specific threat about one's own mortality. If stigmatization associated with abominations of the body (particularly those that indicate ill health) is rooted in threats about mortality, then these types of stigmas may be more similar across cultures and across time than are tribal stigmas, which may be more closely tied to particular social, historical, or economic contexts. Whereas the collective functions of stigmatization based on tribal identities and blemishes of individual character may produce consensual stereotypes, the individual functions of rejection of people with abominations of the body may be accompanied by more socially acceptable personal reactions, such as sympathy (Jones et al., 1984; Katz, 1981).

The relative absence of a strong set of consensual beliefs about individuals with abominations of the body, coupled with strong emotional reactions, may generally make the impact of stereotypes weaker for this type of stigma than for those related to tribal identities or to blemishes of individual character. In terms of the distinction introduced by Dovidio and colleagues in Chapter 1, these latter stigmas are collective and have a stronger cognitive component; abominations of the body are more individually, affectively based.

Research on responses to people with physical disabilities is quite consistent with this proposal. Abominations of the body are generally associated with rejection and avoidance of the marked individuals (see Fine & Asch, 1995), and this treatment is more pronounced for more visible stigmas (Richardson, Ronald, & Kleck, 1974). Across Chinese, Italian, German, Greek, and Australian communities, more concealable conditions such as asthma, diabetes, and heart disease were among the least stigmatized forms of physical disability, whereas less concealable conditions such as mental retardation and cerebral palsy were among the least accepted (Westbrook, Legge, & Pennay, 1993). In interactions that cannot be avoided, people experience high levels of discomfort, anxiety, and physiological arousal with marked individuals (e.g., those presumed to be amputees; Kleck, Ono, & Hastorf, 1966). For example, Lefebvre and Munro (1986) observed that "facial disfigurement elicits anxiety, fear, and a wish to remove it from one's sight" (p. 53). Nonverbal behaviors during interactions with people with disabilities also reflect high levels of tension and greater interpersonal distance (Kleck, 1968, 1969). People with physical disabilities themselves experience anxiety, tension, and discomfort in mixed interactions (Comer & Piliavin, 1972).

However, more cognitive, conscious, and public behaviors show less evidence of negativity by perceivers toward people with physical disabilities. People tend to avoid actions that are readily interpretable as prejudice against disabled people (Snyder, Kleck, Strenta, & Mentzer, 1979). They also tend to evaluate people with physical disabilities generally positively, and more positively than comparable people without such disabilities (Dovidio & Mullen, 1992). These inconsistent responses may reflect different components in the experience of ambivalence involving aversion and sympathy in feelings about disabled persons (Katz, 1981). This ambivalence may also apply to people associated with stigmatized individuals. Partners of physically disabled persons are seen as being relatively nurturant and trustworthy, but as less sociable, intelligent, and athletic (Goldstein & Johnson, 1997). Alternatively, the inconsistency may represent the difference between personal negative feelings and public expressions. Archer (1985) explained, "The mixture of reactions to the handicapped may be less than true ambivalence, however, in the sense that an individual may experience a negative *emotional* reaction to the stigmatized person but also be *intellectually* aware of norms calling for compassion and help toward the disadvantaged" (original emphasis, p. 787) Thus, although responses to people stigmatized with physical disabilities may be complex, they reflect more general and global responses (e.g., aversion, compassion), rather than the effects of an assumed, consensual set of beliefs about specific characteristics (e.g., "irresponsible," "arrogant") of the group—that is, stereotypes.

SUMMARY, IMPLICATIONS, AND CONCLUSIONS

Summary

Stigmatization and stereotyping have much in common. Both involve the recognition of a mark that signifies group or category membership. The meaning of the mark is shaped by individual and collective processes. Furthermore, stereotyping can play a central role in the development, justification, maintenance, and perpetuation of stigmatization. Stereotypes form an associated set of beliefs that guide information processing and attributions and may produce self-fulfilling prophecies. In addition, stereotypes offer coherent explanations that justify more overt forms of treatment in individual actions or institutional policies (i.e., discrimination).

Nevertheless, stereotyping and stigmatization are not always associated. Stereotypes can exist without stigmas. For example, some stereotypes are basically positive (e.g., those about physically attractive people), whereas stigmatization is essentially negative. Stigmatization may also occur largely independent of stereotypes. Stereotypes are consensually held sets of beliefs about a group; they are not simply general negative evaluations, but rather specific semantic associations. Stereotypes may arise from cognitive mechanisms that are triggered by categorization, and they may also emerge as part of an ideology to justify the unequal treatment, resources, and opportunities afforded to different social groups. The more individually and socially functional stereotypes are, the more likely they are to form and persist. As Jones et al. (1984) suggest, more elaborate stereotyping may occur for groups with which people frequently interact, and this may be particularly the case when some threat is involved. However, group threats are more likely to produce consensual stereotypes to justify collective action than are individual threats. Thus threats related to feelings of one's mortality or belongingness may be triggered by exposure to others' abominations of the body, but unless a common social threat is also produced (e.g., by a disease-related cause such as leprosy), this type of stigma may not elicit strong *cultural* stereotypes. The reaction may be one of strong stigmatization, but without an elaborate stereotypic component.

Implications for Reducing Stigmatization

Stereotypes are often considered to be inordinately rigid sets of beliefs, and thus resistant to change. A number of approaches for changing or reducing stereotyping have been proposed. Some aim directly at encouraging conscious suppression of stereotypes, but such attempts may produce unintended rebound effects (Macrae, Bodenhausen, Milne, & Jetten, 1994), the hyperaccessibility of the thoughts (stereotypes) being suppressed (Monteith, Sherman, & Devine, 1998; Wegner & Erber, 1992; see also Smart & Wegner, Chapter 8, this volume); and, because of the effort involved in suppression, relative disregard of nonstereotypic information about individuals (Macrae, Bodenhausen, Milne, & Wheeler, 1996). However, with repeated effort, stereotype suppression may become successful. Monteith and colleagues (1998) observed: "Practice makes perfect. Like other mental processes, though suppression processes may be proceduralized and become relatively automatic" (p. 71; see also Kelly & Kahn, 1994).

Alternative cognitive approaches to change are directed at altering the cognitive schemas that underlie stereotypes. The "bookkeeping" model (Rothbart, 1981) proposes that stereotypes are updated incrementally. Thus exposure to stereotype-inconsistent behavior can change stereotypes gradually, as long as the stereotype-discrepant information is not too extreme (Kunda & Oleson, 1995). The "conversion" model (Rothbart, 1981) posits that stereotypes will change, but in a dramatic rather than an incremental way, after a critical threshold of inconsistency has been reached—and presumably when the stereotype is no longer functional. The "subtyping" model (Brewer, Dull, & Lui, 1981; Hewstone, 1994; Weber & Crocker, 1983) asserts that inconsistent information can lead to recategorization of group members from a superordinate organization to a set of secondary categories. Thus exposure to counterstereotypic group members who deviate extremely from the group and are thus considered highly atypical will have little positive impact on changing group stereotypes, and may even paradoxically strengthen the original stereotypes (Kunda & Oleson, 1997). Research on cross-categorization effects suggests that the consideration of the multiple categories to which an individual belongs may reduce stereotyping based on any one category (see Urban & Miller, 1998, for a review). "Exemplar-based" models argue that stereotypes consist of representations of specific individuals (Smith & Zárate, 1992) and thus can change when new exemplars are added, existing exemplars are strengthened, or new ones are retrieved. In addition, for some stigmas, stereotypes develop primarily through social learning and social influence (Schaller & Conway, 1999) and thus may be unlearned by developing alternative or incompatible associations. Therefore, direct strategies for changing stereotypes by providing counterstereotypic examples may be used to reduce or eliminate stigmatization.

However, as a general strategy, the effectiveness of direct efforts to change stereotypes may be limited by two factors. First, for some types of stigmatization, stereotypes may develop as a *consequence* of stigmatization—in order to justify or rationalize it (e.g., system justification). That is, the assumed causal ordering from stereotyping to stigmatization may be reversed. Thus changing specific stereotypes may have only a weak and indirect influence on the nature or degree of stigmatization. Allport (1954), for instance, argued that stereotypes are "primarily rationalizers. . . . While it does no harm (and may do some good) to combat them in schools and colleges, and to reduce them in mass media of communication, it must not be thought that this attack alone will eradicate the roots of prejudice" (p. 204). Second, attempting to alter stereotypes may be limited in effectiveness for reducing stigmatization that does not have a strong stereotypic component, as in the case of abominations of the body.

An alternative approach, which is not necessarily independent of strategies to change stereotypes, involves the structuring of positive intergroup contact. Intergroup contact has long been psychology's prescription for changing attitudes and stereotypes (Allport, 1954; Williams, 1947), presumably by providing opportunities for people to have positive and productive intergroup experiences, to learn of individuating and personalizing information, and to encounter stereotype-inconsistent information (Rothbart & John, 1985). One way contact can be effective is at the intergroup level—by creating a recategorization of members from separate groups to one superordinate group, thereby harnessing the motives for positive social identity to create new, more positive stereotypes of former outgroup members (Gaertner, Dovidio, Anastasio, Bachman, & Rust, 1993). This effect is more likely to occur when groups can maintain aspects of their separate group identities in a well-differentiated way (Hewstone & Brown, 1986; Dovidio, Gaertner, & Validzic, 1998), and particularly when these previous group identities contribute functionally and in complementary ways to achieving desired outcomes. Cooperative interactions with members of stereotyped groups can also motivate people to form more individualized rather than group-based impressions (Fiske & Neuberg, 1990), allowing them to perceive, process, and accept stereotype-inconsistent information.

Recent theoretical discussions of intergroup contact focus on the individualizing aspects that reduce category-based responses (Wilder, 1981), such as personalizing interactions (Brewer & Miller, 1984) and intimacy (Pettigrew, 1997). Even knowledge that another ingroup member has a close relationship with an outgroup member can help change negative attitudes and stereotypes (Wright, Aron, McLaughlin-Volpe, & Ropp, 1997). These effects seem to occur even when the contact is with members of groups that are socially constructed categories rather than organizationally functioning groups (e.g., people with psychiatric disorders; see Farina, 1998; Kolodziej & Johnson, 1996).

Positive, individuating intergroup contact may be particularly effective for reducing stigmas whose threats are primarily individual (e.g., mortality salience) and whose benefits are personal (esteem enhancement through downward comparison). In these cases, contact may humanize a stigmatized person, produce an adaptation to the person's difference, and permit the development of more differentiated impressions. These effects, in turn, can alter the basis of impression formation from one in which the mark is primary to more complex, individuated responses where the mark is but one aspect of a person's makeup.

In addition, the behaviors and responses of the stigmatized during these interactions can significantly moderate the outcomes of contact situations (Devine & Vasquez, 1998). Although stigmatization can produce self-fulfilling prophecies, people who are aware of their stigmatized status and who are appropriately motivated may engage in compensa-

tory behaviors that can reduce anxiety, undermine stereotypic preconceptions, and emphasize alternative aspects of their personality and appearance (Miller & Myers, 1998; see also Eberhardt & Fiske, 1996).
Perceiving a marked person as a complex individual, with many facets
and characteristics, decreases the salience of the mark and permits other,
individuated factors to become the basis for a relationship to develop.

Conclusions

Stereotyping and stigmatization are separable, yet highly related and
integrated processes. Group stereotypes can exist without stigmatization
of group members, and stigmatization can occur in the absence of structured stereotypes. Nonetheless, stereotypes generally play an integral
role in the devaluation of "marked" persons. Whether stereotypes develop through social learning, influence, and communication, or as rationalizers of the status quo, stereotypes may set in motion biased
attentional and interpretational processing of information about stigmatized persons; trigger affective responses such as disgust, anger, anxiety,
and fear; and contribute to discriminatory actions.

Stereotypes may serve either individual (self-esteem protection, terror management) or collective (positive intergroup differentiation, hierarchy maintenance) functions, and these may determine the precise manner in which stereotypes shape interaction with stigmatized persons.
Specifically, stereotypes serving collective functions are likely to be
consensually shared (even normative) and resistant to change, and therefore particularly likely to produce the kinds of confirmational biases that
sustain and preserve them. Stereotypes serving more individualistic functions, in contrast, may be more readily set aside as threats to the self
wane, thereby increasing the likelihood that individuated rather than
category-based impressions and treatment of a stigmatized person may
emerge.

That stereotypes pose a threat to stigmatized individuals is clear,
but increased research attention needs to be turned to the manner in
which stigmatized persons respond to that threat. Stereotypes may produce a self-fulfilling prophecy, whereby a stigmatized person is inadver-
tently pressed into behavior that confirms a stereotyper's beliefs, or the
prophecy may be invalidated by a target who is aware of the stereotype
and engages in compensatory behavior to disconfirm it (Miller & Myers,
1998). Stereotypes may also lead a stigmatized individual to disengage—
for example, by withdrawing effort or by disidentifying with the stereotyped life domain (Steele, 1998). Although recent research suggests that
outcomes such as these may be moderated by the extent to which the
stigmatized individual is high in "stigma consciousness" (Pinel, 1999),

the conditions under which each of these outcomes will occur has not been fully specified. Nonetheless, in each case stereotypes may contribute to a different, more negative set of experiences and outcomes for stigmatized persons than for nonstigmatized persons. Those stigmas that are less associated with consensual stereotypes (e.g., facial disfigurement) clearly also evoke negative affect and negative outcomes, but in these cases the lack of specific, clear-cut expectations to guide interactions (and to justify negative treatment) removes one avenue of devaluation.

In conclusion, we suggest that considering the role of basic psychological processes and mechanisms, such as stereotyping, can be a productive approach for understanding stigmatization—one that complements the study of particular types of stigmas in isolation from others (e.g., attitudes toward deaf persons, racism, anti-fat attitudes and ideologies). Focusing on general mechanisms offers a dynamic perspective that recognizes the role of common underlying processes across diverse types of stigmatization. At the same time, recognizing the different roles of stereotyping across different types of stigmas places the study of stereotyping in a broader context. From this broader perspective, stereotypes can be seen as both causes and consequences of feeling and behavior toward stigmatized individuals, and their interaction with motives, attitudes, and norms can be better appreciated.

ACKNOWLEDGMENTS

Order of authorship is alphabetical and reflects the joint, collaborative effort that went into this chapter. We are grateful to Amy Eshleman for her helpful comments, and to the editors for their encouragement and support.

NOTES

1. This may be true at both the cultural and individual stereotype level. To the extent that a given person views a stigma as controllable, he or she may develop an idiosyncratic stereotype surrounding that stigma. For a cultural stereotype to form, more consensus on the responsibility attribution (and perhaps more communication about it) is necessary (Schaller & Latané, 1996).
2. Being overweight can certainly also be considered an "abomination of the body." However, research suggests that strong characterological inferences are drawn about fat people (e.g., obesity as sin; see Allon, 1982).
3. However, some research suggests that comparing with a worse-off other may be threatening to the self if the target's conditions or outcomes are perceived to be uncontrollable (Major, Testa, & Bylsma, 1991), or if the self could become like the target in the future (Taylor & Lobel, 1989).

REFERENCES

Abramson, P. R., Goldberg, P. A., Greenberg, J. H., & Abramson, L. M. (1977). The talking platypus phenomenon: Competency ratings as a function of sex and professional status. *Psychology of Women Quarterly, 2,* 114–124.

Allon, N. (1982). The stigma of overweight in everyday life. In B. Wolman (Ed.), *Psychological aspects of obesity: A handbook* (pp. 130–174). New York: Van Nostrand Reinhold.

Allport, G. W. (1954). *The nature of prejudice.* Reading, MA: Addison-Wesley.

Archer, D. (1985). Social deviance. In G. Lindzey & E. Aronson (Eds.), *Handbook of social psychology: Vol. 2. Special fields and applications* (3rd ed., pp. 743–804). New York: Random House.

Bettencourt, B. A., Dill, K. E., Greathouse, S. A., Charlton, K., & Mulholland, A. (1997). Evaluations of ingroup and outgroup members: The role of category-based expectancy violation. *Journal of Experimental Social Psychology, 33,* 244–275.

Biernat, M., & Kobrynowicz, D. (1997) Gender- and race-based standards of competence: Lower minimum standard but higher ability standards for devalued groups. *Journal of Personality and Social Psychology, 72,* 544–557.

Biernat, M., Manis, M., & Nelson, T. (1991). Stereotypes and standards of judgment. *Journal of Personality and Social Psychology, 60,* 485–499.

Bodenhausen, G. V. (1988). Stereotypic biases in social decision making and memory: Testing process models of stereotype use. *Journal of Personality and Social Psychology, 55,* 726–737.

Bodenhausen, G. V., & Macrae, C. N. (1998). Stereotype activation and inhibition. In R. Wyer (Ed.), *Stereotype activation and inhibition: Advances in social cognition* (Vol. 11, pp. 1–52). Mahwah, NJ: Erlbaum.

Borgida, E., & DeBono, K. G. (1989). Social hypothesis testing and the role of expertise. *Personality and Social Psychology Bulletin, 15,* 212–221.

Branscombe, N. R., Schmitt, M. T., & Harvey, R. D. (1999). Perceiving pervasive discrimination among African Americans: Implications for group identification and well being. *Journal of Personality and Social Psychology, 77,* 135–149.

Brewer, M. B. (1996). When stereotypes lead to stereotyping: The use of stereotypes in person perception. In N. Macrae, C. Stangor, & M. Hewstone (Eds.), *Stereotypes and stereotyping* (pp. 254–275). New York: Guilford Press.

Brewer, M. B., Dull, V., & Lui, L. (1981). Perceptions of the elderly: Stereotypes as prototypes. *Journal of Personality and Social Psychology, 41,* 656–670.

Brewer, M. B., & Harasty, A. S. (1996). Seeing groups as entities: The role of perceiver motivation. In R. M. Sorrentino & E. T. Higgins (Eds.), *Handbook of motivation and cognition: Vol. 3: The interpersonal context* (pp. 347–370). New York: Guilford Press.

Brewer, M. B., & Miller, N. (1984). Beyond the contact hypothesis: Theoretical perspectives on desegregation. In N. Miller & M. B. Brewer (Eds.), *Groups in contact: The psychology of desegregation* (pp. 281–302). Orlando, FL: Academic Press.

Brewer, M. B., Weber, J. G., & Carini, B. (1995). Person memory in intergroup contexts: Categorization versus individuation. *Journal of Personality and Social Psychology, 69*, 29–40.

Brigham, J. C. (1971). Ethnic stereotypes. *Psychological Bulletin, 76*, 15–38.

Bruner, J. S. (1957). On perceptual readiness. *Psychological Review, 64*, 123–152.

Calicchia, J. P. (1981). Attitudinal comparison of mental health professionals toward ex-mental patients. *Journal of Psychology, 108*, 35–41.

Campbell, D. T. (1958). Common fate, similarity and other indices of the status of aggregates of persons as social entities. *Behavioral Science, 3*, 14–25.

Cohen, C. E. (1981). Person categories and social perception: Testing some boundaries of the processing effects of prior knowledge. *Journal of Personality and Social Psychology, 40*, 441–452.

Cohen, L. L., & Swim, J. K. (1995). The differential impact of gender ratios on women and men: Tokenism, self-confidence, and expectations. *Personality and Social Psychology Bulletin, 21*, 876–884.

Comer, R. J., & Piliavin, J. A. (1972). The effects of physical deviance upon face-to-face interaction: The other side. *Journal of Personality and Social Psychology, 23*, 33–39.

Corrigan, P. W. (1998). The impact of stigma on severe mental illness. *Cognitive and Behavioral Practice, 5*, 201–222.

Crandall, C. S. (1994). Prejudice against anti-fat people: Ideology and self-interest. *Journal of Personality and Social Psychology, 66*, 882–894.

Crandall, C. S., & Biernat, M. R. (1990). The ideology of anti-fat attitudes. *Journal of Applied Social Psychology, 20*, 227–243.

Crandall, C. S., & Martinez, R. (1996). Culture, ideology, and antifat attitudes. *Personality and Social Psychology Bulletin, 22*, 1165–1176.

Crandall, C. S., & Moriarty, D. (1995). Physical illness stigma and social rejection. *British Journal of Social Psychology, 34*, 67–83.

Crocker, J., & Major, B. (1989). Social stigma and self-esteem: The self-protective properties of stigma. *Psychological Review, 96*, 608–630.

Crocker, J., Major, B., & Steele, C. (1998). Social stigma. In D. T. Gilbert, S. T. Fiske, & G. Lindzey (Eds.), *Handbook of social psychology* (4th ed., Vol. 2, pp. 504–553). Boston: McGraw-Hill.

Crosby, F., Bromley, S., & Saxe, L. (1980). Recent unobtrusive studies of Black and White discrimination and prejudice: A literature review. *Psychological Bulletin, 87*, 546–563.

Crumpton, E., Weinstein, A. D., Acker, C. W., & Annis, A. P. (1967). How patients and normals see the mental patient. *Journal of Clinical Psychology, 23*, 46–49.

DeJong, W., & Kleck, R. E. (1986). The social psychological effects of overweight. In C. P. Herman, M. P. Zanna, & E. T. Higgins (Eds.), *The Ontario Symposium: Vol. 3. Physical appearance, stigma, and social behavior* (pp. 65–88). Hillsdale, NJ: Erlbaum.

Devine, P. G. (1989). Stereotypes and prejudice: Their automatic and controlled components. *Journal of Personality and Social Psychology, 56*, 5–18.

Devine, P. G., & Elliot, A. J. (1995). Are racial stereotypes really fading?: The Princeton trilogy revisited. *Personality and Social Psychology Bulletin, 21*, 1139–1150.

Devine, P. G., & Vasquez, K. (1998). The rocky road to positive intergroup relations. In J. Eberhardt & S. T. Fiske (Eds.), *Confronting racism: The problem and the response* (pp. 234–262). Thousand Oaks, CA: Sage.

Dovidio, J. F., Brigham, J. C., Johnson, B. T., & Gaertner, S. L. (1996). Stereotyping, prejudice, and discrimination: Another look. In N. Macrae, C. Stangor, & M. Hewstone (Eds.), *Stereotypes and stereotyping* (pp. 276–319). New York: Guilford Press.

Dovidio, J. F., Evans, N., & Tyler, R. B. (1986). Racial stereotypes: The contents of their cognitive representations. *Journal of Experimental Social Psychology, 22,* 22–37.

Dovidio, J. F., & Gaertner, S. L. (1986). Prejudice, discrimination, and racism: Historical trends an contemporary approaches. In J. F. Dovidio & S. L. Gaertner (Eds.), *Prejudice, discrimination, and racism* (pp. 1–34). Orlando, FL: Academic Press.

Dovidio, J. F., & Gaertner, S. L. (1991). Changes in the nature and expression of racial prejudice. In H. Knopke, J. Norrell, & R. Rogers (Eds.), *Opening doors: An appraisal of race relations in contemporary America* (pp. 201–241). Tuscaloosa, AL: University of Alabama Press.

Dovidio, J. F., & Gaertner, S. L. (1993). Stereotypes and evaluative intergroup bias. In D. M. Mackie & D. L. Hamilton (Eds.), *Affect, cognition, and stereotyping: Interactive processes in intergroup perception* (pp. 167–193). Orlando, FL: Academic Press.

Dovidio, J. F., & Gaertner, S. L. (1998). On the nature of contemporary prejudice: The causes, consequences, and challenges of aversive racism. In J. Eberhardt & S. T. Fiske (Eds.), *Confronting racism: The problem and the response* (pp. 3–32). Thousand Oaks, CA: Sage.

Dovidio, J. F., Gaertner, S. L., & Validzic, A. (1998). Intergroup bias: Status, differentiation, and a common ingroup identity. *Journal of Personality and Social Psychology, 75,* 109–120.

Dovidio, J. F., Kawakami, K., Johnson, C., Johnson, B., & Howard, A. (1997). On the nature of prejudice: Automatic and controlled processes. *Journal of Experimental Social Psychology, 33,* 510–540.

Dovidio, J. F., & Mullen, B. (1992). *Race, physical handicap, and response amplification.* Unpublished manuscript, Colgate University.

Duncan, B. L. (1976). Differential social perception and attribution of intergroup violence: Testing the lower limits of stereotyping of blacks. *Journal of Personality and Social Psychology, 34,* 590–598.

Dunning, D. (1999). A newer look: Motivated social cognition and the schematic representation of social concepts. *Psychological Inquiry, 10,* 1–11.

Dunning, D., & Sherman, D. A. (1997). Stereotypes and tacit inference. *Journal of Personality and Social Psychology, 73,* 459–471.

Eagly, A. H. (1987). *Sex differences in social behavior: A social-role interpretation.* Hillsdale, NJ: Erlbaum.

Eagly, A. H., & Steffen, V. J. (1984). Gender stereotypes stem from the distribution of women and men into social roles. *Journal of Personality and Social Psychology, 46,* 735–754.

Eberhardt, J. L., & Fiske, S. T. (1996). Motivating individuals to change: What is a target to do? In C. N. Macrae, C. Stangor, & M. Hewstone (Eds.), *Stereotypes and stereotyping* (pp. 369–415). New York. Guilford Press.

Fanon, F. (1967). *Black skins, white masks*. New York: Grove Press. (Original work published 1952)

Fine, M., & Asch, A. (1995). Disability beyond stigma: Social interaction, discrimination, and activism. In N. G. Rule & J. B. Veroff (Eds.), *The culture and psychology reader* (pp. 536–558). New York: New York University Press.

Farina, A. (1998). Stigma. In K. T. Mueser & N. Tarrier (Eds.), *Handbook of social functioning in schizophrenia* (pp. 247–279). Boston: Allyn & Bacon.

Farina, A., Felner, R. D., & Boudreau, L. A. (1973). Reactions of worker to male and female mental patient job applicants. *Journal of Consulting and Clinical Psychology, 41*, 363–372.

Farina, A., Gliha, D., Boudreau, L. A., Allen, J. G., & Sherman, M. (1971). Mental illness and the impact of believing others know about it. *Journal of Abnormal Psychology, 77*, 1–5.

Fazio, R. H., Jackson, J. R., Dunton, B. C., & Williams, C. J. (1995). Variability in automatic activation as an unobtrusive measure of racial attitudes: A bona fide pipeline? *Journal of Personality and Social Psychology, 69*, 1013–1027.

Fein, S., & Spencer, S. J. (1997). Prejudice as self-image maintenance: Affirming the self through negative evaluations of others. *Journal of Personality and Social Psychology, 73*, 31–44.

Fields, B. J. (1990). Slavery, race, and ideology in the United States of America. *New Left Review, 181*, 95–118.

Fisher, K. (1982, August). TV and the mentally ill. *APA Monitor*, pp. 12–13.

Fiske, S. T. (1982). Schema-triggered affect: Applications to social perception. In M. S. Clark & S. T. Fiske (Eds.), *The seventeenth annual Carnegie Symposium on Cognition* (pp. 55–78). Hillsdale, NJ: Erlbaum.

Fiske, S. T. (1989). Examining the role of intent. In J. Uleman & J. Bargh (Eds.), *Unintended thought* (pp. 253–283). New York: Guilford Press.

Fiske, S. T. (1998). Stereotyping, prejudice, and discrimination. In D. T. Gilbert, S. T. Fiske, & G. Lindzey (Eds.), *Handbook of social psychology* (4th ed., Vol. 2, pp. 357–411). Boston: McGraw-Hill.

Fiske, S. T., & Neuberg, S. (1990). A continuum of impression formation from category-based to individuating processes. In M. P. Zanna (Ed.), *Advances in experimental social psychology* (Vol. 23, pp. 1–73). San Diego, CA: Academic Press.

Fiske, S. T., Neuberg, S. L., Beattie, A. E., & Milberg, S. J. (1987). Category-based and attribute-based reactions to others: Some informational conditions of stereotyping and individuating processes. *Journal of Experimental Social Psychology, 23*, 399–427.

Fiske, S. T., & Pavelchak, M. A. (1986). Category-based versus piecemeal-based affective responses: Developments in schema-triggered affect. In R. M. Sorrentino & E. T. Higgins (Eds.), *Handbook of motivation and cognition: Foundations of social behavior* (Vol. 1, pp. 167–203). New York: Guilford Press.

Fiske, S. T., & Taylor, S. E. (1991). *Social cognition*. New York: McGraw-Hill.

Fyock, J., & Stangor, C. (1994). The role of memory biases in stereotype maintenance. *British Journal of Social Psychology, 33,* 331–343.

Gaertner, S. L., Dovidio, J. F., Anastasio, P. A., Bachman, B. A., & Rust, M. C. (1993). The common ingroup identity model: Recategorization and the reduction of intergroup bias. In W. Stroebe & M. Hewstone (Eds.), *European review of social psychology* (Vol. 4, pp. 1–26). Chichester, England: Wiley.

Gibson, J. J. (1979). *The ecological approach to visual perception.* Boston: Houghton Mifflin.

Glick, P., Zion, C., & Nelson, C. (1988). What mediates sex discrimination in hiring decisions? *Journal of Personality and Social Psychology, 55,* 178–186.

Goffman, E. (1963). *Stigma: Notes on the management of spoiled identity.* Englewood Cliffs, NJ: Prentice-Hall.

Goldstein, S. B., & Johnson, V. A. (1997). Stigma by association: Perceptions of the dating partners of college students with physical disabilities. *Basic and Applied Social Psychology, 19,* 495–504.

Greenwald, A. G., & Banaji, M. R. (1995). Implicit social cognition: Attitudes, self-esteem, and stereotypes. *Psychological Review, 102,* 4–27.

Haddock, G., Zanna, M. P., & Esses, V. (1993). Assessing the structure of prejudicial attitudes: The case of attitudes toward homosexuals. *Journal of Personality and Social Psychology, 65,* 1105–1118.

Hamilton, D. L. (1998, May). *Perceiving individuals and groups as units: The social psychology of glue.* Paper presented at the Society for Personality and Social Psychology's Preconference before the annual meeting of the American Psychological Society, Washington, DC.

Hamilton, D. L., & Sherman, J. W. (1994). Stereotypes. In R. S. Wyer, Jr. & T. K. Srull (Eds.), *Handbook of social cognition: Vol. 1* (pp. 1–68). Hillsdale, NJ: Erlbaum.

Hamilton, D. L., & Sherman, S. J. (1996). Perceiving persons and groups. *Psychological Review, 103,* 336–355.

Hamilton, D. L., & Trolier, T. K. (1986). Stereotypes and stereotyping: An overview of the cognitive approach. In J. F. Dovidio & S. L. Gaertner (Eds.), *Prejudice, discrimination, and racism* (pp. 127–163). Orlando, FL: Academic Press.

Harding, J., Proshansky, H., Kutner, B., & Chein, I. (1969). Prejudice and ethnic relations. In G. Lindzey & E. Aronson (Eds.), *Handbook of social psychology: Vol. 5. Applied social psychology* (2nd ed., pp. 1–76). Reading, MA: Addison-Wesley.

Hastie, R., & Kumar, P. A. (1979). Person memory: Personality traits as organizing principles in memory for behaviors. *Journal of Personality and Social Psychology, 37,* 25–38.

Hayward, P., & Bright, J. A. (1997). Stigma and mental illness: A review and critique. *Journal of Mental Health, 6,* 345–354.

Helms, J. E. (1995). An update of Helms' white and people of color racial identity models. In J. G. Ponterotto, J. M. Casas, L. A. Suzuki, & C. M. Alexander (Eds.), *Handbook of multicultural counseling* (pp. 181–198). Thousand Oaks, CA: Sage.

Herek, G. M. (1991). Stigma, prejudice, and violence against lesbians and gay men. In J. C. Gonsiorek & J. D. Weinrich (Eds.), *Homosexuality: Research implications for public policy* (pp. 60–80). Newbury Park, CA: Sage.

Hewstone, M. (1990). The "ultimate attribution error"?: A review of the literature on intergroup attributions. *European Journal of Social Psychology, 20,* 311–335.

Hewstone, M. (1994). Revision and change of stereotypic beliefs: In search of the elusive subtyping model. In W. Stroebe & M. Hewstone (Eds.), *European review of social psychology* (Vol. 5, pp. 69–109). Chichester, England: Wiley.

Hewstone, M., & Brown, R. J. (1986). Contact is not enough: An intergroup perspective on the "contact hypothesis." In M. Hewstone & R. Brown (Eds.), *Contact and conflict in intergroup encounters* (pp. 1–44). Oxford: Blackwell.

Hilton, J. L., & von Hippel, W. (1996). Stereotypes. *Annual Review of Psychology, 47,* 237–271.

Hogg, M. A., & Hains, S. C. (1996). Intergroup relations and group solidarity: Effects of group identification and social beliefs on depersonalized attraction. *Journal of Personality and Social Psychology, 70,* 295–309.

Jones, E. E., Farina, A., Hastorf, A. H., Markus, H., Miller, D. T., & Scott, R. A. (1984). *Social stigma: The psychology of marked relationships.* New York: Freeman.

Jones, J. M. (1986). Racism: A cultural analysis of the problem. In J. F. Dovidio & S. L. Gaertner (Eds.), *Prejudice, discrimination, and racism* (pp. 279–314). Orlando, FL: Academic Press.

Jost, J. T., & Banaji, M. R. (1994). The role of stereotyping in system-justification and the production of false consciousness. *British Journal of Social Psychology, 33,* 1–27.

Jost, J. T., Kruglanski, A. W., & Simon, L. (1999). Effects of epistemic motivation on conservatism, intolerance and other system-justifying attitudes. In L. L. Thompson, J. M. Levine, & D. M. Messick (Eds.), *Shared cognition in organizations: The management of knowledge* (pp. 91–116). Mahwah, NJ: Erlbaum.

Jussim, L. (1991). Social perception and social reality: A reflection-construction model. *Psychological Review, 98,* 54–73.

Jussim, L., Coleman, L. M., & Lerch, L. (1987). The nature of stereotypes: A comparison and integration of three theories. *Journal of Personality and Social Psychology, 52,* 536–546.

Kawakami, K., Dion, K., & Dovidio, J. F. (1998). Racial prejudice and stereotype activation. *Personality and Social Psychology Bulletin, 24,* 407–416.

Karlins, M., Coffman, T. L., & Walters, G. (1969). On the fading of social stereotypes: Studies in three generations of college students. *Journal of Personality and Social Psychology, 13,* 1–16.

Katz, I. (1981). *Stigma: A social psychological analysis.* Hillsdale, NJ: Erlbaum.

Kelly, A. E., & Kahn, J. H. (1994). Effects of suppression of personal intrusive thoughts. *Journal of Personality and Social Psychology, 66,* 998–1006.

Kleck, R. E. (1968). Physical stigma and nonverbal cues emitted in face-to-face interaction. *Human Relations, 21,* 19–28.

Kleck, R. E. (1969). Physical stigma and task-oriented interaction. *Human Relations, 22,* 53–60.

Kleck, R. E., Ono, H., & Hastorf, A. H. (1966). The effect of physical deviance upon face-to-face interaction. *Human Relations, 19,* 425–436.

Klinker, P. A., & Smith, R. M. (1999). *The unsteady march: The rise and decline of American commitments to racial equality.* New York: Free Press.

Kobrynowicz, D., & Biernat, M. (1997). Decoding subjective evaluations: How stereotypes provide shifting standards. *Journal of Experimental Social Psychology, 33,* 579–601.

Kolodziej, M. E., & Johnson, B. T. (1996). Interpersonal acceptance of persons with psychiatric disorders: A research synthesis. *Journal of Consulting and Clinical Psychology, 64,* 1387–1396.

Kunda, Z., & Oleson, K. C. (1995). Maintaining stereotypes in the face of disconfirmation: Constructing grounds for subtyping deviants. *Journal of Personality and Social Psychology, 68,* 565–579.

Kunda, Z., & Oleson, K. C. (1997). When exceptions prove the rule: How extremity of deviance determines the impact of deviant examples on stereotypes. *Journal of Personality and Social Psychology, 72,* 965–979.

Kunda, Z., & Sherman-Williams, B. (1993). Stereotypes and the construal of individuating information. *Personality and Social Psychology Bulletin, 19,* 90–99.

Kunda, Z., & Sinclair, L. (1999). Motivated reasoning with stereotypes: Activation, application, and inhibition. *Psychological Inquiry, 10,* 12–22.

Kunda, Z., Sinclair, L., & Griffin, D. (1997). Equal ratings but separate meanings. *Journal of Personality and Social Psychology, 72,* 720–734.

Kunda, Z., & Thagard, P. (1996). Forming impressions from stereotypes, traits, and behaviors: A parallel constraint satisfaction theory. *Psychological Review, 103,* 284–308.

Lefebvre, A., & Munro, I. R. (1986). Psychological adjustment of patients with craniofacial deformities before and after surgery. In C. P. Herman, M. P. Zanna, & E. T. Higgins (Eds.), *The Ontario Symposium: Vol. 3. Physical appearance, stigma, and social behavior* (pp. 53–64). Hillsdale, NJ: Erlbaum.

Lepore, L., & Brown, R. (1997). Category and stereotype activation: Is prejudice inevitable? *Journal of Personality and Social Psychology, 72,* 275–287.

Lerner, M. (1980). *The belief in a just world: A fundamental delusion.* New York: Plenum Press.

Link, B. G., Struening, E. L., Rahav, M., & Phelan, J. C. (1997). On stigma and its consequences: Evidence from a longitudinal study of men with dual diagnoses of mental illness and substance abuse. *Journal of Health and Social Behavior, 38,* 177–190.

Linville, P. W., Salovey, P., & Fischer, G. W. (1986). Stereotyping and perceived distributions of social characteristics: An application of ingroup–outgroup perception. In J. F. Dovidio & S. L. Gaertner (Eds.), *Prejudice, discrimination, and racism* (pp. 165–208). Orlando, FL: Academic Press.

Lueptow, L. B., Garovich, L., & Lueptow, M. B. (1995). The persistence of gender stereotypes in the face of changing sex roles: Evidence contrary to the sociocultural model. *Ethology and Sociobiology, 16,* 509–530.

Maass, A., & Arcuri, L. (1996). Language and stereotyping. In N. Macrae, C.

Stangor, & M. Hewstone (Eds.), *Stereotypes and stereotyping* (pp. 193–226). New York: Guilford Press.

Mackie, D. M., Hamilton, D. L., Susskind, J., & Rosselli, F. (1996). Social psychological foundations of stereotype formation. In N. Macrae, C. Stangor, & M. Hewstone (Eds.), *Stereotypes and stereotyping* (pp. 41–78) New York: Guilford Press.

Macrae, C. N., Bodenhausen, G. V., Milne, A. B., & Jetten, J. (1994). Out of mind but back in sight: Stereotypes on the rebound. *Journal of Personality and Social Psychology, 67,* 808–817.

Macrae, C. N., Bodenhausen, G. V., Milne, A. B., & Wheeler, V. (1996). On resisting temptation for simplification: Counterintentional effects of stereotype suppression on social memory. *Social Cognition, 14,* 1–20.

Macrae, C. N., Stangor, C., & Milne, A. B. (1994). Activating social stereotypes: A functional analysis. *Journal of Experimental Social Psychology., 30,* 370–389.

Major, B. (1994). From social inequality to personal entitlement: The role of social comparisons, legitimacy appraisals, and group membership. In M. P. Zanna (Ed.), *Advances in experimental social psychology* (Vol. 26, pp. 293–348). San Diego, CA: Academic Press.

Major, B., & Crocker, J. (1993). Social stigma: The affective consequences of attributional ambiguity. In D. M. Mackie & D. L. Hamilton (Eds.), *Affect, cognition, and stereotyping* (pp. 345–370). San Diego, CA: Academic Press.

Major, B., Testa, M., & Bylsma, W. H. (1991). Responses to upward and downward social comparisons: The impact of esteem-relevance and perceived control. In J. Suls & T. A. Wills (Eds.), *Social comparison: Contemporary theory and research* (pp. 237–260). Hillsdale, NJ: Erlbaum.

Martin, C. L., & Parker, S. (1995). Folk theories about sex and race differences. *Personality and Social Psychology Bulletin, 21,* 45–57.

McCauley, C., & Stitt, C. L. (1978). An individual and quantitative measure of stereotypes. *Journal of Personality and Social Psychology, 36,* 929–940.

McConahay, J. B. (1986). Modern racism, ambivalence, and the Modern Racism Scale. In J. F. Dovidio & S. L. Gaertner (Eds.), *Prejudice, discrimination, and racism* (pp. 91–125). Orlando, FL: Academic Press.

McGill, A. L. (1998). Relative use of necessity and sufficiency information in causal judgments about natural categories. *Journal of Personality and Social Psychology, 75,* 70–81.

McGuire, J. M., & Borowy, T. D. (1979). Attitudes toward mental health professionals. *Professional Psychology, 10,* 74–79.

Medin, D. L. (1988). Social categorization: Structures, processes, and purposes. In T. K. Srull & R. S. Wyer, Jr. (Eds.), *Advances in social cognition: Vol. 1. A dual process model of impression formation* (pp. 199–226). Hillsdale, NJ: Erlbaum.

Mehta, S. I., & Farina, A. (1988). Associative stigma: Perceptions of the difficulties of college-aged children of stigmatized fathers. *Journal of Social and Clinical Psychology, 7,* 192–202.

Miller, C. T., & Myers, A. M. (1998). Compensating for prejudice: How heavyweight people (and others) control outcomes despite prejudice. In J. K. Swim

& C. Stangor (Eds.), *Prejudice: The target's perspective* (pp. 191–218). San Diego, CA: Academic Press.

Monteith, M. J., Sherman, J. W., & Devine, P. G. (1998). Suppression as a stereotype control strategy. *Personality and Social Psychology Review, 2,* 63–82.

Neuberg, S. L., Smith, D. M., Hoffman, J. C., & Russell, F. J. (1994). When we observe stigmatized and "normal" individuals interacting: Stigma by association. *Personality and Social Psychology Bulletin, 20,* 196–209.

Oakes, P. J., Haslam, S. J., & Turner, J. C. (Eds.). (1994). *Stereotyping and social reality.* Oxford: Blackwell.

Park, B., & Hastie, R. (1987). Perception of variability in category development: Instance- versus abstraction-based stereotypes. *Journal of Personality and Social Psychology, 53,* 621–635.

Park, B., & Judd, C. M. (1990). Measures and models of perceived group variability. *Journal of Personality and Social Psychology, 59,* 173–191.

Park, B., & Rothbart, M. (1982). Perception of out-group homogeneity and levels of social categorization: Memory for subordinate attributes of in-group and out-group members. *Journal of Personality and Social Psychology, 42,* 1051–1068.

Pettigrew, T. F. (1979). The ultimate attribution error: Extending Allport's cognitive analysis of prejudice. *Personality and Social Psychology Bulletin, 5,* 461–476.

Pettigrew, T. F. (1981). Extending the stereotype concept. In D. L. Hamilton (Ed.), *Cognitive processes in stereotyping and intergroup behavior* (pp. 303–332). Hillsdale, NJ: Erlbaum.

Pettigrew, T. F. (1997). Generalized intergroup contact effects on prejudice. *Personality and Social Psychology Bulletin, 23,* 175–185.

Phelan, J. C., Bromet, E. J., & Link, B. G. (1998). *Schizophrenia Bulletin, 24,* 115–126.

Pinel, E. C. (1999). Stigma consciousness: The psychological legacy of social stereotypes. *Journal of Personality and Social Psychology, 76,* 114–128.

Richardson, S. A., Ronald, L., & Kleck, R. E. (1974). The social status of handicapped and nonhandicapped boys in a field setting. *Journal of Special Education, 8,* 143–152.

Rothbart, M. (1981). Memory processes and social beliefs. In D. L. Hamilton (Ed.), *Cognitive processes in stereotyping and intergroup behavior* (pp. 145–182). Hillsdale, NJ: Erlbaum.

Rothbart, M., Evans, M., & Fulero, S. (1979). Recall for confirming events: Memory processes and the maintenance of social stereotyping. *Journal of Experimental Social Psychology, 15,* 343–355.

Rothbart, M., & John, O. P. (1985). Social categorization and behavioral episodes: A cognitive analysis of the effects of intergroup contact. *Journal of Social Issues, 41*(3), 81–104.

Rothbart, M., & Taylor, M. (1992). Category labels and social reality: Do we view social categories as natural kinds? In G. Semin & K. Fiedler (Eds.), *Language, interaction, and social cognition* (pp. 11–36). Newbury Park, CA: Sage.

Rounds, J. B., & Zevon, M. A. (1993). Cancer stereotypes: A multidimensional scaling analysis. *Journal of Behavioral Medicine, 16,* 485–496.

Ruggiero, K. M., & Taylor, D. M. (1997). Why minority group members perceive or do not perceive discrimination that confronts them: The role of self-esteem and perceived control. *Journal of Personality and Social Psychology, 72,* 373–389.

Saenger, G., & Flowerman, S. (1954). Stereotypes and prejudicial attitudes. *Human Relations, 7,* 217–238.

Sagar, H. A., & Schofield, J. W. (1980). Racial and behavioral cues in black and white children's perceptions of ambiguously aggressive acts. *Journal of Personality and Social Psychology, 39,* 590–598.

Sartre, J.-P. (1965). *Anti-Semite and Jew.* New York: Schocken Books. (Original work published 1946)

Schaller, M., & Conway, G. (1999). Influence of impression-management goals on the emerging content of group stereotypes: Support for a social-evolutionary perspective. *Personality and Social Psychology Bulletin, 25,* 819–833.

Schaller, M., & Latané, B. (1996). Dynamic social impact and the evolution of social representations: A natural history of stereotypes. *Journal of Communication, 46,* 64–77.

Scheff, T. J. (1966). *Being mentally ill: A sociological theory.* Chicago: Aldine.

Sibicky, M., & Dovidio, J. F. (1985, April). *Attitudes toward counseling clients: Subtle stigmatization?* Paper presented at the annual convention of the Eastern Psychological Association, Boston.

Sibicky, M., & Dovidio, J. F. (1986). Stigma of psychological therapy: Stereotypes, interpersonal reactions, and the self-fulfilling prophecy. *Journal of Counseling Psychology, 33,* 148–154.

Simpson, G. E., & Yinger, J. M. (1965). *Racial and cultural minorities.* New York: Harper & Row.

Sinclair, L., & Kunda, Z. (1999). Reactions to a Black professional: Motivated inhibition and activation of conflicting stereotypes. *Journal of Personality and Social Psychology, 77,* 885–904.

Smith, E. R. (1993). Social identity and social emotions: Toward new conceptualizations of prejudice. In D. M. Mackie & D. L. Hamilton (Eds.), *Affect, cognition, and stereotyping* (pp. 297–316). San Diego, CA: Academic Press.

Smith, E. R., & Zárate, M. A. (1992). Exemplar-based model of social judgment. *Psychological Review, 99,* 3–21.

Snyder, M. (1981). On the self-perpetuating nature of social stereotypes. In D. L. Hamilton (Ed.), *Cognitive processes in stereotyping and intergroup behavior* (pp. 183–212). Hillsdale, NJ: Erlbaum.

Snyder, M. L., Kleck, R. E., Strenta, A., & Mentzer, S. J. (1979). Avoidance of the handicapped: An attributional analysis. *Journal of Personality and Social Psychology, 37,* 2297–2306.

Sobel, D. (1981, August 4). Thousands with mental health insurance choose to pay own bill. *The New York Times,* Section 1, p. 1.

Solomon, S., Greenberg, J., & Pyszczynski, T. (1991). A terror management theory of social behavior: The psychological functions of self-esteem and cultural worldviews. In M. P. Zanna (Ed.), *Advances in experimental social psychology* (Vol. 24, pp. 93–159). San Diego, CA: Academic Press.

Spears, R., & Haslam, S. A. (1997). Stereotyping and the burden of cognitive load.

In R. Spears, P. J. Oakes, N. Ellemers, & S. A. Haslam (Eds.), *The social psychology of stereotyping and group life* (pp. 171–207). Oxford: Blackwell.

Spencer, S. J., Fein, S., Wolfe, C. T., Fong, C., & Dunn, M. A. (1998). Automatic activation of stereotypes: The role of self-image threat. *Personality and Social Psychology Bulletin, 24,* 1139–1152.

Spencer, S. J., Steele, C. M., & Quinn, D. M. (1999). Stereotype threat and women's math performance. *Journal of Experimental Social Psychology, 35,* 4–28.

Srull, T. K., Lichtenstein, M., & Rothbart, M. (1985). Associative storage and retrieval processes in person memory. *Journal of Experimental Psychology: Learning, Memory, and Cognition, 7,* 440–462.

Stangor, C., & McMillan, D. (1992). Memory for expectancy-congruent and expectancy-incongruent information: A review of the social and developmental literatures. *Psychological Bulletin, 111,* 42–61.

Stangor, C., & Schaller, M. (1996). Stereotypes as individual and collective representations. In N. Macrae, C. Stangor, & M. Hewstone (Eds.), *Stereotypes and stereotyping* (pp. 3–37). New York: Guilford Press.

Stangor, C., Sullivan, L. A., & Ford, T. E. (1991). Affective and cognitive determinants of prejudice. *Social Cognition, 9,* 359–380.

Steele, C. M. (1992, April). Race and the schooling of Black Americans. *The Atlantic Monthly,* pp. 68–78.

Steele, C. M. (1998). A threat in the air: How stereotypes shape intellectual identity and performance. In J. Eberhardt & S. T. Fiske (Eds.), *Confronting racism: The problem and the response* (pp. 202–233). Thousand Oaks, CA: Sage.

Steele, C. M., & Aronson, J. (1995). Stereotype threat and intellectual test performance of African Americans. *Journal of Personality and Social Psychology, 69,* 797–811.

Stephan, W. G., & Stephan, C. W. (1985). Intergroup anxiety. *Journal of Social Issues, 41*(3), 157–175.

Stephan, W. G., & Stephan, C. W. (1993). Cognition and affect in stereotyping: Parallel interactive networks. In D. M. Mackie & D. L. Hamilton (Eds.), *Affect, cognition, and stereotyping* (pp. 111–136). San Diego, CA: Academic Press.

Stunkard, A. J., & Sobal, J. (1995). Psychosocial consequences of obesity. In K. D. Brownell & C. G. Fairburn (Eds.), *Eating disorders and obesity: A comprehensive handbook* (pp. 417–421). New York: Guilford Press.

Tajfel, H. (1969). Cognitive aspects of prejudice. *Journal of Social Issues, 25*(4), 79–97.

Tajfel, H., & Turner, J. C. (1979). An integrative theory of intergroup conflict. In W. G. Austin & S. Worchel (Eds.), *The social psychology of intergroup relations* (pp. 33–48). Monterey, CA: Brooks/Cole.

Taylor, S. E. (1981). A categorization approach to stereotyping. In D. L. Hamilton (Ed.), *Cognitive processes in stereotyping and intergroup behavior* (pp. 88–114). Hillsdale, NJ: Erlbaum.

Taylor, S. E., & Lobel, M. (1989). Social comparison activity under threat: Downward evaluation and upward contacts. *Psychological Review, 96*(4), 569–575.

Trope, Y., & Thompson, E. P. (1997). Looking for truth in all the wrong places?: Asymmetric search of individuating information about stereotyped group members. *Journal of Personality and Social Psychology, 73*, 229–241.

Urban, L. M., & Miller, N. (1998). A theoretical analysis of crossed categorization effects: A meta-analysis. *Journal of Personality and Social Psychology, 74*, 894–908.

von Hippel, W., Sekaquaptewa, D., & Vargas, P. (1995). On the role of encoding processes in stereotype maintenance. In M. P. Zanna (Ed.), *Advances in experimental social psychology* (Vol. 27, pp. 177–254). San Diego, CA: Academic Press.

Weber, R., & Crocker, J. (1983). Cognitive processes in the revision of stereotypical beliefs. *Journal of Personality and Social Psychology, 45*, 961–977.

Wegner, D. M., & Erber R. (1992). The hyperaccessibility of suppressed thoughts. *Journal of Personality and Social Psychology, 63*, 903–912.

Weiner, B. (1986). *An attributional theory of motivation and emotion.* New York: Springer-Verlag.

Weiner, B. (1993). On sin versus sickness: A theory of perceived responsibility and social motivation. *American Psychologist, 48*, 957–965.

Weiner, B., Perry, R. P., & Magnusson, J. (1988). An attributional analysis of reactions to stigmas. *Journal of Personality and Social Psychology, 55*, 738–748.

Weitz, S. (1972). Attitude, voice, and behavior: A repressed affect model of interracial interaction. *Journal of Personality and Social Psychology, 24*, 14–21.

Westbrook, M. T., Legge, V., & Pennay, M. (1993). Attitudes toward disabilities in a multicultural society. *Social Science and Medicine, 36*, 615–623.

Wilder, D. A. (1981). Perceiving persons as a group: Categorization and intergroup relations. In D. L. Hamilton (Ed.), *Cognitive processes in stereotyping and intergroup behavior* (pp. 213–258). Hillsdale, NJ: Erlbaum.

Williams, J. E., & Best, D. L. (1982). *Measuring sex stereotypes: A thirty nation study.* Beverly Hills, CA: Sage.

Williams, R. M. (1947). *The reduction of intergroup tension.* New York: Social Science Research Council.

Wills, T. A. (1981). Downward comparison principles in social psychology. *Psychological Bulletin, 90*, 245–271.

Wills, T. A. (1983). Social comparison in coping and help-seeking. In B. M. DePaulo, A. Nadler, & J. D. Fisher (Eds.), *New directions in helping: Vol. 2. Help-seeking* (pp. 109–138). New York: Academic Press.

Wittenbrink, B., Judd, C. M., & Park, B. (1997). Evidence for racial prejudice at the implicit level and its relationship with questionnaire measures. *Journal of Personality and Social Psychology, 72*, 262–274.

Word, C. O., Zanna, M. P., & Cooper, J. (1974). The nonverbal mediation of self-fulfilling prophecies in interracial interaction. *Journal of Experimental Social Psychology, 10*, 109–120.

Wright, B. A. (1983). *Physical disability: A psychological approach* (2nd ed.). New York: Harper.

Wright, S. C., Aron, A., McLaughlin-Volpe, T., & Ropp, S. A. (1997). The extended contact effect: Knowledge of cross-racial friendships and prejudice. *Journal of Personality and Social Psychology, 73*, 73–90.

Wyer, R. S., Jr., & Gordon, S. E. (1984). The cognitive representation of social information. In R. S. Wyer, Jr. & T. K. Srull (Eds.), *Handbook of social cognition* (Vol. 2, pp. 73–150). Hillsdale, NJ: Erlbaum.

Wyer, R. S., & Martin, L. L. (1986). Person memory: The role of traits, group stereotypes, and specific behaviors in the cognitive representation of persons.
Journal of Personality and Social Psychology, 50, 661–675.

Yount, K. R. (1986). A theory of productive activity: The relationships among self-
concept, sex role stereotypes, and work-emergent traits. *Psychology of
Women Quarterly, 10,* 63–88.

Yuker, H. E., & Allison, D. B. (1994). Obesity: Sociocultural perspectives. In L.
Alexander-Mott & D. B. Lumsden (Eds.), *Understanding eating disorders:
Anorexia nervosa, bulimia nervosa, and obesity* (pp. 243–270). Washington,
DC: Taylor & Francis.

Yzerbyt, V., Rocher, S., & Schadron, G. (1997). Stereotypes as explanations: A
subjective essentialistic view of group perception. In R. Spears, P. J. Oakes,
N. Ellemers, & S. A. Haslam (Eds.), *The social psychology of stereotyping
and group life* (pp. 20–50). Oxford: Blackwell.

Zebrowitz, L. A. (1996). Physical appearance as a basis of stereotyping. In N.
Macrae, C. Stangor, & M. Hewstone (Eds.), *Stereotypes and stereotyping*
(pp. 79–120). New York: Guilford Press.

5

Ideology and Lay Theories of Stigma: The Justification of Stigmatization

CHRISTIAN S. CRANDALL

The experience of stigma is common. Virtually every person has experienced the alienation, rejection, exclusion, embarrassment, and feeling of separateness that come from being different, devalued, and demeaned. Even though the process is aversive and actively avoided by nearly everyone, nearly everyone also avoids, rejects, and withdraws from people who are stigmatized.

Are stigmatizers oblivious of the effects of rejection? Do people experience a near-total collapse of empathy, unaware of the pain of exclusion while willingly excluding the stigmatized? This is unlikely. Instead, I suggest that people, in the process of stigmatizing others, believe that the rejection, avoidance, and inferior treatment they dole out to stigmatized others are fair, appropriate, judicious—in other words, *justified*. People believe that there are moral, ethical, legal, social, natural, and logical bases—even requirements—for their rejection. As a result of what I call here "justification ideologies," one can continue to treat people as second-class citizens, apply a lower moral standard, and practice exclusion with a clear conscience.

126

THE NEGATIVITY OF STIGMA

A "stigma" is a characteristic that makes a person different, and less desirable, than would normally be expected. A stigma can be a deviant behavior, physical characteristic, group membership, or moral failing that serves to disqualify the stigmatized person from full membership in a society, and cuts him or her off from normal social contact.

The stigmatization process can have a profound effect on stigmatized individuals, and their less-than-ideal treatment has been widely documented (Crocker, Major, & Steele, 1998; Pfuhl & Henry, 1993). Their social relations can be disrupted, awkward, and embarrassing (Goffman, 1963), and this can lead to anxiety, depression, and the avoidance of others (Crandall & Coleman, 1992). Stigmatization can lead to a distorted self-image and low self-esteem (Wright, 1983), although many times it does not (Crocker & Major, 1989). Stigmatized persons are often avoided in stranger interactions (Langer, Fiske, Taylor, & Chanowitz, 1976), receiving fewer smiles and social contacts. Stigmas have long been known to be impediments to romantic relationship and employment (Barker, Wright, Meyerson, & Gonick, 1953; Jones et al., 1984).

JUSTIFICATION IDEOLOGIES

On the surface, this behavior appears to be unjust, unsupportable, and unfair. How is it that people can so cavalierly apply a lower moral standard for their conduct toward the stigmatized? A variety of "justification ideologies" let people feel that discriminatory treatment is natural, sensible, and fair. A justification ideology is a set of (1) beliefs and values about how the world works, and (2) moral standards that serve to create levels of moral value.

A justification ideology is like a secular religion: It is a set of assumptions and background beliefs that are untested and untestable. Such ideologies are beyond the touch of data and experience; they are the very frames and lenses through which we view the world. They are described as "ideologies" because they are often not open to dispassionate discussion, and not based on careful reflection and sifting of evidence by the people who endorse them. In addition, justification ideologies are often part of a complex web of belief, with the separate beliefs and value components bolstering each other and protecting the ideology from outside challenges (Crandall, Britt, & Glor, 1999). When justification ideologies are threatened, the believer can react with anxiety, hostility, and anger (Schutte, 1995).

Suppose for a moment that you are a department store manager, looking to hire a clerk for your men's shoe department. If you learn that an otherwise highly qualified male applicant had a conviction (now legally expunged) for murder, you might decide not to hire him. In anticipating being uncomfortable and perhaps fearful around the applicant, you set out to avoid him. Or, suppose you wish to hire a babysitter for your 5-year-old child, and the apparently most qualified applicant is a man rumored to be a pedophile. You are extremely likely to avoid hiring this applicant.

Is this avoidant and clearly discriminatory behavior justifiable? When presented with this scenario, many people argue that the behaviors described are not discriminatory; they are rational and sensible. The only difference between "rational" treatment and "unjust" treatment of the stigmatized, I argue, is the presence of a justification ideology. The use of justification ideologies may be rational or not, but no sensible parent hires a pedophile as a child care provider. But whether rational or unjust, in each case a justification ideology is easily and rapidly applied to one's aversive reaction, and the discriminatory behavior becomes acceptable, even necessary. The presence of justification ideologies provides both public and private "cover" for otherwise unacceptable treatment, alleviating guilt and releasing prejudice and discrimination that values, social norms, and personal standards would otherwise suppress.

A reader of this chapter might conclude from this argument that prejudice and discrimination against any group are unwarranted; this is not my argument. Instead, I argue, the processes that lead to the justification of stigmatization are the same, whether they serve to justify racial prejudice, discrimination against physically disabled individuals, exclusion of people with criminal convictions from the teaching profession, or the obviously sensible decision to avoid hiring a child molester as a babysitter. The key issue is that justification ideologies serve to make individuals accept their own prejudices, discrimination, and rejection toward people with stigmas. The moral value of these justifications, and the defensibility of them, are outside the scope of this chapter.

How do people come to accept their own unjust treatment of the stigmatized? Ideological commitments lead them to self-justification. A justification ideology exempts stigmatized individuals from full moral inclusion, and as a result, the stigma in conjunction with the ideology can lead to rough treatment.

This chapter revolves around a simple fundamental hypothesis: Certain beliefs "justify" stigmatization. These justification beliefs allow, release, or even *promote* stigmatization responses. In what follows, I look at how two categories of beliefs, based on attributions and acceptance of hierarchy, can allow people to treat some stigmatized people according to a lower moral standard than they would apply to the unstigmatized. Much of the literature on prejudice and discrimination can be considered literature on justifications, with roots in attribution, hierarchy beliefs, or a combination of both. Justification is the flip side of suppression; it is the *releaser* of stigmatization-based prejudice and discrimination, rather than the cause of it. Finally, some of the affective and public policy consequences of justification ideologies are considered.

In the next section, a variety of justification ideologies and belief systems are outlined, and their effects on the perceiver are outlined. The focus is on the perceiver, and the nature of and processes associated with these justification ideologies are described.

TWO KINDS OF JUSTIFICATION IDEOLOGIES

I identify two basic kinds of justification ideologies here. The first kind consists of "attributional" approaches, in which the primary focus of justification is on the use of attributions of causality, judgments of responsibility, and blame to justify stigmatization. The second kind consists of "hierarchical" approaches, in which the focus is on the endorsement of the presence of hierarchy, and the acceptance of superior–inferior relations as necessary, good, inevitable, or "natural." These two categories of justifications can be "blended" in various combinations.

Attributional Approaches

The category of attributional justifications focuses on attributions that make a stigmatized person responsible for his or her stigma. An attribution of internal controllability points the finger of blame directly at stigmatized individuals: Since they are responsible for their fate, they have earned its consequences. These attributions take several forms, and research and theory on attribution-based justification strategies were particularly vigorous in the 1970s and 1980s.

Just-World Beliefs

Probably the best-known attribution-based justification strategy is the "belief in a just world." Lerner (1980) describes a just world as "one in which people 'get what they deserve.' The judgment of deserving is based on the outcome that someone is entitled to receive" (p. 11). If one believes that people get what they deserve (and deserve what they get), then people with stigmas must, by dint of this belief, deserve their fate. Lerner (1980) shows that perceivers will select, distort, or even invent evidence suggesting that stigmatized individuals are deserving of blame. For example, Walster (1966) found that as the severity of an automobile accident increased from trivial to significant, so did attributions of responsibility to the driver of the car. Similarly, when we view a person who has been victimized in some way, we often look for evidence suggesting that he or she was responsible; this is a particular problem with respect to rape, where often the first reaction is to search for evidence suggesting that the victim was in some way responsible for this negative event (Herbert & Dunkel-Schetter, 1992; Struckman-Johnson & Struckman-Johnson, 1992). Just-world beliefs support a tendency to blame the victim—a closely connected concept.

Blaming the Victim

The way that attributions of controllability and judgments of responsibility can justify negative reactions to the stigmatized is illuminated in the powerful and persuasive book *Blaming the Victim* (Ryan, 1971). Ryan reviews the many ways in which people who have been victimized in some way, due to social structure, history, or other cultural processes that lead to stigmatization, are instead held accountable for their own state. Ryan uses the writings and speeches of politicians, journalists, and social scientists, as well as letters to the editor, to show the subtle way in which the stigmatized are blamed for their fate. Some examples of blaming the victim that Ryan (1971) reviews are as follows: (1) Poor people are focused only on the present; (2) Black parents neglect their children, creating a cycle of despair; (3) poor persons seek self-esteem in gambling; (4) single mothers have "strange" and loose sexual mores; and (5) people from the inner city undermine the economic integrity of their neighborhoods through violence and crime.

Although Ryan's book was published in 1971, there is no shortage of evidence that blaming the victim is common practice in current rhetoric. The description of single mothers on public assistance as "welfare queens" suggests that receiving Aid to Families with Dependent Children and food stamps represents a lifestyle choice made willingly and eagerly. Similarly, the recent passing of a California initiative that ended three decades of bilingual instruction in the public schools was promoted in part as a response to the low value placed on education of immigrant Mexicans, and to the perception of their unwillingness to master English rapidly (see Glazer, 1998).

Attributions of Control and Responsibility

Attributions of responsibility for negative outcomes directly support justification processes. Weiner (1995) reviews the evidence that anger comes as a result of making a judgment that a person is responsible for a negative fate. For example, Weiner, Perry, and Magnusson (1988) presented people with vignettes describing people stigmatized with a wide range of stigmas, including blindness, obesity, HIV infection, and so on. When the targets were described as responsible for their fate (e.g., through carelessness, low self-control, or promiscuity), they were met with responses of anger and little willingness to help. On the other hand, when the targets were described as not responsible (e.g., because of the actions of others, a glandular disorder, or a blood transfusion), they were met with a significantly more positive emotional response and a willingness to improve or ameliorate their situation. Similarly, the willingness to express prejudice toward fat people is based on the attribution that fat people are responsible for their weight (Crandall, 1994; DeJong, 1981), and racists are more likely to hold Blacks responsible for their relatively low socioeconomic position (Vescio, 1995) and to express anger and rejection publicly as a result.

The anger that results from this attributional pattern can have a broad impact on a variety of reactions to the stigmatized, including helping, avoidance, discrimination, and its subsequent justification (Weiner, 1986). When perceivers are angry, they tend to make person-focused attributions rather than attributing events to external forces (Keltner, Ellsworth, & Edwards, 1993), which in turn can heighten anger. Blame for a negative outcome can lead to anger, and anger in turn can lead to enhanced blame—a result that can emotionally justify rejection.

The Protestant Work Ethic

Among the fundamental values and beliefs that characterizes traditional American values is the Protestant worth ethic (PWE). This is a set of values about the moral value of work, and the connection between hard work and success. It has been a main theme of the history of modern Western civilization (Parsons, 1937) and a major component of individualism.

The psychology of the PWE has two basic ingredients. The first consists of the repudiation of pleasure, self-abnegation as a component of self-control, and anxiety about gratification and luxury. For example, Katz and Hass's (1988) measure of the PWE includes such items as "I feel uneasy when there is little work for me to do," and "A distaste for hard work usually reflects a weakness of character."

The more germaine second ingredient is the attribution that hard work, determination, and self-control lead to success. Katz and Hass's (1988) PWE measure includes such items as "Most people who don't succeed in life are just plain lazy," and "People who fail at a job usually have not tried hard enough." These items reveal the clear underlying attributional component of the value system: The cause of success is individual action—hard work, determination, persistence.

The more a person endorses PWE values, the more likely he or she is to be willing to express a variety of prejudices. McConahay and Hough (1976) found that PWE values predicted racism in suburbanites and seminarians (see also Kinder & Sears, 1981), and Katz and Hass (1988) found that the PWE predicted anti-Black affect in college students. I (Crandall, 1994) found that PWE values predicted prejudice against fat people, and a group of us (Biernat, Vescio, Theno, & Crandall, 1996) found that the PWE predicted rejection of homosexuals.

Heider: Attributions and Essence

Most of the work on causal attribution can trace its roots directly back to the work of Heider (1944, 1958). Heider's work affected social-psychological research indirectly, through the work of a small handful of interpreters (e.g., Jones et al., 1972). This work was remarkably productive, and has had a profound effect on social, personality, organizational, and clinical psychology. But there is still much to be gained by looking at Heider's original conceptualization of attribution, along with the notions of psychological balance and unit relations. (Heider's thinking is more fully spelled out in his published notebooks, six volumes edited by Marijana Benesh; see also Benesh-Weiner & Weiner, 1982.)

Heider argued that attribution and balance theories are closely connected, as two parts of a more integrated theory of social perception (e.g., Heider, 1976). As Heider saw it, attribution is much more than causal explanation. The perception of causal attribution, especially when an internal or controllable attributions is made, is equivalent to seeing the outcome and the person as a single, harmonious perceptual unit (Heider, 1988); causal attribution leads to the formation of such a perceptual unit. Furthermore, this perception is characterized by a pressure to be balanced, uniform, and affectively consistent (see Crandall, N'Gbala, & Dawson, 1999, for a review).

As a result, when a person is seen to be causally responsible for some aspect of his or her fate, such as a stigma, then the stigma is seen to be a revelation of the person's character—a manifestation of the individual's moral "essence." Because a causal attribution is a unit (part of a larger perception of the person), and because of the pressure for affective uniformity within a perceiver's feelings toward a person, a perception of responsibility for a stigma leads to a negative evaluation of the person. The stigma and the moral value of the person are all of a piece. Accordingly, the stigmatized person is devalued, and a negative affective reaction ensues.

Summary of Attributional Approaches

The attributional approaches are closely related to each other, and make many of the same kinds of predictions. If a person is seen as responsible for his or her own negative fate, then anger and other negative emotional reactions to the person will follow. If stigmatized individuals are perceived as responsible for their victimhood, they are not seen as worthy of help, and rejection, avoidance, and other pernicious affective and behavioral consequences of stigmatization can be heaped on their heads like hot coals—all with a clear conscience, because the bad treatment is *justified* by the perceivers' belief that "it's their own fault."

Hierarchical Approaches

The other kind of approach to justification of bad treatment of the stigmatized is based on the perception of the goodness, naturalness, or necessity of social hierarchies. Various theories suggest that people perceive—and value—hierarchies among people and groups of people. This "natural" hierarchy in turn justifies differential treatment for occupants of various places in the hierarchy: The elite deserve special privileges and very little social control, while the *bas monde* receive little in the way of privilege or opportunity, and are subject to significant social control.

Social Darwinism

One of the most influential styles of hierarchical thinking in Western thought is social Darwinism. Social Darwinism was developed in the late 19th century, notably by Herbert Spencer (Spencer, 1872), based on the application of the biological evolutionary ideas of Charles Darwin to problems of society. Social inequalities were "explained" as inevitable, natural, and even *good*, by appeal to the idea that societal success reflects the "survival of the fittest" (a phrase coined by the social Darwinists).

Social Darwinism can be characterized by five beliefs: (1) All of nature, including humans, is governed by natural biological laws; (2) population and habitat pressure leads to a struggle for existence; (3) physical and intellectual traits that provide a selective advantage will succeed, persist, and spread; (4) genetic inheritance and natural selection produce new species and eliminate others; and (5) all of the preceding arguments apply equally well to human social behavior and social structure (Hawkins, 1997).

According to Hofstadter (1955), American social Darwinism is characterized by laissez-faire economics, militarism, and (most impor-

tant for our purposes) racism and imperialism. Social Darwinism ele-
vates hierarchies to a state in which inferior treatment of stigmatized individuals (those of "inferior" race or culture) is not simply natural, but
morally good and even necessary—an effective way of elevating humanity through natural selection. For example, social Darwinism in psychology was responsible for much of the earlier research in intelligence testing, notably Goddard's measurement of immigrant intellect (see Kamin,
1981). Although straightforward social Darwinism has largely been intellectually discredited, threads of it continue to live on in modern political, social, and scientific thought in an adapted, more modern version.

Modern Social Darwinism

Social Darwinism has persisted successfully for several intellectual generations, and social Darwinist ideas have been influential in public discourse and policy making in the United States in recent decades. "Modern" social Darwinism is a blend of the old-fashioned social Darwinism
of Spencer with a pseudoscientific understanding of race, anthropology,
and genetics.

Some thinkers have adopted the explosion of the field of behavioral
genetics as evidence of the relative superiority–inferiority of different racial groups. The belief that different racial and ethnic groups have a distinct genetic past, and that this past characterizes *essential* differences
between the groups as compared to the human diversity across groups,
characterizes this kind of revised (and racialist) social Darwinist belief.
Thinking along these lines can be found in groups ranging from neo-
Nazi skinhead groups and modern Ku Klux Klan members (Ezekiel,
1995) to academic psychologists (e.g., Rushton, 1995).

A prominent example of modern Social Darwinism in psychology is
the work of Richard Herrnstein, who has argued that the social inferiority of certain groups is a consequence of their genetic inferiority. The
stigma of unemployment, for example, was explained by Herrnstein
(1971) in an article in *The Atlantic Monthly*: "the tendency to be unemployed may run in the genes of a family about as certainly as bad teeth
do now. . . . As the wealth and complexity of human society grow, there
will be precipitated out of the mass of humanity a low-capacity residue
that may be unable to master the common occupations" (p. 53). Together with public policy professor James Q. Wilson, Herrnstein published *Crime and Human Nature* (Wilson & Herrnstein, 1985), which
argued that criminal conduct is based on personality types and traits,
which are genetically transmitted. And the best-known example of
Herrnstein's social Darwinism is his collaboration with Charles Murray,
The Bell Curve (Herrnstein & Murray, 1994). In this book, Herrnstein
and Murray argue that in modern Western society, intelligence is in-

creasingly becoming the single factor by which social selection is made. They argue that IQ, which measures unitary general intelligence (g), is mostly genetically determined, and that families and races that are less well endowed with g must necessarily suffer socially and economically. As a result, attempts at creating social equality are doomed to failure, because the underlying genetic capital is unable to take advantage of education or other social interventions.

Social Dominance Orientation

An important defining component of a culture is the way in which it creates status hierarchies. These hierarchies form the basic skeleton of social structure (Berreman, 1981), and serve to determine access to income, reproduction, education, and other social assets. People within these cultures can differ in the extent to which they are attracted to hierarchical structure, and upon which dimensions hierarchies should be constructed. For example, in the world of finance, income and the extent of fiscal resources are endorsed as means of establishing rank, but in the academic world, intellect and productivity are endorsed as allocation rules for status, grant support, and office size. Each culture and subculture has conventions about status, prestige, and moral value.

Sidanius, Pratto, and their colleagues have conceptualized an individual-difference approach to belief and endorsement of status hierarchies: "social dominance orientation" (SDO). SDO is the degree of one's preference for inequality among social groups. Their SDO scale measures individual differences in the extent to which one believes that one's ingroup should dominate and be superior to outgroups (Pratto, Sidanius, Stallworth, & Malle, 1994; Sidanius & Pratto, 1993). People who score high in SDO are considered to prefer hierarchical relations among groups, as compared to equal relations among groups. Such people are hierarchy-enhancing and support a variety of beliefs that align social groups on a superior–inferior dimension. These ideologies are considered "legitimizing myths"; they include racial and ethnic prejudice, as well as nationalism, patriotism, separation between "high" and "low" culture, sexism, meritocracy, political conservatism, and *noblesse oblige*.

People who are high in SDO endorse a wide variety of beliefs about the goodness, naturalness, efficiency, and moral value of hierarchy. The beliefs in hierarchy in turn serve as straightforward justifications of inferior treatment of people low in a status hierarchy.

System Justification

Hierarchy persists in all cultures, and the vast majority of people tend to believe that hierarchy serves some useful function, whether it is based on race, social class, education, test scores, age, experience, or the fashionableness of one's clothing. Jost and Banaji (1994) have argued that stereotypes can serve a "system justification" function. They write that "stereotypes serve ideological functions, in particular that they justify the exploitation of certain groups over others, and they explain the poverty or powerlessness of some groups and the success of others in ways that make these differences seem legitimate and even natural" (p. 10).

Jost and Banaji argue that people develop stereotypes to serve three functions: ego justification, to feel better about ourselves and our position in society; group justification, to justify the actions of the group, particularly toward outgroups; and system justification, to justify the existing social arrangements, institutions, organizations, government, and so on. The system justification approach hypothesizes that we come to develop stereotypes and expectations about social groups based on our experience with the current social arrangement. We perceive differences in social status among groups and among the roles group members typically inhabit. Subsequent to these observations, we create stereotypes about the groups, which serve to support the status quo, reify group differences, and palliate resentment and irritation about others' or our own low status and poor access to resources. The system justification approach focuses on how an unfair or inequitable system can become legitimized by creating beliefs about groups that explain why such groups deserve their status (see also Allport, 1954, and Katz & Braly, 1935, who make some similar arguments).

Blended Attributional and Hierarchical Phenomena

Some psychological phenomena combine attributional and hierarchical components in the justification of stigmatization. In complex social perception and intergroup relations, a wide variety of more complex psychological processes meld causal attributions with beliefs about the nature of social hierarchy. I categorize these processes as "blended approaches."

Political Orientation

Political ideology and cognition often represent a blend of hierarchy beliefs and attributions. As noted above, political conservatism in the United States has close ties to social Darwinism and beliefs in meritocracy (Hofstadter, 1955), and to endorsement of hierarchical beliefs (Pratto et al., 1994). A significant amount of research has shown that political conservatism is also associated with a tendency to make attributions of responsibility for outcomes (Lane, 1962; Skitka & Tetlock,

1992, 1993; Thomas, 1970; Weiner, 1995; Zucker & Weiner, 1993). As a result, political socialization and political identification in turn can lead to the justification of stigmatization by creating consistent and persistent political ideological styles of attribution, and the endorsement of hierarchical structure in society.

As a result, it is not surprising to discover that in the United States, political conservatism is correlated with the rejection of a wide variety of stigmatized social groups. These groups include Blacks (Bierly, 1985; Hurwitz & Peffley, 1992; Kinder & Sears, 1981; Maranell, 1967; McConahay & Hough, 1976), Jews (Adorno, Frenkel-Brunswik, Levinson, & Sanford, 1950; Maranell, 1967; Petropolous, 1978), homosexuals (Herek & Glunt, 1993; Seltzer, 1992; Strand, 1998), immigrants from Latin America (Ramirez, 1988) and Vietnam (Starr & Roberts, 1982), and fat people (Crandall, 1994, 1995).

Principled Racism

Several psychologists and political scientists have sought to explain the correlation between political ideology and racial attitudes in terms of ideological consistency; that is, they say that some people express "principled racism." The argument of several psychologists and political scientists (Sniderman, Brody, & Tetlock, 1991; Sniderman, Piazza, Tetlock, & Kendrick, 1991) is that the well-established correlation between political conservatism and anti-Black racism is based not on racial antipathy, but rather on commitment to a range of race-blind political and social values and beliefs, which inductively and deductively lead to public policy preferences that some have construed as anti-minority or racist. For example, political opposition to busing and affirmative action may be based not on racial antipathy, but on a firm commitment against government intervention.

As reviewed earlier, however, political principles are associated with attributions for the causes of stigmatization, and these political principles are also consonant with hierarchical justification ideologies. Sidanius, Pratto, and Bobo (1996) showed that opposition to affirmative action among political conservatives can be better accounted for by domination and hierarchy beliefs than by educated commitment to political principle.

Summary of Blended Approaches

This section has briefly covered a small selection of justification beliefs and ideologies that combine both attributions and hierarchy preferences. Some political ideologies combine explanations for social and economic success with a value system that vindicates disparity between the "haves" and "have-nots." When compared to political ideologies, individual and socially shared stereotypes serve many of the same functions (Jost & Banaji, 1994) and can contain a mixture of hierarchy-supporting beliefs as well as attributions; they provide explanations for how the stigmatized earned their fate, and justifications for why some groups deserve their social supremacy. Many of the complex belief systems about other groups are blends of these two kinds of justification ideologies.

In sum, the two underlying components of justification ideologies are (1) attributions, which create anger and rejection, and indicate a perception of persons and their negative stigmas as "units"; and (2) the appreciation and endorsement of hierarchy, and acceptance of a superior–inferior structure of social relations. These two kinds of ideologies can and often do work in close tandem with each other. Working together, these kinds of ideologies can provide a satisfying moral and psychological justification for treating the stigmatized with rough justice and social, economic, and moral exclusion.

JUSTIFICATION *CONTRA* SUPPRESSION

One of the most important developments in social psychology of the last two decades has been research on the suppression of attitudes, beliefs, and prejudice toward stigmatized groups (e.g., Bodenhausen & Macrae, 1998; Wegner, 1989, 1994). Chapter 8 of this volume, by Smart and Wegner, reviews the processes and consequences of suppression in reaction to the stigmatized; this chapter is about the release of negative reactions. But release must be considered to occur only in the presence of some restraining force. I have reviewed a set of processes that exist, to a large extent, as ways to overcome suppression—that allow people to feel and act out their responses to the stigmatized, but without guilt or shame.

I now provide a very brief review of some of the ideological and social bases for the suppression of prejudice and stigmatization, which act in conflict with justification ideologies. The goal is to create a picture of the nature of the tension between justification and suppression, rather than to create an exhaustive review of the causes of suppression (which is well beyond the scope of this chapter).

Suppression Ideologies

A wide range of beliefs and values serve to suppress the expression of stigmatization. The most broad suppression factor is social pressure from norms (e.g., Blanchard, Crandall, Brigham, & Vaughan, 1994). But human values, religious beliefs, and personal standards for behavior (Devine & Monteith, 1993; Devine, Monteith, Zuwerink, & Elliot, 1991; Monteith, Sherman, & Devine, 1998) also represent suppression ideologies.

One important value system that suppresses rejection of the stigmatized is humanitarianism/egalitarianism (HE)—the belief that all people are created equal and deserve treatment as full human beings. Katz and Hass (1988) showed that HE was positively correlated with pro-Black attitudes. We (Biernat et al., 1996) found that HE was negatively correlated with prejudice against fat people, Blacks, and homosexuals; and Cowan, Martinez, and Mendiola (1997) found that HE was negatively correlated with anti-Latino attitudes.

This set of values is associated with establishing one's own high personal standards for intolerance of racism. Monteith, Devine, and their colleagues (e.g., Devine et al., 1991; Monteith et al., 1998) have shown that the endorsement of egalitarian values leads to the intolerance of tolerance, and that the existence of prejudice within one's self leads to feelings of anxiety, guilt, and shame. Thus values create personal standards, which in tandem serve to suppress stigmatization and prejudice.

Religion can also serve to suppress prejudice. Although antipathies based on mere categorization as well as intergroup conflict can lead to prejudice and stigmatization, many religious teachings expressly suppress stigmatization. Allport (1954) argues that the Judeo-Christian ethic is in conflict with the expression of prejudice; the New Testament explicitly proscribes stigmatization and prejudice: "There is neither Jew nor Greek, there is neither slave nor free, there is neither male nor female; for you are all one in Christ Jesus" (Galatians 3:28, Revised Standard Version). Some religious groups are characterized by the apparent absence of stigmatization of the sick (e.g., the work of Mother Teresa among the sick of Calcutta); by anti-discrimination work (e.g., Quakers; see Jennings, 1997); and by anti-prejudice teachings of tolerance and acceptance of all, such as in the Baha'i faith (Universal House of Justice, 1985).

Consequences of Suppression

The suppression of stigmatization responses has a number of affective, behavioral, and cognitive consequences. Affectively, the suppression of stigmatization and prejudice leads to ambivalence, anxiety, tension, and ultimately avoidance of stigmatized individuals, because they are associated with negative affect—which arises not only from the stigmatization process itself, but also from the negative emotions and cognitive effort associated with managing affective expression.

In addition to the negative effects of suppression, in terms of affective response and the usurpation of useful cognitive energy, there is reason to believe that the suppression of prejudice and stigmatization can have the opposite of the intended effect. I suggest that the suppression of stigmatization responses can, in certain circumstances, lead to increased avoidance and enhanced prejudice as a direct result of the suppression. I propose four different pathways by which suppression ideologies can paradoxically lead to more negative emotional and behavioral reactions to the stigmatized.

Ironic "Boomerang" Effects

The first and best-known of these pathways consists of the ironic "boomerang" effects uncovered by Wegner and his colleagues (Wegner, 1989, 1994; Wegner, Erber, & Zanakos, 1992, see also Smart & Wegner, Chapter 8, this volume). Wegner argues that attempts at suppressing a thought often result in the *increase* of the thought in consciousness. Thought suppression requires that one must (1) monitor consciousness for the presence of the thought, and then (2) suppress the thought when it bubbles up into awareness. Thus to monitor consciousness requires some representation of the unwanted thought in consciousness, and the to-be-suppressed thought ends up being more activated, more persistent, and more insistent as the process wears on. As a result, the more one actively seeks to suppress thoughts of stereotyping and prejudice, the more strongly activated the cognitive "node" is, and the more readily available the thought, feeling, or stereotype becomes.

Suppression as Justification

McConahay, Hardy, and Batts (1981) have argued that at the societal level, White Americans' suppression of prejudice may exacerbate racism. The denial of racial prejudice can lead to failure to perceive racism and discrimination. When a person suppresses prejudice, the action may lead the prejudiced person to believe that he or she is not prejudiced (Gaertner & Dovidio, 1986). The suppression of a genuine underlying prejudice can become a moral victory, leading to the self-perception of nonprejudice. With this moral victory in hand, the person may then express prejudice in ambiguous ways, feigning rejection of it but still managing to express it.

The stereotype of the extremely racist person can lead to suppression of racism and to justification of oneself as open-minded, unprejudiced, and nonstigmatizing. Feagin and Vera (1995) note that the stereotype of a "racist person" is someone who is uneducated, hostile, violent,

Southern, coarse and common. This extreme stereotype may provide "cover" for the everyday racist, "If the cultural definition of an unsympathetic or prejudiced person is someone who is so obviously different from *me*, then the rejection of this extreme form of rejection, in combination with a modest amount of suppression of my own prejudice, leaves me with the impression of myself as distinctly nonprejudiced." This self-image can then serve to justify and permit discriminatory behavior in the future (Monin & Miller, 1998).

Reactance to Prevailing "Politically Correct" Social Norms

Although people generally follow explicit norms regarding the expression of stigmatization and prejudice, a psychologically reactant "backlash" against norms of political correctness has been prevalent in recent years. Plant and Devine (1998) show that internal and external pressures to suppress prejudice have different effects on expressions of prejudice; reactance can occur when people feel forced to suppress prejudice. Decreasing such persons' freedom to be prejudiced by enforcing social norms may lead to greater prejudice in response to this reactance.

Rewards of Suppression Release

Suppression requires mental energy and deflects resources from other goal-oriented pursuits. Failing to express emotional states can lead to feelings of anxiety and to an uncomfortable cognitive pressure (Pennebaker, 1989; Wegner, 1989). By contrast, the expression of suppressed emotions reduces this tension and anxiety. Reducing anxiety and releasing tension are inherently pleasurable states.

Because the release of suppressed energy is rewarding, one must consider the possibility that the expression of suppressed stigmatization and prejudice can be accompanied by positive emotions that serve to reinforce the expression of prejudice. This is a tension–release model of stigmatization and prejudice, based on the principles of operant conditioning. Energy and tension build up when opportunities to express underlying prejudices or to avoid and malign the stigmatized are stymied by suppression, social norms, the fear of audience reaction, contrary values, and so on. When an opportunity is taken to express the unadulterated prejudice or negative stereotype, tension is reduced. The pleasant internal state that accompanies the public release acts as a reinforcer, which may enhance the probability of future expression.

To test the idea that prejudice expression can be pleasurable, we (O'Brien & Crandall, 1999) had students freely express negative thoughts about either a suppressed prejudice (against fat people), a nonsuppressed prejudice (against child abusers), or a negative topic unrelated to prejudice (pollution). Compared to the other groups, the suppressed-then-released-prejudice group experienced an elevated mood and enjoyed the group discussion more. Because of this affective reward (elevated mood), suppressors may ultimately express *more* prejudice and stigmatization, and take more pleasure in doing so, than nonsuppressors.

Summary of Suppression Consequences

The suppression of stigmatization responses is costly. It requires energy, it requires cognitive vigilance, and it creates emotional ambivalence and anxiety. It leads to avoidance of the stigmatized. The effects of suppression point to the clear value of a justification ideology: It can reduce ambivalence and anxiety, it relieves tension, and it may thus create a pleasant affect state. Finally, there are several other pathways by which suppression of prejudice and stigmatization responses may paradoxically lead to increased negative affect and discrimination: ironic "boomerang" effects, suppression as justification, and reactance to "political correctness."

CONSEQUENCES OF JUSTIFICATION IDEOLOGIES

The justification of stigmatization has a number of important consequences. First and foremost, the justification ideologies lead to the acceptance of prejudice, discrimination, rejection, and avoidance of people with stigmas. To the extent that negative behavior and emotions can be justified, they can be let free. The freedom to discriminate, without guilt, allows suffering and oppression to continue.

Justification ideologies stand in opposition to the suppression of emotions and thoughts relevant to stigmatization and prejudice. Many people actively seek to suppress prejudice and stereotypes associated with racial, religious, and ethnic groups, as well as physical disabilities and other stigmas.

Justification ideologies also serve to direct public policy. For example, Skitka and Tetlock (1993) have shown that conservatives, who focus attention on attributions of personal responsibility, will provide public assistance to needy people *only* when they are not perceived as personally responsible for their needy state. This is in contrast to liberals, who do not focus so single-mindedly on personal causation and will provide help to any needy claimant when resources are plentiful, but will use responsibility information when resources are scarce.

These ideologies also affect people's preferences for policy on access to welfare benefits. Zucker and Weiner (1993) found that conservatism correlated positively with a belief in the importance of individualistic causes for poverty, and conversely correlated negatively with perceptions of the importance of societal causes. The more their research participants believed in individual causes of poverty, the less they supported policies that offered government assistance to the poor. In addition, judgments about an individual person's suitability for welfare support were a direct function of attributions of responsibility, based in political ideology.

Some of these attributional functions play an important role in actual U.S. domestic policy. For example, the Americans with Disabilities Act of 1990 (1993) specifically protects from discrimination people suffering from alcoholism and people who have sought treatment for alcohol abuse. In this way, the act specifically protects people who abuse alcohol by defining alcoholism as a *disease*, and thus outside of the control of the individual. However, alcohol abuse, including current use and drunkenness, is *not* protected under the law, even though it is the same essential behavior. In this case, the act recharacterizes excessive consumption of alcohol from a medical disease to a personally controllable behavior, for which the person is responsible (see Americans with Disabilities Act Title II Technical Assistance Manual, 1993). When it is viewed as controllable (and in unitary relationship with a person's moral character), alcohol consumption is not protected by law. When it is viewed as uncontrollable (and due to some uncontrollable disease state, rather than individual moral virtue), alcohol consumption is protected as a physical disability.

Hierarchical justification ideologies affect an equally wide array of social and political consequences. Hierarchy-based ideologies tend to support the status quo, and so we are most likely to note their appearance in opposition to programs that alter the status quo. People who endorse hierarchy-based ideologies are likely to actively oppose or subvert social programs that "level the playing field" between the haves and the have-nots.

Much of the recent debate in the United States concerning the role of affirmative action in hiring and education has focused on coded speech that takes for granted the "natural" superiority of one group over another. An example of this is the use of sports and athletics as a contrary example to education and business employment. One form of attack on affirmative action is to assert that the logic of affirmative action suggests that more White players should be brought into professional sports by means of a quota, to make the teams more "racially representative." The barely suppressed subtext of this argument is that

Blacks have a natural advantage in athletic and other physical prowess areas, and that Whites, by contrast, have a natural advantage in matters of intellect and commerce (see, e.g., "Remarks by Packer's," 1998).

Similarly, opposition to equal educational opportunity may be based in perceptions of hierarchy. The single most effective way of raising the income, health, and well-being of a social group is through high-quality education and schools (including free lunch and breakfast programs). However, resistance to equal funding across states and the nation is well organized, well funded, and highly successful. Kozol (1992) has shown that vast disparities in quality of education can be found between wealthy versus poor students, and between Black and Hispanic versus White and Asian students—all within the same district. It is typical to find in large U.S. cities that schools are separate by wealth, race, and social class—and not even remotely equal.

Some organizations serve, as an important purpose, the hierarchical status quo. One function of the uniformed police is to protect goods and property from unauthorized redistribution. One result of this purpose for the police is that they adopt a conflict-based hierarchical structure (Sidanius, Liu, Pratto & Shaw, 1994). In this highly hierarchical structure, it is not surprising to learn that patrol officers who are noted for demarcating superiority through means of physical intimidation and violence are typically given performance ratings that are well above average, even when they face a significant number of citizen complaints for brutality (Human Rights Watch, 1998; *Report of the Independent Commission*, 1991).

These are only a small sample of instances where justification ideologies based on attributions and hierarchy preferences affect public policy. There is no shortage of examples; the section has been kept brief only to avoid tedium. Many different public policies reflect the justification ideologies I have touched on, including the attributional definitions of crime and the sentencing guidelines that follow them; allowances for absences in organizational settings; grading and makeup policies in educational settings; and so on. Justification ideologies proscribe and prescribe rough treatment of the stigmatized, and they even serve to define what is and what is not a stigma (e.g., Pfuhl & Henry, 1993).

GENERAL SUMMARY

Fundamental beliefs that *precede* stigmas generally provide cognitive and emotional cover for negative treatment of stigmatized individuals. The justification of stigmatization can come from various kinds of attributions, from fundamental beliefs about hierarchy, or from some combination of these beliefs. Justifications give cover to rejection and avoidance. Suppressing stigmatization responses can lead to ambivalence and to ultimately the same kinds of behaviors caused by the stigmatization process itself. Stigma theories, and their justification and suppression, determine both public and private policy.

REFERENCES

Adorno, T., Frenkel-Brunswik, E., Levinson, D., & Sanford, R. N. (1950). *The authoritarian personality*. New York: Harper.

Allport, G. W. (1954). *The nature of prejudice*. Garden City, NY: Doubleday.

Americans with Disabilities Act of 1990, 42 U. S. C. A. § 12101 *et seq*. (West 1993).

Americans with Disabilities Act Title II Technical Assistance Manual, 28 C.F.R. §§ 35.102–35.104 (1993).

Barker, R. G., Wright, B. A., Meyerson, L., & Gonick, M. R. (1953). *Adjustment to physical handicap and illness: A survey of the social psychology of physique and disability*. New York: Social Science Research Council.

Benesh-Weiner, M., & Weiner, B. (1982). On motivation and emotion: From the notebooks of Fritz Heider, *American Psychologist, 38*, 887–897.

Berreman, G. D. (Ed.). (1981). *Social inequality: Comparative and developmental approaches*. New York: Academic Press.

Bierly, M. (1985). Prejudice toward contemporary outgroups as a generalized attitude. *Journal of Applied Social Psychology, 15*, 189–199.

Biernat, M., Vescio, T. K., Theno, S. A., & Crandall, C. S. (1996). Values and prejudice: Toward understanding the impact of American values on outgroup attitudes. In C. Seligman, J. Olson, & M. Zanna (Eds.), *The Ontario Symposium: Vol. 8. The psychology of values* (pp. 153–190). Hillsdale, NJ: Erlbaum.

Blanchard, F., Crandall, C., Brigham, J., & Vaughan, L. A. (1994). Condemning and condoning racism: A social context approach to interracial settings. *Journal of Applied Psychology, 79*, 993–997.

Bodenhausen, G. V., & Macrae, C. N. (1998). Stereotype activation and inhibition. In R. S. Wyer (Ed.), *Advances in social cognition* (Vol. 11, pp. 1–52). Mahwah, NJ: Erlbaum.

Cowan, G., Martinez, L., & Mendiola, S. (1997). Predictors of attitudes toward illegal Latino immigrants. *Hispanic Journal of Behavioral Sciences, 19*, 403–415.

Crandall, C. S. (1994). Prejudice against fat people: Ideology and self-interest. *Journal of Personality and Social Psychology, 66*, 882–894.

Crandall, C. S. (1995). Do parents discriminate against their own heavyweight daughters? *Personality and Social Psychology Bulletin, 21*, 724–735.

Crandall, C. S., Britt, T. W., & Glor, J. (1999). *When ideology is challenged: Pediatric AIDS and the belief in the just world*. Manuscript submitted for publication.

Crandall, C. S., & Coleman, R. (1992). AIDS-related stigmatization and the disruption of social relationships. *Journal of Social and Personal Relationships, 9,* 163–177.

Crandall, C. S., N'Gbala, A. N., & Dawson, K. (1999). *Balance theory, unit relations and attribution: Relationships among some of Heider's basic constructs.* Manuscript submitted for publication.

Crocker, J., & Major, B. (1989). Social stigma and self-esteem: The self-protective properties of stigma. *Psychological Review, 96,* 608–630.

Crocker, J., Major, B., & Steele, C. (1998). Social stigma. In D. T. Gilbert, S. T. Fiske, & G. Lindzey (Eds.), *Handbook of social psychology* (4th ed., Vol. 2, pp. 504–553). New York: McGraw-Hill.

DeJong, W. (1980). The stigma of obesity: The consequences of naive assumptions concerning the causes of physical deviance. *Journal of Health and Social Behavior, 21,* 75–87.

Devine, P. G., & Monteith, M. J. (1993). The role of discrepancy-associated affect in prejudice reduction. In D. M. Mackie & D. L. Hamilton (Eds.), *Affect, cognition, and stereotyping: Interactive processes in group perception* (pp. 317–344). New York: Academic Press.

Devine, P. G., Monteith, M. J., Zuwerink, J. R., & Elliot, A. J. (1991). Prejudice with and without compunction. *Journal of Personality and Social Psychology, 60,* 817–830.

Ezekiel, R. S. (1995). *The racist mind: Portraits of American Neo-Nazis and Klansmen.* New York: Penguin.

Feagin, J. R., & Vera, H. (1995). *White racism.* New York: Routledge.

Gaertner, S. L., & Dovidio, J. F. (1986). The aversive form of racism. In J. F. Dovidio & S. L. Gaertner (Eds.), *Prejudice, discrimination, and racism* (pp. 61–89). Orlando, FL: Academic.

Goffman, E. (1963). *Stigma: Notes on the management of spoiled identity.* Englewood Cliffs, NJ: Prentice-Hall.

Hawkins, M. (1997). *Social Darwinism in European and American thought, 1860–1945: Nature as model and nature as threat.* Cambridge, England: Cambridge University Press.

Heider, F. (1944). Social perception and phenomenal causality. *Psychological Review, 6,* 358–374.

Heider, F. (1958). *The psychology of interpersonal relations.* New York: Wiley.

Heider, F. (1976). A conversation with Fritz Heider. In J. H. Harvey, W. J. Ickes, & R. F. Kidd (Eds.), *New directions in attribution research* (Vol. 1, pp. 3–21). Hillsdale, NJ: Erlbaum.

Heider, F. (1988). *The notebooks of Fritz Heider: Vol. 4. Balance theory* (M. Benesh-Weiner, Ed.). Munich: Psycologie Verlags Union.

Herbert, T. B., & Dunkel-Schetter, C. (1992). Negative social reactions to victims: An overview of responses and their determinants. In L. Montada & S.-H. Filipp (Eds.), *Life crises and experiences of loss in adulthood* (pp. 497–518). Hillsdale, NJ: Erlbaum.

Herek, G. M., & Glunt, E. K. (1993). Interpersonal contact and heterosexuals' attitudes toward gay men: Results from a national survey. *Journal of Sex Research, 30,* 239–244.

Herrnstein, R. (1971). IQ. *The Atlantic Monthy, 1,* pp. 43–58, 110.

Herrnstein, R. J., & Murray, C. (1994). *The bell curve: Intelligence and class structure in American life.* New York: Free Press.

Hofstadter, R. (1955). *Social Darwinism in American thought.* Boston: Beacon Press.

Human Rights Watch. (1998). *Shielded from justice: Police brutality and accountability in the United States.* New York: Author.

Hurwitz, J., & Peffley, M. (1992). Traditional versus social values as antecedents of racial stereotyping and policy conservatism. *Political Behavior, 13,* 395–421.

Glazer, N. (1998). *We are all multiculturalists now.* Cambridge, MA: Harvard University Press.

Jennings, J. (Ed.). (1997). *The business of abolishing the British slave trade, 1783–1807.* London: Cass.

Jones, E. E., Farina, A., Hastorf, A. H., Markus, H., Miller, D. T., & Scott, R. A. (1984). *Social stigma: The psychology of marked relationships.* New York: Freeman.

Jones, E. E., Kanouse, D., Kelley, H. H., Nisbett, R. E., Valins, S., & Weiner, B. (1972). *Attribution: Perceiving the causes of behavior.* Morristown, NJ: General Learning Press.

Jost, J. T., & Banaji, M. R. (1994). The role of stereotyping in system-justification and the production of false consciousness. *British Journal of Social Psychology, 33,* 1–27.

Kamin, L. J. (1981). Mental testing and immigration. *American Psychologist 37,* 97–98.

Katz, D., & Braly, K. (1935). Racial prejudice and racial stereotypes. *Journal of Abnormal and Social Psychology, 30,* 175–193.

Katz, I., & Hass, R. G. (1988). Racial ambivalence and American value conflict: Correlational and priming studies of dual cognitive structures. *Journal of Personality and Social Psychology, 55,* 893–905.

Keltner, D., Ellsworth, P. C., & Edwards, K. (1993). Beyond simple pessimism: Effects of sadness and anger on social perception. *Journal of Personality and Social Psychology, 64,* 740–752.

Kinder, D. R., & Sears, D. O. (1981). Prejudice and politics: Symbolic racism versus racial threats to the good life. *Journal of Personality and Social Psychology, 40,* 414–431.

Kozol, J. (1992). *Savage inequalities: Children in America's schools.* New York: Harper Perennial.

Lane, R. E. (1962). *Political ideology.* New York: Free Press.

Langer, E. J., Fiske, S., Taylor, S. E., & Chanowitz, B. (1976). Stigma, staring and discomfort: A novel-stimulus hypothesis. *Journal of Experimental Social Psychology, 12,* 451–463.

Lerner, M. (1980). *The belief in a just world: A fundamental delusion.* New York: Plenum Press.

Maranell, G. M. (1967). An examination of some religious and political attitude correlates of bigotry. *Social Forces, 45,* 356–362.

McConahay, J. B., Hardee, B. B., & Batts, V. (1981). Has racism declined in America? It depends on who is asking and what is asked. *Journal of Conflict Resolution, 25,* 563–579.

McConahay, J. B., & Hough, J. C. (1976). Symbolic racism. *Journal of Social Issues, 32,* 23–45.

Monin, B., & Miller, D. T. (1998, May). *Getting away with prejudice by asserting one's lack thereof.* Paper presented at the 10th Annual Convention of the American Psychological Society, Washington, DC.

Monteith, M. J., Sherman, J. W., & Devine, P. G. (1998). Suppression as a stereotype control strategy. *Personality and Social Psychology Review, 2,* 63–82.

O'Brien, L., & Crandall, C. S. (1999). *A tension-reduction model of prejudice expression: Mood improves when suppressed prejudice is released.* Manuscript submitted for publication.

Parsons, T. (1937). *The structure of social action.* New York: McGraw-Hill.

Pennebaker, J. W. (1989). Confession, inhibition, and disease. In L. Berkowitz (Ed.), *Advances in experimental social psychology, Vol. 22* (pp. 211–244). San Diego, CA: Academic.

Petropolous, N. P. (1978). Prejudice: The status politics of Spiro Agnew. *International Journal of Intercultural Relations, 2,* 225–247.

Pfuhl, E. H., & Henry, S. (1993). *The deviance process* (3rd ed.). New York: Aldine de Gruyter.

Plant, E. A., & Devine, P. G. (1998). Internal and external motivation to respond without prejudice. *Journal of Personality and Social Psychology, 75,* 811–832.

Pratto, F., Sidanius, J., Stallworth, L. M., & Malle, B. F. (1994). Social dominance orientation: A personality variable predicting social and political attitudes. *Journal of Personality and Social Psychology, 67,* 741–763.

Ramirez, A. (1988). Racism toward Hispanics: The culturally monolithic society. In P. A. Katz & D. A. Taylor (Eds.), *Eliminating racism* (pp. 137–157). New York: Plenum Press.

Remarks by Packers' White draw criticism in Wisconsin. (1998, March 25). *The New York Times,* p. C3.

Report of the Independent Commission on the Los Angeles Police Department [The Christopher Commission]. (1991). Los Angeles: Independent Commission on the Los Angeles Police Department.

Rushton, J. P. (1995). *Race, evolution, and behavior: A life history perspective.* New Brunswick, NJ: Transaction.

Ryan, W. (1971). *Blaming the victim.* New York: Vintage.

Schutte, G. (1995). *What racists believe: Race relations in South Africa and the United States.* Thousand Oaks, CA: Sage.

Seltzer, R. (1992). The social location of those holding antihomosexual attitudes. *Sex Roles, 26,* 391–398.

Sidanius, J., Liu, J., Pratto, F., & Shaw, J. (1994). Social dominance orientation, hierarchy-attenuators and hierarchy-enhancers: Social dominance theory and the criminal justice system. *Journal of Applied Social Psychology, 24,* 338–366.

Sidanius, J., & Pratto, J. (1993). The inevitability of oppression and the dynamics of social dominance. In P. M. Sniderman, P. E. Tetlock, & E. G. Carmines

(Eds.), *Prejudice, politics and the American dilemma* (pp. 173–211). Stanford, CA: Stanford University Press.

Sidanius, J., Pratto, J., & Bobo, L. (1996). Racism, conservatism, affirmative action, and intellectual sophistication: A matter of principled conservatism or group dominance? *Journal of Personality and Social Psychology, 70,* 476–490.

Skitka, L., & Tetlock, P. E. (1992). Allocating scarce resources: A contingency model of distributive justice. *Journal of Experimental Social Psychology, 28,* 491–522.

Skitka, L., & Tetlock, P. E. (1993). Providing public assistance: Cognitive and motivational processes underlying liberal and conservative policy preferences. *Journal of Personality and Social Psychology, 65,* 1205–1223.

Sniderman, P. M., Brody, R. A., & Tetlock, P. E. (1991). *Reasoning and choice: Explorations in political psychology.* New York: Cambridge University Press.

Sniderman, P. M., Piazza, T., Tetlock, P. E., & Kendrick, A. (1991). The new racism. *American Journal of Political Science, 35,* 423–447.

Spencer, H. (1872). *Social statics; or, the conditions essential to human happiness specified, and the first of them developed.* New York: Appleton.

Starr, P. D., & Roberts, A. E. (1982). Attitudes toward new Americans: Perceptions of Indo-Chinese in nine cities. *Research in Race and Ethnic Relations, 3,* 165–186.

Strand, D. A. (1998). Civil liberties, civil rights, and stigma: Voter attitudes and behavior in the politics of homosexuality. In G. M. Herek (Ed.), *Psychological perspectives on lesbian and gay issues: Vol. 4. Stigma and sexual orientation: Understanding prejudice against lesbians, gay men, and bisexuals* (pp. 108–137). Thousand Oaks, CA: Sage.

Struckman-Johnson, C., & Struckman-Johnson, D. (1992). Acceptance of male rape myths among college men and women. *Sex Roles, 27,* 85–100.

Thomas, L. E. (1970). The I-E Scale, ideological bias, and political participation. *Journal of Personality, 38,* 273–286.

Universal House of Justice. (1985). *The promise of world peace.* Wilmette, IL: Baha'i Public Trust.

Vescio, T. K. (1995). *The attributional underpinnings of stereotyping and prejudice.* Unpublished doctoral dissertation, University of Kansas.

Walster, E. (1966). Assignment of responsibility for an accident. *Journal of Personality and Social Psychology, 3,* 73–79.

Wegner, D. M. (1989). *White bears and other unwanted thoughts.* New York: Viking.

Wegner, D. M. (1994). Ironic processes of mental control. *Psychological Review, 101,* 34–52.

Wegner, D. M., Erber, R., & Zanakos, S. (1993). Ironic processes in the mental control of mood and mood-related thought. *Journal of Personality and Social Psychology, 65,* 1093–1104.

Weiner, B. (1986). *An attributional theory of motivation and emotion.* New York: Springer-Verlag.

Weiner, B. (1995). *Judgments of responsibility.* New York: Guilford Press.

Weiner, B., Perry, R. P., & Magnusson, J. (1988). An attributional analysis of reactions to stigmas. *Journal of Personality and Social Psychology, 55,* 738–748.

Wilson, J. Q., & Herrnstein, R. J. (1985). *Crime and human nature.* New York: Simon & Schuster.

Wright, B. A. (1983). *Physical disability: A psychological approach* (2nd ed.). New York: Harper & Row.

Zucker, G. S., & Weiner, B. (1993). Conservatism and perception of poverty: An attributional analysis. *Journal of Applied Social Psychology, 23,* 925–943.

II

THE STIGMATIZED

6

Social Stigma and the Self: Meanings, Situations, and Self-esteem

JENNIFER CROCKER
DIANE M. QUINN

To be "stigmatized" is to have a social identity, or membership in some social category, that raises doubts about one's full humanity: One is devalued, spoiled, or flawed in the eyes of others (Crocker, Major, & Steele, 1998; Goffman, 1963; Jones et al., 1984). Stigmatized individuals are often the targets of negative stereotypes, and elicit emotional reactions such as pity, anger, anxiety or disgust, but the central feature of social stigma is devaluation and dehumanization by others.

In this chapter, we consider the consequences of social stigma for the self-esteem of those whose social identities are devalued. We first consider the historical context of research on social stigma and self-esteem, and how it happened that the established wisdom of social psychology suggested that social stigma results in low self-esteem for the stigmatized. We then briefly consider the empirical evidence for this claim, which is at best inconsistent and at worst contradictory. We suggest that this contradiction is related to a central problem in the way that self-esteem is conceptualized in much of this literature: namely, as a stable trait that is consistent across social situations and contexts. We suggest an alternative view of self-esteem, arguing that self-esteem is constructed at the moment, in the situation, as a function of the meanings

153

that individuals bring with them to the situation, and features of the situation that make those meanings relevant or irrelevant. We then consider the implications of this view for the effects of social stigma on self-esteem. We consider the various meanings that stigmatized individuals bring with them to situations, and the important features of situations that can make those meanings relevant or irrelevant to the self; we also describe some research that is consistent with our claim.

HISTORICAL CONTEXT

For most of its history, social psychology has been concerned with the ways in which stigmatized individuals are devalued, stereotyped, and discriminated against. Although metatheoretical perspectives, such as learning theory, psychodynamic theory, consistency theories, and cognitive theories, have waxed and waned in popularity over the decades, the topics of prejudice and stereotyping have held the enduring attention of social psychologists. In contrast, relatively little theoretical or empirical attention has been paid to the experience of those who are devalued, and who are often the targets of prejudice and negative stereotypes. Until recently, research and theory on the consequences of social stigma for stigmatized persons themselves were relatively scarce.

The major exception to this inattention to the experience of stigmatized individuals has been a focus on the consequences of having a devalued identity for self-esteem. Hundreds if not thousands of studies have measured the self-esteem of people with a stigmatized identity (such as African Americans and persons with obesity or facial disfigurement), and compared their self-esteem to that of people without that stigmatized identity. The reasons for this intense focus on the self-esteem of people with stigmatized identities are no doubt complex, involving both theoretical and practical issues.

In part, interest in the effects of stigma on self-esteem is explained by the fact that the self and self-esteem have been of interest to social psychologists since the publication of William James's *Principles of Psychology* in 1890. Self-esteem is powerfully related to variables that influence the affective quality of one's daily experience, with individuals high in self-esteem reporting, for example, more positive affect (Pelham & Swann, 1989), more life satisfaction (Diener, 1984; Myers & Diener, 1995), less hopelessness (Crocker, Luhtanen, Blaine, & Broadnax, 1994) and fewer depressive symptoms (e.g., Crandall, 1973) than individuals low in self-esteem. Indeed, in a review of the literature, Diener (1984) concluded that self-esteem is the strongest predictor of life satisfaction in the United States, outstripping all demographic and objective outcomes (such as age, income, education, physical health, and marital status) and all other psychological variables. Thus researchers have focused on the effects of having a stigmatized identity on self-esteem, because self-esteem is a central aspect of psychological well-being and mental health.

In addition, however, theoretical developments began to suggest how one's position in the social order, and particularly having a devalued social identity, might affect self-esteem. In the first half of the 20th century, symbolic interactionists such as Mead (1934) and Cooley (1902/1956) proposed that the self is a social construction, and that we humans develop our sense of who and what we are from our observation and interpretation of the responses we receive from others. According to this view, we cannot understand the self without understanding the social context in which it functions. This viewpoint is articulated in the "looking-glass self" hypothesis, which argues that one of the most important ways we come to know ourselves is through the reactions of others to us. Other people provide the "looking glass" in which we see ourselves reflected. We then incorporate those reflections into our own self-views. Mead argued that the looking-glass self is a product of, and essential to, social interaction. To interact smoothly and effectively with others, we need to anticipate how others will react to us, and so we need to learn to see ourselves through the eyes of others. Those "others" may be either the specific individuals with whom we are interacting, or a generalized view of how most people see us—a "generalized other." This representation of how others view us guides our behavior, even when no specific other is present. The implication of this analysis for the stigmatized is clear: Being stigmatized or devalued by others should lead to low self-esteem.

Empirical research on the consequences of devaluation, prejudice, and negative stereotypes on the self-esteem of members of minority racial and ethnic groups also dates to the first half of the 20th century, with Clark and Clark's (1939) demonstration that African American children preferred White dolls to Black dolls. This finding has since been replicated many times (see Banks, 1976, and Brand, Ruiz, & Padilla, 1974, for reviews). The preference of White dolls over Black dolls was interpreted as revealing low self-esteem in African American children, and led to the conclusion that the devaluation of African Americans had been internalized by African American children.

By the 1950s this view was so widely accepted by social psychologists that it was regarded as truth. Cartwright (1950) argued, "The group to which a person belongs serves as primary determinants of his self-esteem. To a considerable extent, personal feelings of worth depend on the social evaluation of the group with which a person is identified. Self-hatred and feelings of worthlessness tend to arise from membership in underprivileged or outcast groups" (p. 440). Erikson (1956) claimed that "There is ample evidence of inferiority feelings and of morbid self-hate in all minority groups" (p. 155). And in his classic book *The Nature of Prejudice*, Allport (1954/1979) recognized that responses to oppression vary widely, but suggested that a common consequence was low self-esteem: "Group oppression may destroy the integrity of the ego entirely, and reverse its normal pride, and create a groveling self-image" (p. 152).

These strong claims about the damaging effects of social stigma on self-esteem were no doubt related to early legal challenges to desegregation in education (Scott, 1997). Social science evidence played a major role in the U.S. Supreme Court's decision in *Brown v. Board of Education*, which found that "separate but equal" educational systems for Blacks and Whites were unconstitutional. The Clarks' research, suggesting that one consequence of separate but equal treatment was low self-esteem in African Americans, was cited as key evidence regarding the harm caused by such treatment. Thus social-psychological theory and research about the harmful effects of stigma on self-esteem were joined with the effort to overturn legal but discriminatory laws and customs and achieve a measure of social justice for African Americans.

Through the 1950s, empirical evidence for the damaging effects of social stigma on self-esteem was primarily based on the "doll preference" paradigm developed by the Clarks. This resulted mainly from the absence of alternative, standardized, and validated methods for assessing self-esteem. In the 1950s and 1960s, however, researchers developed face-valid self-report questionnaire measures of self-esteem. Some of these measures were idiosyncratic to particular studies or particular researchers, but some of them had good psychometric properties such as high internal consistency and high test–retest reliability, and were validated in a large number of studies (see Wylie, 1974, and Blascovich & Tomaka, 1991, for reviews). The development of self-report questionnaire measures of self-esteem provided a huge boost to research on self-esteem, in part because of the ease of administration of these measures. Self-esteem could be assessed in just a few moments via paper-and-pencil questionnaires, telephone interviews, or surveys.

With the development of self-report measures of self-esteem, research on self-esteem differences between stigmatized and nonstigmatized individuals burgeoned. Hundreds of studies assessed self-esteem differences associated with race, gender, weight status, physical attractiveness, physical disabilities, sexual orientation, cognitive disabilities, disfigurement, various illnesses, and so on (see Crocker & Major, 1989, for a brief review). This research provides a test of the looking-glass self hypothesis that having a stigmatized social identity is associated with low self-esteem.

Support for this hypothesis is mixed at best. Comparisons of average levels of self-esteem among stigmatized and nonstigmatized groups have yielded conflicting results (Crocker & Major, 1989). For example, studies comparing the self-esteem of African Americans to that of Americans of European descent typically report either no difference, or higher self-esteem in African Americans (Gray-Little & Hafdahl, 2000; Porter & Washington, 1979; Rosenberg, 1965). Studies of gender differences in self-esteem typically find either no differences, or very small differences favoring males (Maccoby & Jacklin, 1974; Major, Barr, Zubek, & Babey, 1999). Studies comparing self-esteem in obese and nonobese populations also typically find no differences or very small differences (Friedman & Brownell, 1995; Miller & Downey, 1999).

SITUATIONAL CONSTRUCTION OF SELF-ESTEEM

A little over 10 years ago, Crocker and Major (1989) noted that the empirical evidence regarding levels of self-esteem among people with a wide variety of devalued social identities has provided only occasional support for the looking-glass self hypothesis. Over the last decade, researchers have proposed a number of resolutions of this apparent paradox. In this chapter, we propose that part of the problem for research on self-esteem among people with stigmatized identities has been the tendency to conceptualize self-esteem as a stable trait that individuals carry with them from situation to situation. This tendency on the part of researchers reflects the assumption that the stigmatized internalize the devaluation, negative images, and stereotypes about them that are pervasive in the culture (Crocker et al., 1998; Steele, 1997; see Scott, 1997, for a historical overview). This internalization of devaluation was assumed to affect stable aspects of personality, especially levels of trait self-esteem. Allport (1954/1979), for example, began his analysis of the psychological consequences of stigma by asking, "What would happen to your personality if you heard it said over and over again that you are lazy and had inferior blood?" (p. 42). This assumption has been so pervasive that studies of the effects of stigma on self-esteem have almost always used trait measures of self-esteem administered at a single time in a single situation, and have assumed that the resulting self-esteem scores reflect a stable characteristic of individuals.

In contrast, we, like a number of other researchers (e.g., Heatherton & Polivy, 1991), argue that self-esteem is constructed in the situation, as a function of the meaning the situation has for the self. Several types of evidence have led us to this view. First, research on self-esteem in the stigmatized has demonstrated enormous individual differences among people with the same stigmatized social identity (e.g., Quinn & Crocker, 1998; Twenge & Crocker, 1997; Major et al., 1999), indicating that the stigmatized are not, en masse, internalizing negative cultural images of them. Second, research by Kernis and his colleagues has demonstrated that at least some people have self-esteem that is unstable over time (see Kernis & Waschull, 1995, for a review). For example, when their self-esteem was measured once a day for 5 days, some college students had self-esteem that was relatively stable over time, whereas others had self-esteem that fluctuated over time (Kernis, Cornell, Sun, Berry, & Harlow, 1993; Kernis, Grannemann, & Barclay, 1989). Third, research suggests that manipulating the salience of self-relevant information can lead to changes in self-esteem. For example, recalling a positive (or negative) achievement or interpersonal experience leads to increased (or decreased) global self-esteem (Levine, Wyer, & Schwarz, 1994).

Further evidence that levels of self-esteem depend on the meaning of the situation for the self was provided by a recent study by Sommers and Crocker (1999). In that study, 32 college seniors applying to PhD programs completed a measure of global state self-esteem (the Rosenberg [1965] self-esteem scale, with items modified to reflect how participants felt that day) twice a week, plus any day that they heard from a graduate program they had applied to, for the period from February 15 through April 1. At the beginning of the study, all participants completed a measure of the extent to which their self-esteem depended on being competent at school. The investigators analyzed the data by computing indexes of average self-esteem on days when students received acceptances from graduate schools, days they received rejections, and baseline days. The results showed that the more students' self-esteem was contingent on their school competency, the greater the increases in self-esteem on acceptance days (over baseline), and the greater the decreases in self-esteem on rejection days. Thus, on any particular day, level of global self-esteem depended in part on whether students heard good news, bad news, or no news from the graduate programs they had applied to, and this effect depended on how relevant school competency was to the students' self-esteem (see Crocker & Wolfe, in press, for an extended discussion of this perspective on self-esteem).

Based on these and other data, we suggest that self-esteem is not a stable characteristic individuals bring with them to situations, but rather that feelings of self-worth, self-regard, and self-respect are constructed in the situation. People bring sets of beliefs, attitudes, and values to the situations in which they find themselves. When positive or negative events happen, self-esteem depends on the meaning those events have for an individual, which depends in turn on the individual's chronically accessible beliefs, attitudes, and values. Even when no positive or negative events happen, however, feelings of self-worth may depend on the chronic beliefs and values that individual brings with him or her, in combination with features of the situation that make those beliefs and values relevant or irrelevant to the self. Note that our analysis does not imply that self-esteem is never stable across time and situations. Rather, it suggests that self-esteem will be stable when the situations in which a person finds him- or herself have consistently positive (or consistently negative) implications for the self.

SITUATIONAL CONSTRUCTION OF SELF-ESTEEM IN STIGMATIZED INDIVIDUALS

Based on this view that self-esteem is constructed in the situation, we argue that the effects of stigma on the self are negotiated, created, and acted upon *in the situation*. We propose that self-worth, or the lack of it, in stigmatized individuals is not a stable, deep-seated personality characteristic. Rather, it emerges in the situation and is a function of the meaning given to that situation for the self. Meaning is partly shaped by idiosyncratic meanings that individuals bring to the situation. These idiosyncratic meanings may stem from early childhood experiences, or from other personal experiences that shape individuals' construals of situations. Meaning is also shaped by the "collective representations," or shared beliefs, values, and attitudes, that stigmatized persons bring to the situation. To understand differences in self-esteem between those with stigmatized and those with nonstigmatized identities, it is particularly important to understand shared meanings, or collective representations, that can lead to consistent differences between groups of people.

These collective representations are sometimes broadly known and shared by both stigmatized and nonstigmatized persons, sometimes shared by individuals with a particular social identity but not by people with another social identity, and sometimes shared by only some of those individuals with a particular stigmatized identity. These collective representations may lead the *same situation* to have different meanings, and different implications for self-worth, for stigmatized and nonstigmatized people. When collective representations are not shared by all people with a particular stigmatized identity, the situation may have negative implications for self-worth for some stigmatized people but not others. Thus, to understand the effects of having a devalued identity on the self, we must understand both the collective representations that stigmatized individuals bring to situations, and the features of the situation (often very subtle features) that make those collective representations relevant or irrelevant in that situation.

COLLECTIVE REPRESENTATIONS
OF STIGMATIZED INDIVIDUALS

Although it is too early in our research and thinking about this issue to identify all of the collective representations that are important to the self-esteem of stigmatized individuals, and all of the features of situations that can make those collective representations relevant to the self, we can suggest a few that clearly matter.

Beliefs about Prejudice and Discrimination

One collective representation shared by members of many stigmatized groups is the belief that others are prejudiced against them. This belief may affect the meaning that positive and negative events have for stigmatized persons, and the implications of those events for the self (Crocker & Major, 1989; Major & Crocker, 1994). In general, stigmatized individuals seem to be aware of prejudice against people with their social identity. For example, Rosenberg (1979) found that African Americans past the age of 14 are generally aware that others are prejudiced against their group. Mexican Americans believe that Anglo Americans hold negative views of their group (Casas, Ponterotto, & Sweeney, 1987). Most women believe that women are discriminated against (Crosby, 1982). Mentally retarded persons are aware of the negative consequences of their label (Gibbons, 1981), as are blind persons (Scott, 1969), obese individuals (Harris, Waschull, & Walters, 1990; Jarvie, Lahey, Graziano, & Framer, 1983; Millman, 1980), persons with mental illness (Link, 1987), and homosexuals (D'Emilio, 1983). The age at which this awareness develops is not always clear, but it is likely to be well established by adolescence (Jarvie et al., 1983; Rosenberg, 1979). People with different devalued identities differ in the extent to which they believe that their groups are discriminated against, or that others are prejudiced against their groups. For example, South Asian and Haitian women in Montreal believe more strongly that their groups are discriminated against than Inuit people do (Taylor, Wright, & Porter, 1994). Furthermore, there are differences among individuals who share a devalued social identity in their beliefs about discrimination against their group. For example, Taylor and colleagues (1994) showed that undergraduate women at a university are more likely than nonuniversity women to believe that women are targets of discrimination.

Although many stigmatized people believe that others are prejudiced against their group, they do not always believe that they personally have experienced prejudice and discrimination. In general, people believe that their group is discriminated against more than they personally are discriminated against (see Taylor et al., 1994, for a review). For example, Crosby (1982) found that employed women tended to believe that women in general are discriminated against, but did not believe that they personally had been discriminated against—a phenomenon she labeled "denial of discrimination." Denial of personal discrimination is not always found in members of stigmatized groups, however (Taylor et al., 1994).

Black students' collective representations include the belief that Blacks are frequently the targets of racial discrimination. Crocker and her colleagues (Crocker et al., 1994; Crocker, Luhtanen, Broadnax, & Blaine, 1999) investigated self-esteem and collective representations about prejudice and discrimination in a sample of 91 Black and 96 White college students at a large public university. Consistent with previous research, they found that Black students were nonsignificantly higher in self-esteem ($M = 33.70$) than were White students ($M = 32.58$, n.s.) (see Crocker & Blanton, 1999). Black students were more likely to believe that they personally had been discriminated against ($M = 4.45$) than were Whites ($M = 1.61$, $p < .05$). In results from the same study reported elsewhere (Crocker et al., 1999), they also found that Black students had very different understandings of the plight of Black Americans than did White students: They were higher in system blame (i.e., more likely to believe that problems confronting the Black community are caused by prejudice and discrimination) ($M = 4.91$) than were Whites ($M = 3.58$, $p < .0001$), and more likely to believe that the U.S. government conspires to harm Black Americans ($M= 4.16$) than were Whites ($M= 1.67$, $p < .0001$). Thus the collective representations of Black students clearly include the beliefs that Blacks in general, and they personally, are targets of racial prejudice. These beliefs are not widely shared by White students, regarding either their own experiences with racial prejudice, or their understanding of Blacks' experiences with racial prejudice.

Are these collective representations about prejudice and discrimination associated with self-esteem? Crocker and Major (1989) argued that recognizing that one's negative outcomes may be the result of prejudice, rather than of one's own personal shortcomings, can protect self-esteem. Consistent with this view, Crocker and Blanton (1999) reported that among Black students, beliefs about personal experiences with racial discrimination were positively correlated with personal self-esteem ($r = .23$), whereas for Whites they were negatively correlated ($r = -.10$). Similarly, Crocker and colleagues (1999) found that "system blame" (i.e., blaming the problems of Black Americans on prejudice and discrimination, and on a racist system) was positively correlated with self-esteem for Blacks ($r = .16$) and negatively correlated for Whites ($r = -.39$), and that belief in government conspiracies against Blacks was positively correlated with self-esteem for Blacks ($r = .27$) and negatively correlated for Whites ($r = -.28$). In all of these cases, the correlations differed significantly for Blacks and Whites.

These data indicate that Black and White college students have different collective representations about prejudice and discrimination, and that these collective representations have different associations with the self-esteem of Black and White students. One limitation of this research, however, is that it represents a snapshot of the link between collective representations and self-esteem at a single moment, in a single situation. Thus, like a great deal of research on stigma and self-esteem, these survey data convey a static picture; they cannot capture how self-esteem is constructed in situations, as a function of both collective representations about prejudice and features of the situation.

What features of situations might make these beliefs about prejudice and discrimination relevant or irrelevant to the self? One situational feature that might be important is whether or not a stigmatized person believes that the specific person or people in the situation are prejudiced, regardless of his or her beliefs about the prejudice of others in general. Even when one generally believes that others are prejudiced against one's group, knowledge that a specific person is not prejudiced may render those beliefs irrelevant to interpreting the meaning of that person's behavior, and consequently may affect the implications of that person's behavior for self-evaluation.

An example of this can be seen in a study by Crocker, Voelkl, Testa, and Major (1991, Study 1). In that study, each of a group of women wrote an essay that she was told would be evaluated by a man seated in the next room. After writing their essays, the women heard the man describe their essays in positive or negative terms. Subsequently, the women completed measures of self-esteem and affect, as well as evaluations of the male who critiqued their essays. Prior to writing their essays, the women read an "opinion questionnaire" ostensibly completed by their male evaluator. For half of the women, his responses indicated generally sexist attitudes toward women (e.g., he agreed with the suggestion that men should be paid more than women for the same work because they have families to support); for the other half, his responses indicated nonsexist attitudes. The results showed that women whose essays were negatively evaluated experienced more depressed mood when they believed that the man who evaluated their essays did not have sexist attitudes ($M = 11.53$) than when they believed he had sexist attitudes ($M = 8.54$), or had evaluated their essays favorably (M's = 8.77 and 9.59 for the nonsexist and sexist evaluator, respectively). In addition, women who received a negative evaluation from a nonsexist evaluator tended to have lower self-esteem than women in the other three groups, although this effect did not reach significance. Crocker and colleagues (1991) argued that knowing the man was prejudiced against women gave the women an explanation for the negative evaluation (his sexism) that was unrelated to the quality of their essays.

In light of our analysis of the situational construction of self-esteem, we suggest that the women in this study had collective representations, or beliefs, that some men are prejudiced against women and that this can affect such men's behavior and evaluations of women. These beliefs affected the meaning of the negative evaluation the women received, and particularly its implications for self-evaluation, when they learned that the man had endorsed sexist attitudes toward women. Specifically, a negative evaluation from a sexist man had few implications for mood and self-esteem. On the other hand, when a man who was known not to be sexist gave an essay a negative evaluation, his comments were interpreted as reflecting on the quality of the essay, and hence did have implications for mood and self-esteem.

Knowing that a potentially prejudiced person is aware or unaware of one's social identity is a second feature of situations that may make beliefs about prejudice and discrimination relevant or irrelevant to interpreting the meaning of a situation for the self. When a stigmatized person believes that others are unaware of his or her devalued identity, then beliefs about their possible prejudice should become irrelevant to interpreting their behavior. A second study by Crocker and colleagues (1991) was designed to examine this hypothesis. In that study, 38 Black and 45 White college students were recruited for a study they were told concerned the development of same-race and cross-race friendships. Students came to the laboratory individually, and each one was seated in a room with a one-way mirror. All students were told that a White, same-sex peer evaluator was seated on the other side of the one-way mirror. For half of the students, the blinds on the one-way mirror were down, and the experimenter explained that this was to ensure that factors such as appearance and race could not affect the other students' reaction to them. For the other half of the students, the blinds were up, and the experimenter explained that this was because factors such as appearance and race were known to affect the development of friendships. All students completed a pretest measure of self-esteem, and then wrote a brief self-descriptive paragraph, which was then ostensibly shown to the evaluator (who did not actually exist). The experimenter later returned with a form supposedly completed by the evaluator, which indicated either that the other student thought they could become friends (positive-feedback condition) or did not think so (negative-feedback condition). Participants then completed several dependent measures, including attributions for the evaluator's response to them and a posttest measure of self-esteem, administered in a different format and embedded in another questionnaire to dis-

guise the fact that the same items were asked before and after the rejection or acceptance experience.

Means on the attribution-to-prejudice measure are presented in Table 6.1. Analyses revealed that White students did not see the other person's prejudice or racism as a likely explanation for the evaluator's reaction. Neither the type of feedback (acceptance vs. rejection) nor the
manipulation of the blinds (leaving them up or down) significantly affected White students' attributions to prejudice. This is unsurprising, as
the research described previously clearly shows that most White students
do not share a collective representation that they are targets of racial
prejudice, and being visible to a White evaluator does not change this.
Black students overall made more attributions to prejudice, $F(1, 74) =$
11.30, $p < .002$. Both the type of feedback and the manipulation of the
blinds affected their attributions to prejudice. Black students were more
likely to attribute the feedback to prejudice when the feedback was rejection rather than acceptance, $F(1, 36) = 24.12$, $p < .0001$, and they were
more likely to attribute the feedback to prejudice when the blinds were
up (and they believed the other student could see them) than when the
blinds were down, $F(1, 36) = 5.97$, $p < .02$. Thus, by manipulating a
subtle feature of the situation (whether the blinds on the one-way mirror
were up or down), Crocker and colleagues (1991, Study 2) were able to
alter the meaning of the feedback to Black students.

Means for the change in self-esteem from pretest to posttest (com-
puted after standardizing each measure) are also presented in Table 6.1.
Again, the type of feedback and the manipulation of the blinds had no significant effects on the self-esteem of White students. However, the effects
of receiving acceptance or rejection feedback on Black students' self-
esteem depended on whether the blinds on the one-way mirror were up or
down, $F(1, 35) = 6.20$, $p < .02$. When the blinds were down, the feedback
had predictable effects: Self-esteem went up following acceptance and
went down following rejection ($p < .05$). When the blinds were up, however, self-esteem went down following acceptance and was unchanged
following rejection, although this difference was not significant ($p > .10$).

Thus, when the blinds were down, Black students apparently
thought that the feedback they received had very little to do with their
race—and, as one might expect, rejection by the White evaluator hurt
their self-esteem and acceptance helped it. When the blinds were up,
however, it appears that Black students' collective representations about
prejudice and discrimination against Blacks affected their attributions
for the feedback, and its meaning for self-evaluation. Negative feedback
was attributed to prejudice and had no effect on self-esteem. Positive
feedback was also attributed to prejudice, perhaps reflecting the assumption that the evaluator was positive to avoid appearing prejudiced. Posi-

TABLE 6.1. Attributions to Prejudice and Change in Self-Esteem as a Function of Race of Participant, Feedback, and Visibility

Race	Feedback	Visibility	
		Blinds up	Blinds down
	Attributions to prejudice		
White	Positive	4.70	4.40
	Negative	5.63	4.81
Black	Positive	5.62	3.40
	Negative	9.58	7.70
	Change in self-esteem		
White	Positive	0.38	0.04
	Negative	0.07	−0.03
Black	Positive	−0.50	0.40
	Negative	0.06	−0.47

Note. The data are from Crocker, Voelkl, Testa, and Major (1991). Attributions to prejudice fell on a scale ranging from "not at all due to prejudice" (3) to "very much due to prejudice" (15). Change in self-esteem was the difference between standardized pretest and posttest self-esteem scores, with positive numbers indicating an increase in self-esteem and negative numbers indicating a decrease.

tive feedback given this meaning had no benefits for self-esteem. On the contrary, self-esteem declined in this condition.

Although there are many interesting implications of these results (see Crocker et al., 1991, and Major & Crocker, 1994, for discussions), the important point here is that the self-esteem of Black students following positive and negative feedback depended both on the collective representations about prejudice that they brought with them to the situation, and on a subtle feature of the situation—whether the blinds on the mirror were up or down—that rendered those collective representations relevant or irrelevant for interpreting their experience. When the blinds were down, Black students thought it was unlikely that prejudice could account for the other person's reaction to them; when the blinds were up, however, prejudice was a more plausible explanation for both positive and negative feedback, and altered the implications of the feedback for self-esteem. Because White students came to this situation with no collective representations about prejudice against their group (especially from a White evaluator), whether the blinds on the mirror were up or down had no effect on their self-esteem.

Awareness of Stereotypes

A second, somewhat related collective representation that stigmatized persons may bring to situations is awareness of the specific stereotypes about their group that could be applied to them in that situation. Because these stereotypes are often pervasive in the culture, it may be inevitable that members of stigmatized groups know the content of those stereotypes (Devine, 1989; Gaertner & Dovidio, 1986). That is not to say that stigmatized individuals inevitably accept the validity of these stereotypes, although some do (see Jost & Banaji, 1994). Rather, stigmatized individuals are aware of the accusations against them that are contained in those stereotypes. African Americans, for example, are likely to be well aware that stereotypes accuse them of being intellectually inferior and aggressive; women are well aware that stereotypes accuse them of being emotional, bad at math, and lacking in leadership aptitude; gay men are aware that stereotypes accuse them of being flamboyant, effeminate, and promiscuous; overweight individuals are aware that stereotypes accuse them of lacking self-control and being inwardly miserable, even if they present a jolly face to the world (Allon, 1982; Jones et al., 1984).

Research suggests that African Americans are aware of negative stereotypes that others hold of them (Leiberson, 1995); that Mexican Americans are aware of the negative stereotypes that Anglo Americans hold of their appearance, personality, and social class (Casas et al., 1987); that Asian students are aware of both the positive and negative aspects of stereotypes about their group (Lee, 1994); that girls as young as 3 years old are aware of some sex stereotypes (Best et al., 1977); and that overweight people are aware of the negative stereotypes that others hold of them (Harris et al., 1990).

What features of the situation might make knowledge of the stereotypes affect feelings about the self? When members of a stereotyped group are in situations in which the stereotype could be applied to them—used to judge them or their ability in some way—their knowledge of the stereotype and the features of the situation may combine to affect feelings about themselves, as well as stereotype-relevant performance. Steele and his colleagues have called this "stereotype threat" (Spencer, Steele, & Quinn, 1999; Steele, 1997; Steele & Aronson, 1995). When negative stereotypes concern abilities, such as the stereotypes that women are bad at math, that elderly people are bad at remembering, and that African Americans are lacking in intellectual ability, awareness of the stereotypes may affect the meaning of performance in settings where the negative stereotypes apply.

Thus people who are stigmatized as intellectually inferior in one domain or many may experience doubts about their ability, which are related to, if not identical with, low state self-esteem. Steele and Aronson (1995) have demonstrated this by placing African American and European American students in a testing context in which they anticipated taking a very difficult test. For some of the students, the test was presented as diagnostic of ability. A group of control students did not anticipate taking a test at all. According to the stereotype threat hypothesis, for African American students but not for European American students, anticipating taking a test that is diagnostic of ability should increase the salience of stereotypes about the intellectual limitations of African Americans, and being in this situation should cause self-doubts about ability. Dependent measures included the number of word fragments students completed with words related to self-doubt (e.g., completing "_ERIOR" with "inferior"). African American students completed more word fragments with self-doubt-related words than did European American students when they anticipated taking a test that was diagnostic of ability, but not when the test was thought to be nondiagnostic. Thus knowledge of the negative stereotype about intellectual ability combined with the type of situation—whether African American students believed that their abilities could be judged by an upcoming test— to affect feelings about the self.

These stereotype threat studies demonstrated that one type of collective representation—awareness of stereotypes about the intellectual inferiority of people with one's social identity—can lead to self-doubts about one's own ability. Although stigmatized and nonstigmatized persons share these collective representations, they are relevant to self-evaluation for stigmatized but not nonstigmatized individuals. Furthermore, subtle features of the situation, such as whether the test is described as a test of intellectual ability or just as a laboratory exercise, can make these collective representations relevant or irrelevant to evaluating the self.

Ideologies

"Ideologies," or widely shared cultural values, are another type of collective representation that may affect the meaning of situations for stigmatized and nonstigmatized individuals. The values may be so widely shared and unquestioned that people are not even aware that they represent ideologies, or are not shared by people in different cultures. Nonetheless, these ideologies provide an important standard against which the self is evaluated, and hence can be a source of high or low self-esteem (Greenberg, Pyszczynski, & Solomon, 1986). Stigmatized individuals are particularly likely to fall short when evaluated in the context of these ideologies. Indeed, people with particular social identities may be stigmatized *because* they are perceived as not measuring up to these ideologies (see Crocker et al., 1998, for a discussion).

One of the dominant ideologies in the United States is individualism (Kleugel & Smith, 1981, 1986). Individualism encompasses a variety of beliefs and values, all focused on personal responsibility, freedom, and the power of individuals to work autonomously and achieve their goals. America's focus on individualism can be traced in part to its Protestant work ethic roots (Weber, 1904–1905/1958). Indeed, the Protestant work ethic has been called one of America's core values (Hsu, 1972; Katz & Hass, 1988). It includes the belief that individual work is virtuous and leads to success, and that lack of success is caused by the moral failings of self-indulgence and lack of self-discipline. Thus those who receive positive outcomes deserve them because they worked hard and are morally superior, whereas those who receive negative outcomes deserve them because they are self-indulgent, lack self-discipline, and are morally flawed.

Although this ideology is widely shared in North American culture, it has different implications for the worth or value of stigmatized and nonstigmatized individuals. People who endorse individualism may be particularly likely to devalue members of stigmatized groups who fall short according to its percepts. Consistent with this view, research has demonstrated that endorsement of the Protestant ethic is related to negative attitudes toward African Americans (Katz & Hass, 1988), those on welfare (Furnham, 1985), those who are overweight (Crandall, 1994; Quinn & Crocker, 1998), those with alcoholism, and those who are unemployed (Quinn, 1999). However, virtually no research has examined the implications of these ideologies for stigmatized persons. Ideologies have implications for the meaning of one's position in the world, especially how much that position is due to one's character as opposed to the social structure or the system (e.g., Sidanius, 1993). Consequently, they are likely to play an important role in the construction of self-esteem among stigmatized individuals. We suggest that members of stigmatized groups who endorse individualistic ideologies such as the Protestant ethic may devalue themselves, and hence may have low self-esteem. We have explored this hypothesis in the context of the self-esteem of overweight people.

Although this ideology, on the face of it, has nothing to do with body shape or size, endorsement of the Protestant ethic and related notions of personal responsibility are associated with attitudes toward overweight individuals. Crandall (1994) demonstrated that the belief that being fat results from a lack of willpower is part of a larger system of beliefs about personal responsibility, including conservative political leanings, belief in a just world, and endorsement of the Protestant ethic. This link between individualistic ideology and anti-fat attitudes, especially willpower beliefs, suggests that individualistic ideologies may provide a frame by which overweight individuals evaluate themselves, and consequently may affect their self-esteem. Although endorsement of individualism may be positively related to self-esteem among those who are relatively successful, it may be negatively related to self-esteem in those who are overweight. To examine this link between individualistic ideology and self-esteem, we (Quinn & Crocker, 1999, Study 1) had 257 female undergraduates at the University of Michigan indicate their weight status, and complete a Protestant ethic scale and trait measures of psychological well-being. A modified version of the Protestant ethic scale from Katz and Hass (1988) was used as a measure of individualistic ideology. The scale measures the extent to which people endorse hard work, self-discipline, and personal responsibility (e.g., "A distaste for hard work usually reflects a weakness of character"). Psychological well-being was assessed with the Rosenberg (1965) measure of global self-esteem, the Center for Epidemiologic Studies Depression scale (Radloff, 1977), and the Trait Anxiety Scale of the Spielberger State–Trait Anxiety Inventory (Spielberger, Vagg, Barker, Donham, & Westberry, 1980). The order of the scales within the questionnaire packet was counterbalanced, so that some participants received the psychological well-being measures first and the ideology and attitude measures second, whereas the rest of the participants received the scales in the reverse order.

Of the 257 participants, no women rated themselves as very underweight, 8 women rated themselves as somewhat underweight, 116 felt themselves to be of normal weight, 114 felt somewhat overweight, and 19 felt very overweight. Very overweight women were significantly lower in psychological well-being (a composite of high self-esteem, low anxiety, and low depression) than normal-weight or somewhat overweight women (see Table 6.2). There were no significant differences in endorsement of the Protestant ethic by weight. More interesting, for our purposes, is the link between endorsement of the Protestant ethic and psychological well-being for normal-weight and overweight women. To examine this link, we conducted regression analyses in which well-being was predicted by self-perceived weight, Protestant ethic scores, and their interaction. The interaction between weight status and Protestant ethic was significant ($\beta = -.15$, $p < .02$). The pattern of this interaction, depicted in Figure 6.1, shows that endorsement of the Protestant ethic was positively related to well-being for normal-weight women, unrelated for women who rated themselves as somewhat overweight, and negatively related for women who rated themselves as very overweight.

It appears that believing that one is overweight has different implications for self-esteem, depending on whether one is high or low in endorsement of the Protestant ethic. We suspect that for normal-weight women, endorsement of the Protestant ethic implies that one is responsible for one's success. For women who feel very overweight, however, endorsement of the Protestant ethic implies a moral failure. This study pro-

TABLE 6.2. Means (and Standard Deviations) for Self-Perceived Normal-Weight, Somewhat Overweight, and Very Overweight Women

	Perceived normal-weight	Perceived somewhat overweight	Perceived very overweight
Psychological well-being	0.39 (2.68)[a]	−0.25 (2.37)[a]	−1.81 (3.08)[b]
Protestant ethic	4.25 (0.65)[a]	4.37 (0.66)[a]	4.47 (0.56)[a]

Note. The data are from Quinn and Crocker (1999). Means with different subscripts differed significantly at $p < .05$.

vides intriguing evidence of the link between collective representations such as the Protestant ethic and the psychological well-being of stigmatized individuals. However, it provides a static picture of this link, and does not permit an examination of how this link may depend on features of the situation that make those ideologies relevant or irrelevant.

Although ideologies such as the Protestant ethic may be endorsed by many people in our culture, competing ideologies, such as egalitarianism, are also widely endorsed (e.g., Katz, 1981). Consequently, whether the Protestant ethic is used as a standard against which the stigmatized

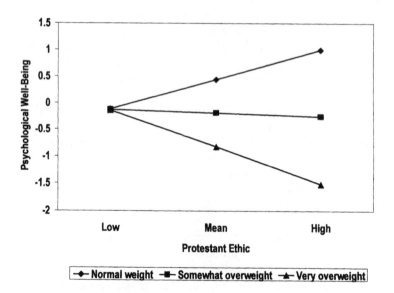

FIGURE 6.1. Predicted values for the interaction between weight status and Protestant ethic beliefs on psychological well-being at the mean and one standard deviation above and below the mean on Protestant ethic. Adapted from Quinn and Crocker (1999).

evaluate themselves may depend on features of the situation that make the Protestant ethic or competing, more inclusive ideologies salient. We again investigated this hypothesis in the context of the stigma of being overweight (Quinn & Crocker, 1999, Study 2).

In this study, women who rated themselves as overweight or normal-weight in a pretest at the beginning of the semester were recruited for a study of comprehension and mood effects of media messages (Quinn & Crocker, 1999, Study 2). The salience of the Protestant ethic was manip-ulated by having women read a political speech. For half of the women, the speech emphasized the values of the Protestant ethic (e.g., "America is a country where people can stand proud on their accomplishments. Self-reliance and self-discipline are the cornerstones of this country"). For the remaining women, the speech emphasized inclusiveness (e.g., "America is a country in which we strive to combine our differences into unity. . . . A country whose divergent but harmonizing communities are a reflection of our deeper community values. . . ."); this speech was based on Ronald Reagan's 1988 State of the Union address. After read-ing the speech, women rated it on a number of measures included to sup-port the cover story. Then all women read a "newspaper article" about the negative social experiences of overweight individuals. This latter message was included to ensure that all women were focused on their weight and on the negative consequences of being overweight. Depend-ent measures included several state measures of psychological well-being, including the Rosenberg (1965) self-esteem inventory modified to reflect momentary feelings about the self, and the Anxiety, Hostility, and Depression subscales of the Multiple Affect Adjective Checklist (Zuckerman & Lubin, 1965).

Analyses of ratings of the two messages indicated that the political speeches were rated as equally powerful. The message about the negative social consequences of being overweight was rated as more powerful by women who had read the Protestant ethic message than by women who had read the inclusive message, $F(1, 114) = 7.61, p < .01$. Examining the effects of weight status and the manipulation on state psychological well-being revealed a marginally significant interaction, $F(1, 113) = 2.95, p = .09$. In the Protestant ethic condition, overweight women had lower psychological well-being ($M = -1.11$) than did normal-weight women ($M = -0.21, p < .01$), whereas in the inclusive condition, the dif-ference between overweight ($M = 0.98$) and normal-weight ($M = 0.35$) women did not approach significance. This pattern was also obtained on self-esteem when it was analyzed separately.

Taken together, these studies on ideology and the psychological well-being of overweight women indicate that the self-esteem of women who are overweight, or think they are, depends on the collective representations that are salient. The survey shows that for some women, individualistic ideologies such as the Protestant ethic are highly endorsed and probably chronically salient or easily activated. When such women think they are very overweight, they tend to have low levels of self-esteem and other aspects of psychological well-being. Interestingly, among women who do not endorse the Protestant ethic, there are no differences between overweight and normal-weight women in well-being.

The experiment shows that differences between overweight and normal-weight women in state psychological well-being depend on the ideology that is salient at the moment. In our research context, when an inclusive ideology was made salient, overweight and normal-weight women did not differ in well-being. When the Protestant ethic was made salient, however, overweight women were lower in psychological well-being. Again, these results are consistent with the argument that low self-esteem among overweight women is not internalized and stable, reflecting a pathology caused by being stigmatized. Rather, they are consistent with the view that negative self-evaluations are constructed in the situation as a result of collective representations that provide standards by which one can be judged. When features of the situation render alternative, less judgmental collective representations salient, then overweight and normal-weight women do not differ in self-esteem or other aspects of psychological well-being.

Controllability of Stigma

Another type of collective representation that may affect the meaning of situations for self-evaluation consists of beliefs about the controllability of stigmatizing conditions. These collective representations are clearly related to endorsement of individualistic ideologies, such as the Protestant ethic and the belief that the world is just (Crandall, 1994; Quinn & Crocker, 1999). However, stigmatized identities vary widely in how controllable they are perceived to be. For example, whereas a person's racial group or skin color is uncontrollable, in North American culture weight is perceived to be under a person's control, and being overweight is believed to reflect a lack of willpower or self-discipline (e.g., Crandall, 1994; DeJong & Kleck, 1986; Jones et al., 1984; Weiner, Perry, & Magnusson, 1988). Overweight and normal-weight people are equally likely to endorse these willpower beliefs (Crandall, 1994). Furthermore, for both overweight and normal-weight people, the belief that being overweight results from a lack of willpower is related to dislike of overweight people (Crandall, 1994).

These collective representations about the causes of overweight may affect the self-esteem of women who are, or believe they are, overweight, especially when they experience a rejection. Because their weight is perceived to be their fault, and to reflect badly on their characters, overweight women may believe that they deserve to be rejected (Crocker & Major, 1994). Consequently, although they may attribute the rejection to their weight and to the evaluator's concern with appearance, this may not be interpreted as prejudice. According to this reasoning, altering the situation so that uncontrollable causes of weight are salient might lead women to see rejection as reflecting prejudice, and consequently protect their self-esteem.

To test this hypothesis, Amato and Crocker (1995) recruited overweight and normal-weight women for a study of "dating relationships." When each woman arrived alone at the laboratory, the experimenter measured her height and weight, consulted an insurance table of height and weight, and told the woman whether she was classified according to the table as overweight or normal weight. This procedure ensured that an overweight or normal-weight designation would be salient to all participants. Each woman was seated in a room with a one-way mirror, although in this study the blinds on the mirror were always down. Each woman was told that she was participating in a study of the early stages of dating relationships, that there was a male student in the next room, and that he would decide whether he was interested in dating her after learning more about her. The woman completed a self-description form indicating her height and weight, her year in college, her major, and whether she was currently involved in a romantic relationship. This form was ostensibly shown to the male evaluator. Each woman received a similar form ostensibly filled out by the man, indicating that he was 5'10", 170 pounds, a junior in college, a pre-med major, and not currently involved in a romantic relationship (pretesting indicated that these qualities would make him attractive to most female students). The woman then completed the Rosenberg (1965) self-esteem scale as a pretest measure of self-esteem, and a self-description questionnaire on which she answered questions about her personal likes and dislikes, which was then shown to the fictional male subject. The salience of beliefs about the controllability of weight was manipulated by having all of the women in the study read an "article" about the scientific evidence on the causes of overweight, supposedly written by the Surgeon General of the United States. For half of the participants, the article presented scientific evidence that weight is controllable through proper diet and exercise. For the other half of the participants, the article presented scientific evidence that weight is a function of genetics and other biological processes, and is very difficult to control through diet and exercise. Participants were told that they were to read the article and answer questions about it as part of a test of cognitive abilities. After reading the article and answering questions about it, all participants learned that the male evaluator was not interested in dating them. The women then completed several measures, including a manipulation check for the controllability manipulation, attributions for the rejection, and a measure of trait self-esteem (the Rosenberg self-esteem scale). All participants were fully debriefed at the conclusion of the study.

The manipulation checks showed that women who read the "weight is controllable" article did believe that weight was more controllable than the women who read the "weight is not controllable" article. As predicted, an interaction between weight status and the controllability manipulation indicated that overweight women in the weight-uncontrollable condition were more likely to attribute the rejection to the evaluator's prejudice ($M = 4.11$) than either overweight women in the weight-controllable condition ($M = 3.3$), or normal-weight women in the weight-uncontrollable ($M = 2.45$) or weight-controllable ($M = 2.75$) condition. Analysis of the self-esteem measure, with initial self-esteem as a covariate, revealed only an interaction between weight and the controllability manipulation. Overweight women in the weight-uncontrollable condition ($M = 3.19$) and normal-weight women in the weight-controllable condition ($M = 3.29$) had higher self-esteem than overweight women in the weight-controllable condition ($M = 2.97$) or normal-weight women in the weight-uncontrollable condition ($M = 3.03$), who did not differ from each other. Thus, in the context of being rejected for a date, the self-esteem of overweight and normal-weight women depends on the salience of information about the controllability of weight. For normal-weight women, self-esteem is higher when they have recently read that weight is controllable, perhaps because they can take personal credit for being thin. For overweight women, however, self-esteem is higher when they have recently read that weight is uncontrollable; this encourages them to see their weight as not their fault, and to attribute the rejection to prejudice.

These results suggest that overweight women have not internalized the negative images of them portrayed in the mass media and conveyed by many people in their lives. Rather, their self-esteem depends on the beliefs about the causes of overweight, and the implications of those beliefs for the self when others are rejecting. Collective representations about the controllability of weight lead overweight women to attribute rejection to their weight, and to see that rejection as deserved. However, when features of the situation (in this case, reading an article) make uncontrollable causes of overweight salient, overweight women are more likely to attribute rejection to prejudice, and to have relatively high self-esteem. Again, the results of these studies are consistent with the argument that the stigmatized do not have stable, internalized low self-esteem. Rather, their self-esteem depends at least in part on the shared beliefs and meanings they bring to the situation (especially beliefs about the controllability of weight), and on features of the situation that make those beliefs relevant or irrelevant to interpreting their experience and its implications for the self.

Contingencies of Self-Esteem

A final collective representation that the stigmatized bring with them to situations is a set of beliefs about what makes a person worthwhile—beliefs that Crocker and Wolfe (in press) have called "contingencies of self-esteem." The prediction that people who are members of stigmatized or devalued racial or ethnic groups suffer from low self-esteem derives, as noted previously, from the notion of the looking-glass self. In this view, self-esteem depends on a process of reflected appraisals, in which the self-concept is based on one's beliefs about the views that others have of the self. From this perspective, self-esteem is not only socially constructed; it is constructed in the same way for all people. In contrast, we argue that there are differences in the degree to which people base their self-esteem on the real or imagined approval and regard of others. Specifically, Crocker and Wolfe (in press) have proposed that there are both individual differences and differences between groups with different social identities in the extent to which people derive their self-esteem from a process of reflected appraisals. People who base their self-esteem on reflected appraisals, or approval from others, and who have a devalued social identity should be vulnerable to low self-esteem.

We have investigated this issue in the context of the stigma associated with being, or feeling, overweight (Quinn & Crocker, 1998). As part of the study of the Protestant ethic and self-esteem described earlier (Quinn & Crocker, 1999, Study 1), we had overweight and normal-weight women complete a measure of basing self-esteem on approval from others, developed by Wolfe, Crocker, Coon, and Luhtanen (1999). This measure includes items such as "I can't respect myself if others don't respect me," and "Being criticized by others really takes a toll on my self-respect." We conducted a set of regression analyses in which we predicted self-esteem from self-perceived weight and the extent to which self-esteem is based on reflected appraisals. The analysis indicated that both feeling overweight ($\beta = -.13$, $p < .05$) and basing self-esteem on reflected appraisals ($\beta = -.38$, $p < .0001$) were significantly related to low self-esteem among all women. Adding the interaction between self-perceived weight and reflected appraisals increased the amount of variance explained ($p < .06$).

To examine the nature of this interaction, we calculated the rela tionship between basing self-esteem on reflected appraisals and self-esteem separately for women who felt normal-weight and those who felt overweight. Among women who felt normal-weight, basing self-esteem on reflected appraisals was related to being low in self-esteem ($r = -.28$, $p < .01$), but this relationship was even stronger among women who felt overweight ($r = -.46$, $p < .01$). Thus basing self-esteem on reflected appraisals did appear to be a risk factor for low self-esteem for all of the women in our sample, but especially for those women who felt over-weight. This research supports our view that people differ in the degree to which they base their self-esteem on approval from others, and that basing self-esteem on approval from others is a risk factor for low self-esteem among those who are stigmatized.

In the Quinn and Crocker (1998) study, basing self-esteem on others' approval was more an individual, idiosyncratic source of meaning than a collective representation. However, Crocker and Wolfe (in press) have proposed that there are reliable differences between identity groups in basing self-esteem on others' approval. To test this idea, Wolfe and colleagues (1999) gave their measure of basing self-esteem on others' approval to a sample of 87 European American, 84 African American, and 82 Asian American college students. Scores on the measure indicated that European American students were most likely to base their self-esteem on approval from others ($M = 4.78$), followed by Asian American students ($M = 4.43$); African American students were least likely to base their self-esteem on approval from others ($M = 3.83$), $F (2, 250) = 21.04$, $p < .001$. These group differences in basing self-esteem on others' approval have since been replicated in a number of college student samples.

This disengagement of self-esteem from the approval of others may be one factor that inoculates the self-esteem of African American students from the negative consequences of devaluation. Asian American students, on the other hand, seem to have self-esteem that is more contingent on approval from others; this may increase their vulnerability to low self-esteem. This assumes, of course, that basing self-esteem on approval is related to having low self-esteem among individuals who are devalued, disadvantaged, and discriminated against. Consistent with this assumption, basing self-esteem on approval was correlated with lower levels of self-esteem for African American ($r = -.41$, $p < . 001$) and Asian American ($r = -.41$, $p < .001$) students, but not for European American students ($r = -.04$, n.s.). Thus self-esteem that is contingent on others' approval appears to be a vulnerability factor for low self-esteem among both African American and Asian American students. The different levels of self-esteem characterizing these two groups—African Americans tend to have higher self-esteem than Asian Americans (Twenge & Crocker, 1999)— is explained, at least in part, by the fact that African

American students are less likely to base their self-esteem on what others think of them.

These studies of stigma and contingencies of self-esteem again do not take into account features of situations that may make these contingencies relevant or irrelevant to evaluating the self. Although contingencies of self-esteem appear to be relatively stable characteristics of individuals (Sommers & Crocker, 1999; Wolfe et al., 1999), situations differ in the degree to which others' evaluations are salient. For example, making a public speech is a situation in which others' evaluations may be particularly salient, whereas others' evaluations may be nonsalient when one is working alone on a computer card game. Research examining features of the situation that make these contingencies relevant to evaluating the self is only in the planning stages. However, we hypothesize that in situations in which evaluation by others is particularly salient, stigmatized individuals, who know they have an identity that is devalued by others, may be low in self-esteem; the more their self-esteem is based on others' approval, the more this should be true.

IMPLICATIONS AND CONCLUSIONS

The studies described here were not designed to test the notion that the effects of stigma on self-esteem depend on the collective representations that the stigmatized bring to the situation, and on features of the situation that make those collective representations relevant or not. Nonetheless, the pattern of results across these studies seems very consistent with this view. Some important implications for the study of social stigma follow from this perspective.

First, understanding the experience of stigmatized people requires that we understand the collective representations that these people bring with them to situations. Whether collective representations held by members of devalued groups are shared by those in valued or advantaged groups (such as individualism), or are not shared (such as beliefs about prejudice and discrimination), they may cause situations to have different meaning for different groups. This suggests that research on the experience of stigmatized persons should not only document the collective representations that stigmatized and nonstigmatized individuals bring with them to situations, but should also explore how those collective representations affect the meaning of situations for these two groups. We cannot assume that the same situation will mean the same thing for stigmatized and nonstigmatized people.

Second, our analysis suggests that the experience of disadvantaged, devalued, or stigmatized groups cannot be understood by creating stigmatized identities or minimal groups in the laboratory. Such studies strip away the shared beliefs and values that stigmatized individuals bring with them that give situations their meaning. In the present analysis, the effects of stigma are crucially dependent on those collective representations.

Third, this analysis suggests that stigmatization and its consequences do not require the presence of prejudiced individuals. Because collective representations are widely known and shared among stigmatized people, it is not necessary for a prejudiced individual to communicate the devaluation of these people for that devaluation to be felt. Stigmatized individuals bring with them to situations collective representations that may devalue them, as the Protestant ethic devalues overweight persons, or that deflect devaluation, as awareness of prejudice and system blame may for African American students.

Like the "looking-glass self" perspective of the symbolic interactionists, this perspective views the self *as* a social construction. However, in this view it is not only the "imagination of our appearance to the other person" and "the imagination of his judgment of that appearance" (Cooley, 1902/1956, p. 184) that affect the self-esteem of the stigmatized. Rather, collective representations such as the Protestant ethic may directly affect inferences about self-worth, without mediation by beliefs about how others judge the self.

ACKNOWLEDGMENTS

The research reported in this chapter was supported by National Science Foundation Grant Nos. BNS 9596226 and BNS9010487. Preparation of this chapter was supported by National Institute of Mental Health (NIMH) Grant No. 1 R01 MH58869-01 to Jennifer Crocker, and by an NIMH traineeship to Diane M. Quinn.

REFERENCES

Allon, N. (1982). The stigma of overweight in everyday life. In B. Wolman (Ed.), *Psychological aspects of obesity: A handbook* (pp. 130–174). New York: Van Nostrand Reinhold.

Allport, G. (1979). *The nature of prejudice.* New York: Doubleday/Anchor. (Original work published 1954)

Amato, M., & Crocker, J. (1995, August). *Perceived controllability of weight and women's reactions to rejection.* Paper presented at the annual meeting of the American Psychological Association, New York.

Banks, W. C. (1976). White preference in Blacks: A paradigm in search of a phenomenon. *Psychological Bulletin, 83,* 179–186.

Best, D. L., Williams, J. E., Cloud, J. M., Davis, S. W., Robertson, L. S., Edwards, J. R., Giles, H., & Fowles, J. (1977). Development of sex-trait stereotypes among young children in the United States, England, and Ireland. *Child Development, 48*, 1375–1394.

Blascovich, J., & Tomaka, J. (1991). Measures of self-esteem. In J. P. Robinson, P. R. Shaver, & L. S. Wrightsman (Eds.), *Measures of personality and social psychological attitudes* (pp. 115–160). San Diego, CA: Academic Press.

Brand, E. S., Ruiz, R. A., & Padilla, A. M. (1974). Ethnic identification and preference: A review. *Psychological Bulletin, 81*, 860–890.

Cartwright, D. (1950). Emotional dimensions of group life. In M. L. Raymert (Ed.), *Feelings and emotions* (pp. 439–447). New York: McGraw-Hill.

Casas, J. M., Ponterotto, J. G., & Sweeney, M. (1987). Stereotyping the stereotyper: A Mexican American perspective. *Journal of Cross-Cultural Psychology, 18*, 45–57.

Clark, K. B., & Clark, M. P. (1939). Skin color as a factor in racial identification of Negro preschool children. *Journal of Social Psychology, 11*, 159–169.

Cooley, C. H. (1956). *Human nature and the social order*. New York: Free Press. (Original work published 1902)

Crandall, C. S. (1994). Prejudice against fat people: Ideology and self-interest. *Journal of Personality and Social Psychology, 66*, 882–894.

Crandall, C. S., & Biernat, M. (1990). The ideology of anti-fat attitudes. *Journal of Applied Social Psychology, 20*, 227–243.

Crandall, R. (1973). The measurement of self-esteem and related constructs. In J. Robinson & P. Shaver (Eds.), *Measures of social psychological attitudes*. Ann Arbor, MI: Institute for Social Research.

Crocker, J., & Blanton, H. (1999). Social stigma: Vulnerabilities for low self-esteem. In T. Tyler, R. Kramer, & O. John (Eds.), *The social self* (pp. 171–191). Mahwah, NJ: Erlbaum.

Crocker, J., Luhtanen, R., Blaine, B., & Broadnax, S. (1994). Collective self-esteem and psychological well-being among White, Black, and Asian college students. *Personality and Social Psychology Bulletin, 20*, 502–513.

Crocker, J., Luhtanen, R., Broadnax, S., & Blaine, B. (1999). Belief in U. S. government conspiracies against Blacks: Powerlessness or system blame. *Personality and Social Psychology Bulletin, 25*, 941–953.

Crocker, J., & Major, B. (1989). Social stigma and self-esteem: The self-protective properties of stigma. *Psychological Review, 96*, 608–630.

Crocker, J., & Major, B. (1994). Reactions to stigma: The moderating role of justifications. In M. P. Zanna & J. M. Olson (Eds.), *The Ontario Symposium: Vol. 7. The psychology of prejudice* (pp. 289–314). Hillsdale, NJ: Erlbaum.

Crocker, J., Major, B., & Steele, C. (1998). Social stigma. In D. Gilbert, S. T. Fiske, & G. Lindzey (Eds.), *Handbook of social psychology* (4th ed., Vol. 2, pp. 504–553). Boston: McGraw-Hill.

Crocker, J., Voelkl, K., Testa, M., & Major, B. (1991). Social stigma: The affective consequences of attributional ambiguity. *Journal of Personality and Social Psychology, 60*, 218–228.

Crocker, J., & Wolfe, C. T. (in press). Contingencies of self-worth. *Psychological Review*.

Crosby, F. (1982). *Relative deprivation and working women.* New York: Oxford University Press.

D'Emilio, J. (1983). *Sexual politics, sexual communities: The making of a homosexual minority in the United States, 1940–1979.* Chicago: University of Chicago Press.

Diener, E. (1984). Subjective well-being. *Psychological Bulletin, 95,* 542–575.

DeJong, W., & Kleck, R. E. (1986). The social psychological effects of overweight. In C. P. Herman, M. P. Zanna, & E. T. Higgins (Eds.), *The Ontario Symposium: Vol. 3. Physical appearance, stigma, and social behavior* (pp. 65–87). Hillsdale, NJ: Erlbaum.

Devine, P. G. (1989). Stereotypes and prejudice: Their automatic and controlled components. *Journal of Personality and Social Psychology, 56,* 5–18.

Erikson, E. (1956). The problem of ego-identity. *Journal of the American Psychoanalytic Association, 4,* 56–121.

Friedman, M. A., & Brownell, K. D. (1995). Psychological correlates to obesity: Moving to the next research generation. *Psychological Bulletin, 117,* 3–20.

Furnham, A. (1985). The determinants of attitudes towards Social Security recipients. *British Journal of Social Psychology, 24,* 19–27.

Gaertner, S. L., & Dovidio, J. F. (1986). The aversive form of racism. In J. F. Dovidio & S. L. Gaertner (Eds.), *Prejudice, discrimination, and racism* (pp. 61–89). Orlando, FL: Academic Press.

Gibbons, F. X. (1981). The social psychology of mental retardation: What's in a label? In S. S. Brehm, S. M. Kassin, & F. X. Gibbons (Eds.), *Developmental social psychology* (pp. 249–270). New York: Oxford University Press.

Goffman, E. (1963). *Stigma: Notes on the management of spoiled identity.* Englewood Cliffs, NJ: Prentice-Hall.

Gray-Little, B., & Hafdahl, A. R. (2000). Factors influencing racial comparisons of self-esteem: A quantitative review. *Psychological Bulletin, 126,* 26–54.

Greenberg, J., Pyszczynski, T., & Solomon, S. (1986). The causes and consequences of the need for self-esteem: A terror management theory. In R. F. Baumeister (Ed.), *Public self and private self* (pp. 189–207). New York: Springer-Verlag.

Harris, M. B., Waschull, S., & Walters, L. (1990). Feeling fat: Motivations, knowledge, and attitudes of overweight women and men. *Psychological Reports, 67,* 1191–1202.

Heatherton, T. F., & Polivy, J. (1991). Development and validation of a scale for measuring state self-esteem. *Journal of Personality and Social Psychology, 60,* 895–910.

Hsu, F. L. K. (1972). American core values and national character. In F. L. K. Hsu (Ed.), *Psychological anthropology* (pp. 241–262). Cambridge, MA: Schenkman.

James, W. (1890). *Principles of psychology* (2 vols.). New York: Henry Holt.

Jarvie, G. J., Lahey, B., Graziano, W., & Framer, E. (1983). Childhood obesity and social stigma: What we know and what we don't know. *Developmental Review, 3,* 237–273.

Jones, E. E., Farina, A., Hastorf, A. H., Markus, H., Miller, D. T., & Scott, R. A. (1984). *Social stigma: The psychology of marked relationships.* New York: Freeman.

Jost, J. T., & Banaji, M. R. (1994). The role of stereotyping in system-justification and the production of false consciousness. *British Journal of Social Psychology, 33,* 1–27.

Katz, I. (1981). *Stigma: A social-psychological perspective.* Hillsdale, NJ: Erlbaum.

Katz, I., & Hass, R. G. (1988). Racial ambivalence and American value conflict: Correlational and priming studies of dual cognitive structures. *Journal of Personality and Social Psychology, 55,* 893–905.

Kernis, M. H., Cornell, D. P., Sun, C., Berry, A., & Harlow, T. (1993). There's more to self-esteem than whether it is high or low: The importance of stability of self-esteem. *Journal of Personality and Social Psychology, 65,* 1190–1204.

Kernis, M. H., Grannemann, B. D., & Barclay, L. C. (1989). Stability and level of self-esteem as predictors of anger arousal and hostility. *Journal of Personality and Social Psychology, 56,* 1013–1022.

Kernis, M. H., & Waschull, S. B. (1995). The interactive roles of stability and level of self-esteem: Research and theory. In M. P. Zanna (Ed.), *Advances in experimental social psychology* (Vol. 27, pp. 93–141). San Diego, CA: Academic Press.

Kluegel, J. R., & Smith, E. R. (1981). Beliefs about stratification. *Annual Review of Sociology, 7,* 29–56.

Kluegel, J. R., & Smith, E. R. (1986). *Beliefs about inequality: Americans' view of what is and what ought to be.* New York: Aldine de Gruyer.

Lee, S. J. (1994). Behind the model-minority stereotype: Voices of high- and low-achieving Asian American students. *Anthropology and Education Quarterly, 25,* 413–429.

Leiberson, S. (1995). Stereotypes: Their consequences for race and ethnic interaction. *Research in Race and Ethnic Relations, 4,* 113–137.

Levine, S. R., Wyer, R. S., & Schwarz, N. (1994). Are you what you feel?: The affective and cognitive determinants of self-judgments. *European Journal of Social Psychology, 24,* 63–77.

Link, B. G. (1987). Understanding labeling effects in the area of mental disorders: An assessment of the effects of expectations of rejection. *American Sociological Review, 52,* 96–112.

Maccoby, E. E., & Jacklin, C. N. (1974). *The psychology of sex differences.* Stanford, CA: Stanford University Press.

Major, B., Barr, L., Zubek, J., & Babey, S. H. (1999). Gender and self-esteem: A meta-analysis. In W. B. Swan, J. H. Langlois, & L. A. Gilbert (Eds.), *Sexism and stereotypes in modern society: The gender science of Janet Taylor Spence* (pp. 223–254). Washington, DC: American Psychological Association.

Major, B., & Crocker, J. (1994). Social stigma: The affective consequences of attributional ambiguity. In D. M. Mackie & D. L. Hamilton (Eds.), *Affect, cognition, and stereotyping: Interactive processes in intergroup perception* (pp. 345–370). New York: Academic Press.

Mead, G. H. (1934). *Mind, self, and society.* Chicago: University of Chicago Press.

Miller, C. T., & Downey, K. T. (1999). A meta-analysis of heavyweight and self-esteem. *Personality and Social Psychology Review, 3,* 68–84.

Millman, M. (1980). *Such a pretty face: Being fat in America.* New York: Norton.

Myers, D. G., & Diener, E. (1995). Who is happy? *Psychological Science*, 6(1), 10–19.

Pelham, B. W., & Swann, W. B. Jr. (1989). From self-conceptions to self-worth: On the sources and structure of global self-esteem. *Journal of Personality and Social Psychology*, 57, 672–680.

Porter, J. R., & Washington, R. E. (1979). Black identity and self-esteem: A few studies of Black self–concept, 1968–1978. *Annual Review of Sociology*, 5, 5–34.

Quinn, D. M. (1999). [Protestant ethic and judgments of stigmatized groups]. Unpublished raw data, University of Michigan.

Quinn, D. M., & Crocker, J. (1998). Vulnerability to the affective consequences of the stigma of overweight. In J. Swim & C. Stangor (Eds.), *Social stigma: The target's perspective* (pp. 125–143). San Diego, CA: Academic Press.

Quinn, D. M., & Crocker, J. (1999). When ideology hurts: Effects of feeling fat and the Protestant ethic on the psychological well-being of women. *Journal of Personality and Social Psychology*, 77, 402–414.

Radloff, L. S. (1977). The CES-D scale: A self-report depression scale for research in the general population. *Applied Psychological Measurement*, 1, 385–401.

Rosenberg, M. (1965). *Society and the adolescent self-image*. Princeton, NJ: Princeton University Press.

Rosenberg, M. (1979). *Conceiving the self*. New York: Basic Books.

Scott, D. M. (1997). *Contempt and pity: Social policy and the image of the damaged Black psyche 1880–1996*. Chapel Hill, NC: University of North Carolina Press.

Scott, R. A. (1969). *The making of blind men: A study of adult socialization*. New York: Russell Sage Foundation.

Sidanius, J. (1993). The psychology of group conflict and the dynamics of oppression: A social dominance perspective. In W. McGuire & S. Iyengar (Eds.), *Current approaches to political psychology* (pp. 183–219). Durham, NC: Duke University Press.

Sommers, S., & Crocker, J. (1999, April). *Hopes dashed and dreams fulfilled: Contingencies and stability of self-esteem among graduate school applicants*. Paper presented at the annual meeting of the Midwestern Psychological Association, Chicago.

Spencer, S. J., Steele, C. M., & Quinn, D. M. (1999). Stereotype threat and women's math performance. *Journal of Experimental Social Psychology*, 35, 4–28.

Spielberger, C. D., Vagg, P. R., Barker, L. R., Donham, G. W., & Westberry, L. G. (1980). The factor structure of the State–Trait Anxiety Inventory. In C. D. Spielberger & I. G. Sarason (Eds.), *Stress and anxiety* (Vol. 7, pp. 95–109). Washington, DC: Hemisphere.

Steele, C. M. (1997). A threat in the air: How stereotypes shape intellectual identity and performance. *American Psychologist*, 52, 613–629.

Steele, C. M., & Aronson, J. (1995). Stereotype vulnerability and the intellectual test performance of African-Americans. *Journal of Personality and Social Psychology*, 69, 797–811.

Taylor, D. M., Wright, S. C., & Porter, L. E. (1994). Dimensions of perceived discrimination: The personal/group discrimination discrepancy. In M. P. Zanna & J. M. Olson (Eds.), *The Ontario Symposium: Vol. 7. The psychology of prejudice* (pp. 23–355). Hillsdale, NJ: Erlbaum.

Twenge, J., & Crocker, J. (1999). *Race, ethnicity, and self-esteem: Meta-analyses of self-esteem differences among Whites, Blacks, Hispanics, Asians, and Native Americans.* Manuscript in preparation.

Weber, M. (1958). *The Protestant ethic and the spirit of capitalism.* New York: Scribner. (Original work published 1904–1905)

Weiner, B., Perry, R. P., & Magnusson, J. (1988). An attributional analysis of reactions to stigmas. *Journal of Personality and Social Psychology, 55,* 738–748.

Wolfe, C. T., Crocker, J., Coon, H., & Luhtanen, R. K. (1999). *Reflected and deflected appraisals: Race differences in basing self-esteem on others' regard.* Manuscript submitted for publication.

Wylie, R. (1974). *The self-concept.* Lincoln: University of Nebraska Press.

Zuckerman, M., & Lubin, B. (1965). *Manual for the Multiple Affect Adjective Checklist.* San Diego, CA: Educational & Industrial Testing Service.

7

The Looking-Glass Self Revisited: Behavior Choice and Self-Perception in the Social Token

DELIA CIOFFI

The subjective seamlessness of everyday social life is testament to the routinized nature of many common interactions. In a search committee meeting, we spontaneously join our colleagues in evaluating various job candidates; at a social gathering, we listen to others' gossip and readily contribute our own; in the corporate meeting, we signal allegiance to our favored intraoffice camp with a fluent vocabulary of affiliation and distance. Often we also emerge from these interactions knowing a bit more about who we are and what we believe. We feel more certain about the various candidates after evaluating them in committee; we infer that we are natural wits from the ease with which we delivered our party jokes; we have a better sense of our boardroom savvy by the end of the corporate meeting. In this way, the communication between our public and private selves often runs like a well-oiled machine—operating without much explicit supervision, and producing many social experiences that are straightforward and smooth.

But some, of course, are not. Some of us have had the experience of being the only X in such a gathering—the only woman, Hispanic, or homosexual, for example—when at some point our X-ness comes into high relief (if it hasn't been from the start): An X applicant comes before the hiring committee; party talk turns to strained X-Y relations in the neighborhood; the boss mentions the new corporate guidelines to recruit more X's. At the moment when the dimension of X-ness becomes relevant to the interaction at hand—when one of us is no longer just "Sally" or "Sam," but also an "X"—everything seems to change. In short, we have become social tokens, and the social world is suddenly a far more complicated place than it was just a moment ago.

Two things in particular change. First, our sense of social scrutiny intensifies, bringing with it greater evaluative pressure on our behavior. We have the distinct impression that ears now strain in our direction, glances sidle our way, bodies stiffen in anticipation of our next action or reaction. We may suddenly feel moved (or compelled) to represent the X point of view; we may feel responsible for discerning and then correcting for others' preconceptions about X's; we may become more acutely aware of status or power dynamics of the group; we may find that our primary "audience" is no longer simply our immediate coactors, but now includes other X's in our minds' eyes. In short, we may think about, edit, second-guess, or hesitate about doing or saying what a moment ago or in another setting we might have done or said with relatively little thought.

The second change occurs in our processes of self-inference—that is, in using how we have behaved in front of others to inform who we privately believe ourselves to be. This too becomes a more complicated and labored calculus, if for no other reason than that there are now more variables in the equation. Under which of several plausible social pressures did I express that opinion? Which of my identities, loyalties, or "inner" selves" motivated the position I espoused? What did my frown or my shrug or even my silence convey about my values, goals, motives, and skills—about who I am and what I believe? For people in situations such as these, the commute between one's public and private self no longer rides on a relatively smooth and silent road, but now on a noisy and potholed path.

This chapter is about that social traveler: "the social token," who navigates the commute between public acts and private self-views. In particular, I consider the dynamics of token status in light of the relationship between the strategies of self-presentation and the processes of behavior-based self-inference. The picture emerging from this discussion begins to resemble another revision of the "looking-glass self" metaphor for the influence of social interaction on one's privately held self-views. The term originally referred to the idea that we often see ourselves as others see us (Cooley, 1902; Mead, 1934). It was initially modified by the notion that we see ourselves as we *think* others see us, and next by the idea that these reflected appraisals stem as much from our own views of ourselves than from either the real or the presumed views of others

(Felson, 1993; Kenny & DePaulo, 1993; Shrauger & Schoeneman, 1979; Stryker, 1981; Tice, 1992). When these ideas are merged with several recent literatures concerning the dynamic nature of self-concepts and identities (e.g., Markus & Cross, 1990), self-perception (e.g., Olson & Zanna, 1990), impression management (e.g., Leary & Kowalski, 1990), and the relationship between social interaction and social perception (e.g., Levine, Resnik, & Higgins, 1993), we see yet another social pathway by which an actor comes to know him- or herself: Social dynamics help shape public behavior, while simultaneously affecting some of the social-cognitive processes that guide behavior-based self-inference. Thus reflections of today's looking-glass self bounce off many surfaces—some of which are constructed by the actor, some of which are constructed by others, and some of which reflect portraits of the social engagement between the images from the other two.

DEFINITIONS AND CONCEPTS

What Is a "Social Token"?

I operationally define the "social token" as *a salient representative of a social category among coactors who believes that these others hold generalized and at least partially negative expectations of him or her because of this group membership*. I suggest that this definition, expanded upon below, accurately describes most if not all actors who possess a social stigma (Crocker, Major, & Steele, 1998). For the purposes of this analysis, then, the "social token" and the "socially stigmatized individual" serve as functional synonyms.

To illustrate my definitional terms, I quote from several dialogues with African American students at small and predominantly European American schools, who described the situations in which they felt tokenized (Davidson & Cioffi, 1993; Stewart, 1993):

A: [Speaking about her academic advisor] He didn't think I should declare pre-med. He didn't think I could cut it, I could tell—a little Black girl from down South . . .

B: Could you tell? I mean, how do you know that's racist? How do you know?

C: I know some advisors who push Black kids into pre-med, like they're trying to make some political point or something . . .

A: I declared [pre-med] anyway. (*Plaintively*) Who knows? I don't even know what I want any more . . .

D: There are three of us [African-Americans in the literature class]. We
    got to Toni Morrison, and all of a sudden we're the experts. I can
    feel everybody waiting for my opinions and watching for my reac-
    tions. And forget it if we [the African-American students] disagree!
    Damn . . . I'm just figuring this stuff out myself! I'm tired of being
    asked to speak for the whole Black race, like I know what that is
    anyway. I didn't apply for this job . . .

E: What job?

D: To educate everybody about "the Black experience."

F: It's like I'm expected to jump up when they [European American
    sorority sisters] play Queen Latifah [a rap musician].

G: Right, like you should give 'em a prize or something . . .

F: . . . or just love it. I used to like the Queen. Now I just cringe . . .

A Perceived Social Categorization by Others

The most obvious feature uniting the three dialogues above is that the
speakers felt that others had identified them according to their membership in a social group, and this categorization had become salient to the
targets themselves because they believed that it was salient to others
(McGuire & McGuire, 1981; Turner, Hogg, Oakes, Reicher, & Wetherell, 1987). Such a salient categorization may be relatively chronic, as it
was for these Black students in predominantly White schools. But this is
also a "situated" salience; that is, it can intensify when the context or
content of an interaction implicates category-relevant topics (Brown,
1998; Steele, 1997).

A State of Reflective Expectancy

Because social stereotypes have content, membership in various groups
will be associated with *particular* social expectations (e.g., Gardner,
1994). This leads to a second defining feature of social tokenization:
particular expectancies concerning what one's social category implies to
others about who one is, what one believes, and how one will behave.
This means that the social token will operate in a state of "reflective expectancy," believing not only *that* others hold general expectancies
about him or her, but holding some belief about the *content* of those expectancies as well (Crocker et al., 1998; Frable, Blackstone, & Scherbaum, 1990; Kenny & DePaulo, 1993; Major & Crocker, 1993). Thus
the students quoted above believed that others expected them to have
particular tastes in music and in literature, to hold particular political

views, to have had particular cultural experiences, and to possess particular proficiencies (or lack thereof) in academic pursuits. In this way, social tokens often feel that their future actions are foregone conclusions in the eyes of their coactors, and that their skills, opinions, preferences, personalities, and beliefs may have already been presumed.

Negative Social Relevance

Third, the contents of these presumed expectancies are socially relevant on a valenced continuum that is defined in part by one's coactors. Although not all socially relevant categorizations carry a connotation of negative evaluation or disparagement, many do; visibility, social relevance, and social negativity are naturally confounded in many societies, since the most salient marks of difference between individuals are often those that are more socially devalued and also most socially meaningful (Archer, 1985; Brewer, Manzi, & Shaw, 1993). Thus many socially relevant distinctions carry a cultural meaning, which results in tokens' feeling socially stigmatized rather than socially valued (Crocker et al., 1998; Jones et al., 1984).

Representativeness

So far, my definition of the social token shares many features with various other definitions: those of being "stereotyped" (e.g., Crocker et al., 1998), being "vulnerable" to the stereotypic views of others (Steele, 1997), becoming the target of "tribal" or "ethnic" stigma (Goffman, 1963), or possessing a "socially negative master status" (Frable, 1993), most of which derive in some measure from Allport's (1954) description of the person who is the target of social prejudice (see also Dovidio, Brigham, Johnson, & Gaertner, 1996). One additional feature is needed to complete the present definition: the feeling that one is a *representative* of a social category in the eyes of one's coactors (Tajfel & Turner, 1986). Several of the students quoted above, for example, often felt called upon—implicitly or explicitly—to deliver "the Black point of view" on certain social issues or events, because they felt they were the only (or one of the few) individuals who would or could do so. Similarly, the angst of the pre-med student in the first dialogue came in part from feeling that her curricular choice (and her subsequent performance) might affect how the Black students following her would be treated and perceived. In this and many other examples of social tokenism and social stigma, the targets feel as though others' perceptions of their social group will be affected by the impressions that they, personally, will make.

There is a close relationship between feeling that one is representing others and the presence of reflective expectancies, because the content of one's reflective expectancies will identify the representative burden in any particular social context. For Black college students who believe that others presume deficient intellectual achievement from their race, academic performance is a dimension on which they will feel the representative pressure (Steele, 1997); for homosexuals in the Army, bravery on the battlefield and sexual aggression in the barracks are some likely representation domains (Shilts, 1993).

In sum, the stigmatized token is a possibly unique but certainly a salient representative of a disparaged social category among his or her coactors, and believes that these coactors hold particular and at least partially negative expectations (and/or discrediting judgments) of him or her because of this group membership.

The Amplification of Public–Private Comparisons

All of these features of social tokenism are well reflected in the three student dialogues above. But the students' reports reveal another striking characteristic of the experience, which, while not a defining feature of tokenization, is at the heart of the present discussion: Feeling tokenized often seems to imply a complication in behavioral choice *as it relates to private self-identification*, either by compelling a conscious and mindful attention to the relationship between the private and the public self, or (if behavior itself is strategically altered) by creating some noticeable chasm between the two. That is, the additional consideration given to one's behavioral options also extends to one's private views, values, and beliefs—and occasionally this mindfulness results in some particular inflection in the behavior's self-relevant meaning (Gibbons, 1990; Leary, 1993; Schlenker & Leary, 1982). The pre-med student in the first dialogue, for instance, suspected that her curricular choice might reflect her own intrinsic values, the desire to "make a point" to her advisor and others, or a bit of both—and she puzzled over how to weigh these possibilities in interpreting her choice to herself. Similarly, the students who felt pressured to "deliver a verdict" on the writing of Toni Morrison felt compelled to form opinions about this work earlier than they might have under other social conditions—and in particular evaluative directions as well—and this seems to have affected their private views in one way or another. One of these students reported that she didn't particularly believe the opinion she stated in class, in part because she was aware of the social pressures under which it was formed (Cioffi, 1995; Jones & Davis, 1965). In contrast, another student felt extremely certain of her expressed view—although we can plausibly wonder whether she would have felt as committed to that opinion had she been called upon to state it under less social scrutiny and "group obligation" (Cialdini, 1993, Ch. 3). In other words, feeling like a social token often puts pressure on how one acts while simultaneously affecting—straining, strengthening, testing, or revealing—the linkage between how one acts and what one believes.

The "Episodic Construal": Mediator of Behavioral Choice and Self-Perception

A multitude of factors can shape the choice of public behavior—such as one's social situation, audience, self-views, and behavioral repertoire (see Banaji & Prentice, 1994; Baumeister, 1982; Jones & Pittman, 1982; Leary & Kowalski, 1990; Schlenker, 1986). Behavior-based self-inference likewise rests on an equally extensive (and apparently different) set of psychosocial factors—such as the value and strength of one's prior views, the perceived social consequences of the act, and the actor's perceptions of the forces that shaped it (see Fazio, 1987, and the volume by Olson & Zanna, 1990). Thus any compound question about tokenism's effect on behavioral choice and subsequent self-perception is bound to be especially knotty. Will being tokenized change behavior? And to what degree will behavior, whether altered or not, come to affect self-views? When the questions are posed this way, our best answer must be "It depends." This is because the mediators of social behavior and the processes of self-inference each seem to rely on an extensive and apparently different set of psychosocial variables, and, moreover, less on the value of any single psychosocial variable than on the interactions between them.

I propose, however, that the mediators of behavioral choice and self-perception are not different conceptual variables, but rather are different referents to the same higher-order psychological source: the actor's understanding of his or her public behavior and of its context. The factors that guide social behavior and those that guide its degree of internalization both derive from the actor's perception of the meaning, purpose, and effect of the public act being considered: from perceptions of what behavior is presented, where it is presented, to whom it is presented, and why it is presented. This "episodic construal"—the actor's simultaneous and integrated understanding of the self, situation, audience, and act, each derived in the context of the others—can in theory predict both behavioral choice and the self-inference that might result from it. At the episodic construal level of analysis, questions of how a token might behave in a given social situation and questions of what effect (if any) that chosen behavior will have on subsequent self-inference point to the same root: Both will be based on the individual's integrated perception of where he or she is and of what he or she does, to whom, and why.

Figure 7.1 represents the three assumptions of the episodic construal construct.

1. *The social episode is subjectively construed.* The first assumption represented by Figure 7.1 is that nearly everything occurring in the social world passes through the filter of subjective interpretation before it affects social behavior (line "a" at the top of the figure). Within some limits (e.g., McArthur & Baron, 1983), people react to social stimuli as they perceive them, and the most influential features of one's social milieu are subjectively apprehended, not objectively defined (Ross, 1990).

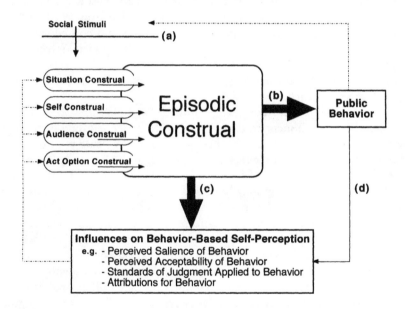

FIGURE 7.1. The "episodic construal" is the actor's simultaneous and integrated understanding of the self, situation, audience, and act, each derived in the context of the others. This unobserved construct mediates between component perceptions of a social interaction (left-hand ovoids) and the choice of public behavior (path "b"). It can therefore affect behavior-based self-inference through one or both of two pathways: first, by creating a particular behavioral history upon which to draw in any process of behavior-based self-inference (path "d"); and, second, by simultaneously affecting the factors that guide the self-inferential process itself (path "c").

2. *There are four basic construal classes.* Subjective interpretations of a social interaction can be organized into the classes represented by the four left-hand ovoids of Figure 7.1. I have chosen these divisions because they parallel those commonly used to discuss the factors that guide strategic public behavior, and each is discussed more fully in the sections that follow. The "situational construal" is a basic identification of the social venue, including the goals and behaviors that seem most relevant in it (e.g., a classroom, social gathering, workplace, or rock concert each suggests prototypic and "appropriate" behaviors in that situation). The "self construal" includes one's self-views (e.g., self-esteem, efficacies, perceived skills), as well as one's prepotent goals and motivations, either instrumental or social (e.g., to gain favor or acceptance; to acquire or deflect sympathy or aid). The "audience construal" defines the nonself others who are witnessing one's behavior or who might hear about it (e.g., one's immediate coactors and/or significant others in the mind's eye), and one's relationship to them, both anticipated and past (e.g., including such factors as status, interdependency, and goal relevance). The "act option construal" represents the perceived causes and consequences of one's behavioral options, and what motives, goals, or social effects each option would serve, further, or create (e.g., why one might verbally disagree with a colleague vs. merely frown at him or her, and the anticipated effects of each).

3. *Any component construal is fully defined only in relation to the others.* Each component construal is truly, fully defined only in context with all the others. The perceived consequences of voicing your true political opinion, for example (act option construal), will in part depend on whether your boss or your friend is listening (audience construal); the effect that this relationship may have on your behavioral choice (audience construal's effect on act option construal) will in part depend on your perceptions of what is generally appropriate in the current social setting (situation construal); perceptions of what is appropriate in this setting (situation construal) will be influenced by various personal variables, such as your self-esteem, social goals, and prepotent self-identities (self construal); and many of these personal variables (self construals) are themselves shaped or activated by your reading of all the other episodic features—such as who is listening (audience construal), where you are (situation construal), and the perceived social effect of various possible behaviors (act option construals). In other words, construals of the "self" are really construals of the self-in-this-situation; construals of the situation are construals of the situation, given this self and this audience; and construals of the audience are formed, given one's act options for this self in this situation.

I refer to this integrated configuration of perceptions as the actor's "episodic construal" of the social interaction: a level of experience that subsumes the actor's subjective understanding of self, behavior, audience, and situation as they relate to and are defined by one another in the present social moment. The box at the center of Figure 7.1 represents this unobserved construct, which mediates between the actor's component perceptions of an interaction episode (four left-hand ovoids) and his or her eventual choice of public behavior (path "b").

This contextual sensibility is central to much research on the phenomenal self, which illustrates how various situational and motivational cues can determine which "self-concept"—out of a repertoire of many potential self-concepts—will emerge as the most accessible and the one that will exert the most influence on public behavior (Jones, 1990; Rhodewalt, 1986). It is also apparent in the work of Schlenker and colleagues, in which any "individual" influence on public behavior (such as the perceived desirability of a social act) is explicitly defined relative to the configuration of other perceptions (such as the likelihood that the act will be credible to the audience who will witness it) (e.g., Schlenker, 1986; Schlenker, Dlugolecki & Doherty, 1994; Schlenker & Weigold, 1992).

Although the notion of an episodic construal may not be new conceptually, the following sections illustrate its utility in the context of the present discussion: that of a linking concept between theories of self-presentation and theories of behavior-based self-inference. I describe this linkage in two parts. First, I discuss how the component construals affecting the choice of public behavior (such as self-views, situational identification, perceived audience, and evaluation of one's act options) are fully described only in configuration with one another—that is, from within the actor's episodic construal (path "b" of Figure 7.1). I illustrate this point by considering how the token and the nontoken may hold systematically different episodic construals within the "same" social situation, largely because of the psychosocial conditions that produce token status in the first place. Second, and again using token status as an illustration, I discuss how one's episodic construal also defines conceptual variables such as the perceived cause, function, and effect of one's behavior (path "c" in Figure 7.1)—all factors that determine whether and how one's public act will subsequently affect one's private self-views (see Fazio, 1987; Jones, 1990; Leary, 1993; Schlenker, 1986). Thus the construct of episodic construal serves as a mediational mapping point between models of self-presentation and theories of behavior-based self-inference (see the volumes by Baumeister, 1986, and Olson & Zanna, 1990). It highlights how the "same" behavior in the "same" situation can take on different functional meanings to the actor—can be perceived to have different social effects, can serve different goals, and can be enacted for different reasons.

HOW DO WE CHOOSE WHAT TO DO?: THE EPISODIC CONSTRUAL AFFECTS THE CHOICE OF PUBLIC BEHAVIOR

Situation Construals: Selecting the Relevant Social Script

"Self-presentation" refers to the process by which individuals try to affect the impression that others form of them; it is an implicit, ubiquitous, and automatic subprocess of almost every interaction with others (see Banaji & Prentice, 1994; Baumeister, 1982; Jones & Pittman, 1982; Leary & Kowalski, 1990; Schlenker & Weigold, 1992).The self-presentational process necessarily includes a basic identification of the social venue. How do people decide where they "are" and what is happening to and around them? To which of many potential social categories or types does the current situation belong?

People commonly rely on scripts and schemas for this sort of decision, assessing the goodness of fit between features of the immediate social topology and common or available interaction "maps" (Abelson, 1981; Baldwin, 1992). Presenting a report in front of one's classmates is commonly seen as an occasion for evaluation—an identification that suggests which behaviors are relevant to that social dimension, effective toward that end, and appropriate in that situation. In contrast, a sorority party is commonly seen as an occasion for assessing sociability and attractiveness, thus also suggesting which behaviors will convey this information in an effective and appropriate way. These schemas and scripts have evolved in part because they are usually "accurate" and "right": Certain cues or configurations of social features come to activate particular situational categories because those categories have been reliable, effective, and adaptive guides to behavior in our social past (e.g., McArthur & Baron, 1983).

But people can differ in the behaviors they judge to be reliable, effective, and adaptive in any given situation, in part because people have accumulated different social pasts. The categorization of a situation as one "thing" rather than another flows in large part from interpretive proclivities and guides, personal self-views, and social expectancies. Thus one perceiver may view a sorority party as an occasion for loss or threat, and another may see a chance to win allies, while a third faces yet one more gauntlet of social hostility. These are sometimes called chronic proclivities—a "person" effect on situational categorization—but they are at least "person × situation" effects: Certain *contextual cues* trigger particular interpretations of the situation, because those cues are of some personal significance to that individual (Higgins, 1990; McArthur & Baron, 1983; Shoda, Mischel, & Wright, 1993; Smith, 1990). Thus even the "chronically X-ed" person is more "X-ed" in some social situations than in others, and the perceived similarities or distinctions between these situations depend on how the actor construes the episode as a whole.

McArthur and Baron's (1983) notion of "attunements" also expresses the idea that different perceivers see different self-relevant opportunities, based on their integrated perceptions of the situation (see also Niemann & Secord, 1995). The perceived affordances offered by a social occasion—that is, the very identification of what kind of situation this is—emerges from the interaction between qualities of the environment and those of the perceiver. Thus even the most elementary stages of self-presentational choice actually subsume perceptions about others, about the self, and about the context in which they meet.

The dynamics of token status illustrate this contextual nature of a situational identification particularly well. The person who believes that others have specific beliefs about him or her may be drawing from a loaded library of situational scripts. For example, if an African American student attending a predominantly European American college presumes an audience with some skepticism about his or her intellectual capabilities (Crocker et al., 1998; Steele, 1997), this presumption might well direct the identification of many situations, including the weekend party, as occasions for evaluation by others on dimensions of intelligence. Likewise, if the lone corporate woman expects that others think she is "too sensitive" for cutthroat company politics, she may perceive many social venues—the water cooler and the Christmas party no less than the board meeting—as occasions for evaluation on some dimension of emotional toughness (Tedeschi & Norman, 1985). In turn, these perceptions might well influence (if not determine) her self-presentational goals in each situation, and also identify what behaviors are likely to be used to meet them (Leary & Kowalski, 1990).

Self Construals: Self-Views, Goals, Motivations, and Sensitivities

Given some basic categorization of the social venue, what is *this* person *particularly* motivated to do in it? Another class of variables that shapes public behavior relates to several "self" dimensions, such as personal needs, motives, goals, traits, and other self-relevant views.

People may seek to leave impressions that are favorable, those that match the people's views of themselves, those that deflect high expectations, or those that facilitate smooth social interactions (see reviews by Banaji & Prentice, 1994; Leary & Kowalski, 1990). Although some people may show a relatively stable proclivity toward some motives over others, here again the phenomenon is less a function of any single perception than of the integration over many perceptions. That is, a "proclivity" for some social motive is not so much a goal faucet that is locked in an open position than it is a biased governor on the spigot—a partisan reading of certain episodic features, due either to some particular triggering contextual cue or to a tendency to hold some particular episodic construal. Thus, for example, the person low in self-esteem may seek to protect against loss or threat across many different situations (Baumeister, 1993), but there is some systematic variability in that motive due to the actor's perceptions of the episode as a whole (e.g., whether this audience poses a threat, given this particular presentational act concerning this particular self-relevant domain, and in this particular social context). These evaluations may well tend toward particular conclusions, but this tendency refers to a bias in one's perception of the episode as a whole rather than to some single, static motive or some portable, dynamic-insensitive belief (e.g., Higgins, 1990; Pittman & Heller, 1987).

Again, the token example illustrates how "self" influences on public presentation are both situated and configural. For example, tokens' global self-esteem is probably no lower than that of nontokens, in part due to mechanisms that buffer against potential threats to their self-views (Crocker & Major, 1989). But all social actors are subject to powerful situational variations in these self-views (Baumeister, 1993), and factors affecting this variability are those under which a social token is especially likely to be placed and that the token would be especially likely to notice (Crocker et al., 1998). Moreover, domain-specific self-doubts often motivate particular self-presentational strategies and occasionally create conflicts between them (LaRonde & Swann, 1993; Schlenker & Leary, 1982; Tice, 1993). When combined with a token's common sensitivity to what is socially desirable and expected by others (e.g., Saenz, 1994), there are several ways in which the token may differ from the nontoken in what "self variables" will influence presentational goals in any given situation.

Audience Construals: Who Is Listening?

Another critical factor guiding public behavior is one's audience for it. Who is watching? Who will know? And what is the actor's relationship to the watchers and listeners? Audiences guide behavior through several routes (see Schlenker & Weigold, 1992), and an explication of each route is really a statement of the behavior-shaping muscle of the actor's episodic construal. For instance, audiences can affect behavior because they serve as communication targets, thus defining what in particular must be done or said to meet one's communication goal (Clark & Brennan, 1991; McCann & Higgins, 1992). But one is only able to "tailor a communication" by weighing who is listening with what is being said, how it is being said, in what context, with what predicted effect, and why—in other words, by weighing audience characteristics, self-efficacies and motives, situational affordances, and evaluations of one's act options in some concurrent, coordinated way. A similar analysis can be applied to the other paths by which an audience shapes behavior. Audiences can serve as cues that activate particular self-schemas or group loyalties; that provide particular standards of self-judgment, social comparisons, or evaluative orientations; or that activate particular social motives based on the relationship between audience and actor (see Schlenker & Weigold, 1992, for a review). None of these "audience" factors can be segregated from the actor's perceptions of the social dynamic as a whole. Thus, for example, a mostly European American audience may serve as a strong racial identity cue for an African American only (or especially) when the communication is race-relevant (e.g., it consists of an argument before an affirmative action hiring board), when the act options are socially risky (e.g., they might affect the individual's standing in the group), or when the audience inspires multiple communication goals (e.g., it contains other people of color, who might activate additional self-presentational aims).

Indeed, the phenomenon of the self-presentational dilemma—in which one holds different, conflicting social motives within the same episode—describes a particular (and particularly uncomfortable) episodic construal (Baumeister & Kenneth, 1992; Emmons, King, & Sheldon, 1993). The token may encounter such dilemmas more often than the average social actor. For instance, although most employees at an office party have a wide set of "potential selves" or identities that might guide their behavior, a large repertoire of behavioral options, and many different relationships with their coactors, the lone homosexual at this party may pay more attention to these options, perceive more potential conflicts between them, and feel that there is more riding on an eventual behavioral choice.

Act Option Construals: Evaluating One's Behavioral Options

The factors that influence how one's behavioral options are weighed depend on how other episodic features have been weighed. Will repeatedly going to the net convince my occasional tennis partner that I am a gutsy, assertive player (thereby increasing her estimation of me), or just an unnecessarily malevolent competitor (thereby merely antagonizing her)? My answer will depend on how I read my partner's skill relative to mine, my perception of her inferential proclivities, my categorization of today's game as either a casual workout or a competitive set, and my estimate of the probability that I will be caught flat-footed in a half-volley instead. Were I to profess a sudden intense interest in golf, would senior colleagues see me as a more *simpatico* coworker or as a mere sycophant? My answer will depend on how I think this group of people will perceive this action (as I believe I can execute it) in this situation, and on whether I value that most likely social result above any one of several others I also cherish. Should I frown, help, ingratiate, opine, demand, clown, or do absolutely nothing in the next social moment? My answer will depend on my episodic construal as a whole, because, depending on my episodic construal, the "same" act—going to the net, talking golf, frowning, helping, or doing nothing—can be performed for different reasons, serve different goals, leave different impressions, and carry different costs. In other words, I can understand it to *be* any one of potentially several very different social acts.

Tokens may systematically differ from nontokens in these episodic construals within the "same" social situation. This idea provides a caution against overly glib interpretations of the "different social values" we may think we observe among various cultural groups, or between those who are versus those who are not the targets of some stigmatizing "mark"—say, when we observe token Sally and nontoken Sam in the "same" situation but acting differently. It is possible, of course, that Sally and Sam do in fact hold entirely different social goals or value different social outcomes (for example). However, an alternative explanation is that Sally and Sam share exactly the same social goals and values, but because they hold different episodic construals (i.e., they are actually *in* different situations), the goals and values that they share will best be met by different overt behaviors by each. Likewise, interpreting apparent "similarities" in the social behavior of tokens and nontokens will benefit from the same caution. It could well be that Sally's and Sam's identical public acts indicate identical social goals (for example), but they may also have entirely different goals. However, because they hold different episodic construals, each may happen to judge the "same" (observed) behavior as best suited for meeting them.

Summary

This brief review has considered some of the variables that can direct an actor's public behavior in response to perceived social demands and in service of various motives and goals. Three major points have been advanced. First, these variables spring largely from subjective assessments of several different aspects of the social interaction. Second, these subjective assessments are relational: The actor experiences an episode—not an inventory of discrete or sequential perceptions—and, by extension, it is the overall construal of this episode that shapes public behavior. Finally, given the "same" objective situation—such as the classroom, the boardroom, or the weekend party—episodic construals of the token may well differ from those of the nontoken, due to the very psychosocial factors that define token status to begin with.

SELF-INFERENCE BASED ON PUBLIC ACTS: THE EPISODIC CONSTRUAL AFFECTS THE INTERNALIZATION OF BEHAVIOR

The same episodic construal that shapes an actor's behavioral choice will also affect that behavior's impact on the actor's private beliefs and self-views. This is because the actor's episodic construal also functionally defines many parameters of behavior-based self-inference. The question "What are the self-inferential consequences of behavior X?" may be answered by resolving another: "What configuration of perceptions shaped that behavior in the first place?" In this section I illustrate how the notion of episodic construal also describes the mediators and moderators of behavior-based self-inference.

Multiple Processes of Behavior-Based Self-Inference

Several different terms have been used to refer to the processes by which one's behavior comes to affect one's private beliefs or self-views. "Self-persuasion" is a common phrase in the attitude literature, where it is argued that certain public acts, such as signing a political petition, tend to strengthen the attitudes implied by them (e.g., Wilson, 1990). "Self-perception" often refers to the process by which social behavior affects self-inference about one's traits, skills, or abilities, as when the joke teller at a party infers that he or she is socially skilled (e.g., Fazio, 1987). "Internalization" refers to a shift in private values or self-identification after some behavior, as when a child values piano playing more if he or she practices without a salient external reward (e.g., Lepper, 1983; see also Schlenker, 1986). These literatures differ in the dependent variables of interest and in the social domains to which they are usually applied (see the volume by Olson & Zanna, 1990).

They also differ in the process by which private views will change. Some refer to situations where "people act contrary to beliefs because of an external constraint . . . [and] because people do not fully appreciate

the fact that their behavior has been constrained . . . assume that it reflects their true nature or beliefs" (Wilson, 1990, p. 44). But questions of
behavior-based self-inference are relevant not only when behavior and
private self-views clash, but also when they match—that is, when one's
behavior and one's beliefs are in perfect accord. Acting on one's true beliefs often serves to strengthen, polarize, or otherwise reinforce them
(e.g., Cialdini, 1993; Schlenker & Trudeau, 1990; Tice, 1992). If, however, the actor's attribution for this behavior can be subtly misdirected,
such reinforcement may not occur or may even result in reinforcement of
the opposite self-inference (Fazio, 1987; Lepper, 1983). Thus, in one
type of self-inference, public but self-discrepant behavior alters private
beliefs because of a particular attributional configuration: The person is
"acted into believing" what he or she would not have otherwise believed. Another type of self-inference occurs when a subtle attributional
configuration causes the act to be taken as relatively less diagnostic of
the person's true beliefs: The person is "acted into unbelieving" what he
or she would have otherwise believed even more. Analysis of the token
situation illustrates how episodic construal can affect both these processes of behavior-based self-inference.

The Social Salience of the Behavior

Behavior that is *public, salient, and indelible* often has a substantial impact on self-inference. Public, noticeable, and irrevocable behavior activates several cognitive, social, and motivational forces that can move
self-views in line with the attitudes and attributes implied by the act.
This may occur because the behavior launches a selective and confirmatory scan of one's past experience, or because of a drive to appear consistent to oneself and to others (see Fazio, 1987; Jones, 1990; Tice,
1992). Certainly, some situations are modally considered more "public"
than others. Most people would agree that delivering a speech at a national conference is more public than is practicing it in front of one's departmental colleagues, all other things being equal. Similarly, most people would probably agree that scheduling a specific time for a volunteer
activity is more of an "indelible commitment" than is a verbal agreement
to that effect, all other things being equal.

   However, "all other things" are very rarely equal. People who *feel*
themselves to be under greater scrutiny by others may *feel* that their
behavior is more public, salient, and indelible than if such scrutiny were
absent, and this feeling of scrutiny is determined not only by objective
features of the social situation (e.g., a departmental vs. a national audience for an editorial speech), but by the actor's contextual interpretation
of it. Thus, although perceived scrutiny may be greater on average when

one signs a pro-choice petition in the presence of 10 acquaintances than in the presence of 10 strangers, an audience of 9 strangers and 1 acquaintance might produce the most perceived scrutiny of all if that single acquaintance is one's socially conservative boss. On the other hand, precisely this same audience may produce relatively less perceived scrutiny if the petition concerns a municipal recycling program. Thus, it is not the presence of (or the number of people in) an audience per se that determines "public scrutiny" and the "indelible" or "salient" nature of one's behavior. Rather, these parameters are derived from the actor's perception of the episode as a whole: self, context, audience, and act .

Token status probably exerts a main effect on several parameters of social scrutiny. Perhaps the most defining feature of social distinctiveness is the heightened sense of attention and evaluation it engenders (e.g., Saenz, 1994). This same perceived scrutiny may also increase the press toward consistency in one's behaviors (Cialdini, 1993). One of my physically disabled first-year students described her experience during a first-term campus election when campaign literature and posters appeared in study rooms and dorm lounges. She reported three different situations in which she felt that her behavior was particularly "public"—all for slightly different reasons, but all related to her perceived token status. First, she felt that others were paying close attention to all of her responses, regardless of the campaign issue or the candidate involved—apparently indicating an awareness that her "mere salience" exerted a main effect in capturing the attentions of others (Mullen, 1991). Second, this chronic sense of social salience made baseline presses toward consistency even more clamant. When some pamphlet or petition made the rounds, this student carefully surveyed her present coactors; if any of them had also been present at a similar occasion in the past, she deliberately recalled her behavior in that earlier episode so that she could act consistently with it now (or so that she could weigh the costs of not doing so). Finally, both of these phenomena were intensified when she thought that the topic of the campaign literature would be construed by *others* as relevant to her stigma category. A pamphlet concerning the college's policy on "need-blind" admissions, for example, engendered particular perceived scrutiny on her part because she believed that "everyone thinks that all the disabled students here are on full financial aid," and she felt that others expected she would have a vested interest in the issue.

Thus several dimensions of token status may serve to make the token's behavior more subjectively "public" on several different fronts. Although this might seem to predict that the token will tend toward more internalization of public behavior than one who feels (or is) under less social scrutiny (e.g., Tice, 1992), this again is based on only one situational perception rather than on a configuration of perceptions. As the following subsections show, other beliefs that may accompany token status predict a *resistance* to behavior-based self-inference, even given (or indeed because of) the perceived salience of one's very public act.

Discrepancy between Behavior and Existing Beliefs

Several key mediators of the internalization process pertain to the match between the values one publicly airs and the values one privately holds. Whether an induced or counterattitudinal behavior falls within one's "latitude of acceptance" or "latitude of rejection"—that is, whether it is near or distant from one's true beliefs or opinions—can determine whether and how it will affect subsequent self-views. If the induced behavior is within one's latitude of acceptance (i.e., is close to one's private views), then any subsequent effect on self-perception is likely to depend on the attributions one eventually makes for one's behavior. But if the behavior falls within one's latitude of rejection (i.e., is highly discrepant from one's private views), any subsequent internalization will occur according to the principles of dissonance reduction, or if the chance to reaffirm one's true values is available (Fazio, 1987; Jones, 1990; Schlenker & Trudeau, 1990; Steele, 1988).

In the experimental lab, the constructs of the latitudes of acceptance and rejection are relatively static terms—as when socially undesirable behavior is presumed to fall within subjects' latitude of rejection (e.g., Jones, 1990; Rhodewalt & Agustsdottir, 1986), or when a subject's attitude on a topic is measured, and the induced or assigned behavior is constructed to represent a stance either close to or grossly discrepant from that value (e.g., Schlenker & Trudeau, 1990). However, the identical utterance may move in or out of one's latitude of acceptance across different situations, because the very notion of the "acceptability" of that view to oneself is based in part on one's understanding of the contingencies of the situation as a whole. For example, a mild radicalization of one's support of affirmative action may fall within one's latitude of acceptance during a meeting of the NAACP (where it may be encouraged and socially rewarded, and, if uttered, will imply particular things about oneself), but may fall outside one's latitude of acceptance if expressed to one's socially conservative supervisors at work (where it may be discouraged or socially punished). This shifting in one's latitude of acceptance is also implied by research showing how the social negativity of a social act and the actor's sensitivity to social norms can moderate the private acceptance of the induced expression (see Jones, 1990). Thus, because the same act can serve different goals, be shaped by different social antecedents, or produce different social effects, it can take on differ-

ent meanings for the actor and thereby functionally define different latitudes of acceptance for that behavior across different social contexts.

Tokens evince a common (and probably necessary) sensitivity to dynamics of power and status, and a sharp vigilance for potential social
sanctions (Saenz, 1994; Tedeschi & Norman, 1985). When paired with
reflective expectancies about the beliefs of one's coactors, shifts in the
latitude of acceptance for any given act might be expected for the token
across different social contexts. Sam and Sue may hold exactly the same
private opinion on issue X as measured on a questionnaire, but whether
that opinion falls within their latitude of acceptance or rejection will depend on the social situation in which that opinion is voiced—for instance, if that situation does or does not make a token of them. Moreover, the *range* of a token's latitude of acceptance may also change—in
particular, it may narrow—when the content of the interaction is related
to one's social category. Tokens may often feel called upon to inflate the
confidence with which they express group-related opinions, or feel pressure to present a "unified front" on issues related to their social group:
"I'll certainly consider how O. J. Simpson might be guilty when we're
hanging out in the [African-American student union]," one student told
me, "but otherwise . . . no way!" It is an interesting empirical question
whether, how, and under what conditions such strategic and issue-ori-
ented public communications affect a token's private self-views (e.g.,
Fleming & Rudman, 1993).

Standards of Self-Judgment and Social Identity

Another parameter of behavior-based self-inference is the standard
against which one compares one's public act—a parameter that parallels
many of the "audience" factors affecting the choice of public behavior.
The people around one, one's relationships with them, the social context, and the content of one's communication can activate particular
comparisons between self and others (Mullen, 1991), can highlight discrepancies between various self-views (Higgins, 1987; Schlenker, 1986;
Schlenker & Leary, 1982), and can bring particular social identities to
the fore (Brewer, 1991; Cheek, 1989; Tajfel & Turner, 1986). These
evaluative anchors can affect behavior-based self-inference because they
affect perceptions of the discrepancy between one's behavior and one's
private views, the behavior's agreement with social norms, its relevance
to oneself, and its perceived social effect—all potential mediators of the
self-perception process (e.g., Fazio, 1987; Jones, 1990; Schlenker, 1986).

It is an empirical question whether tokens and nontokens systematically differ in *which* evaluative standards will dominate in any given situation, and what (if any) effect those standards will have on subsequent

self-perception. At the very least, however, such standards are likely to be more *variable* for the token than for the nontoken across different social episodes, and along the same dimensions that define token status itself (Crocker et al., 1998). The notion of episodic construal may be useful for exploring the complex relationships among social comparison standards, cultural and social status, and group composition (e.g., Brewer et al., 1993; Markus & Kitayama, 1991; Oyserman & Markus, 1993), because it represents the ways in which these variables can be configured in particular social situations. An obese student may have different standards of self-judgment in the dining hall or the gym than in the study group or the classroom, but even his or her standards in the study group may differ from those in the classroom, depending on what topic is being discussed, the specific others who are present, and his or her relationship to them.

Attributional Processes

Several of the self-perception processes discussed above speak to how actors construe the forces and constraints on their behavior. Indeed, several other mediators and moderators of the internalization process explicitly rest on an actor's attributional analysis for his or her behavior. For example, acts that are perceived to be *self-generated* and feel *freely chosen,* and those that are judged *self-relevant* and that implicate personal *responsibility*, are more likely to affect self-views than are behaviors attributed to less self-implicating or more external sources (see Fazio, 1987; Tice, 1992; and the volumes by Baumeister, 1986, and Olson & Zanna, 1990).

The token example illustrates how the same behavior under one episodic construal can produce attributions supporting internalization, but under another episodic construal can produce attributions supporting resistance to internalization. Consider, for example, token Sue, a junior executive who generally supports the affirmative action hiring principles that her corporation vigorously pursues. Now imagine that during a corporate conference she expresses a somewhat stronger support for the practice than she privately holds. All other things being equal, this would represent a "within-latitude-of-acceptance" public stance that, if it were induced in the lab under the proper conditions, could strengthen her private support for the policy. Will this happen for Sue?

It depends. If she attributes her slightly radicalized statement to the tendency of any speaker to polarize or "boost volume" on one's views when facing a large and arousing crowd (Bond, 1982), or, indeed, if she is unaware that her behavior has even been affected at all (Vorauer & Miller, 1997), then her private opinion will probably not change. If, on the other hand, she feels (as a function of her salient token status) that her behavior is more public and indelible (i.e., under particular scrutiny by others and evoking expectations of consistency), then her private support for the policy may well strengthen (Tice, 1992). However, the same salient token status that predicts this internalization also invites a host of salient *external* attributions for her behavior—attributions that may result in *resistance* to an alteration in self-views. For instance, if she believes that others already expect her to hold this "stereotypic" opinion, if she feels compelled because of some gender loyalty or responsibility to espouse it, or if she can clearly identify the forces that compel her as a vulnerable token to conform publicly with her boss—in other words, if she feels she has acted *as* a token—then she may take her public action as due to these social constraints and as that much less diagnostic of her inner values and beliefs (Cialdini, Green, & Rusch, 1992; Jones & Davis, 1965). In this example, what might be considered a single communication in the laboratory can predict three different effects on private views when expressed in different social contexts: polarization, discounting, or no effect at all.

Hypotheses about this situation may be generated by two principles of behavior-based self-inference. The first is that the perceived self-diagnosticity of one's behavior may erode to the extent that one can cite a clear external reason for it (e.g., Fazio, 1987; Jones, 1990; Lepper, 1983; Schlenker, 1986; Schlenker & Trudeau, 1990). Thus, if token junior executive Sue expresses a sentiment that "those of her gender" are stereotypically expected to hold, she may discount some degree of this expression as at least partially due to her spokesperson role. The second principle, however, is that this potential discounting cue is more likely to be used as such in the absence of a strong internal justification for one's public stance—in Sue's case, for instance, if she is somewhat uncertain about the issue to begin with (e.g., Fazio, 1987; Schlenker, 1986; Swann & Ely, 1984). Thus it is when intrinsic justification for the "group interest" aspect of one's public expression is relatively weak that one may chalk up some portion of it to one's role as group representative (Cioffi, 1995). Even a truthful, self-generated statement of opinion can take on different meanings to the actor—and therefore have different self-inferential effects—when it is expressed under the mantle of different social roles.[1]

THE RELENTLESS SPOTLIGHT: SOME PROCESS EFFECTS

A defining experience for the stigmatized token is feeling caught by a bright and relentless social spotlight: on stage, distinguished, and observed. On the beams of this spotlight ride two potential saboteurs of smooth social interaction: intense self-focus and social anxiety. Substantial literatures exist on the effects of these twin tariffs on various self-regulatory processes (see reviews by Gibbons, 1990, and Schlenker & Leary, 1982), and this work generates many questions crosscutting the issues of behavioral choice and self-inference for the social token. Although exploration of these issues deserves another discussion entirely, a few are outlined here. Of particular interest is how self-attention and social anxiety may affect the *processes* of behavioral choice and self-perception in ways that imply a particular liability for the social token. Anxiety and self-focus exact a cost from all social actors, but the cost may be especially high for those who most value the very outcomes likely to be disrupted—smooth social interactions, competent performance, and fine-grained control of self-presentational behavior.

Cognitive Effects

A social token is a preoccupied and absorbed social actor, acutely aware of the attentions and the evaluations of others. These and other concerns can encumber attention and drain cognitive resources, producing deficits of various sorts in memory, judgment, and inference (see Saenz, 1994). But the same token status that encumbers cognitive resources also pulls for extra vigilance or "mindfulness" of the social dynamic and of what one does and says (Baumeister & Kenneth, 1992; Frable et al., 1990; Schlenker & Leary, 1982). This is because tokens' preoccupation with "self" subsumes an acute sensitivity to self-relevant aspects of the environment—in other words, to the evaluations others are making of them (Wicklund & Gollwitzer, 1987). What are the consequences for tokens, who operate under both a strong motive for social vigilance and a significant attentional tax? With a few exceptions (e.g., Lord, Saenz, & Godfrey, 1987; Pendry & Macrae, 1994; Saenz, 1994), this question remains largely unexplored and is ripe for future study. Research on the effect of cognitive load on the attributional process suggests that some consequences spell a relative immunity to shifts in private beliefs, while other consequences spell a particular susceptibility to them (Chaiken, Liberman, & Eagly, 1989; Doherty & Schlenker, 1991; Gilbert, Pelham, & Krull, 1988; Tedeschi, 1986).

The arousal and vigilance that bloom under the spotlight can affect not only the type of attributions one makes for one's behavior, but the effort one expends on the diagnostic. High personal involvement, the need for predictability and control, and the anticipation of negative social outcomes—all possible if not common concerns for the token—usually intensify one's attributional analyses (see Gibbons, 1990). Yet it is ironic that some conditions that would normally release one from this attributional vigilance (such as positive social feedback) may be those that tokens are most likely to distrust or discount (e.g., Crocker & Major, 1989). Another irony germinates if the token situation induces doubts about one's competencies and worth; normally such self-doubts induce an avoidance of self-focusing at all costs (Baumeister & Heatherton, 1996), but this regulatory response may be blocked for the token, who also feels compelled to monitor thoughts and behaviors (Saenz, 1994). Intense attributional analysis is not always maladaptive, of course; effective problem solving and successful self-regulation sometimes rely on it. If, however, tokens attribute their social arousal to token status—that is, if they use a salient and ready environmental (social) attribution for any social anxiety they may feel—then an attributional vigilance that might be adaptive in that situation may be replaced by attributional disengagement instead (e.g., Pittman & Heller, 1987).

Cognitive preoccupation and attentional drain can affect self-presentational processes in a number of ways and through a number of pathways (see Doherty & Schlenker, 1991; Neuberg, 1994; Schlenker & Leary, 1982). These effects may become more significant—and potentially self-perpetuating—when paired with the multiple or conflicting self-presentational goals that tokens may commonly experience: The more one is preoccupied with presentational concerns, the fewer resources one can dedicate to successful impression management tasks, and with less success in the task comes even more preoccupation with it (Baumeister & Kenneth, 1992; LaRonde & Swann, 1993; Schlenker & Leary, 1982). Anxious self-focus and a narrowing of attention may also decouple the token's actions from higher goals and plans, disrupting goal-directed behavior and subverting emotional regulation (Baumeister, 1990; Baumeister & Heatherton, 1996; Martin, Tesser, & McIntosh, 1993; Scheier & Carver, 1988; Wegner & Vallacher, 1986). One intriguing question is how the disregulation of social action plus heavy cognitive load may increase the probability that an actor will behaviorally confirm the stereotypes of others—an irony that, if true, would be particularly cruel in the case of the social token (see Neuberg, 1994; Vallacher, Wegner, McMahan, & Cotter, 1992).

Behavioral Inhibition

Social tokens often report that they worry about disconfirming the expectancies of others, and about being "fairly" and accurately perceived. When coupled with social anxiety and a risk-aversive stance, which often accompany token status, behavioral inhibition may be a common response (DePaulo, Epstein, & Lemay, 1990; Josephs, Larrick, Steele, &

Nisbett, 1992; Schlenker & Leary, 1982). A preliminary pilot study from my lab explored this situation and its possible impact on subsequent self-views (Cioffi & Jaffe, 1993). We found that female "tokens" in small discussion groups were most anxious (based on later self-reports) and behaviorally inhibited (based on codes of amount of time spent talking) when the assigned topic of discussion was gender-related (e.g., whether the college had done an adequate job of hiring and promoting women faculty members). Moreover, tokens reported they believed their coactors thought they "already knew" (or guessed) what they "really" thought on these topics. Thus, when the topics under discussion were those on which they expected their coactors to hold stereotypic beliefs about their opinions, token women felt anxious and prejudged, and many of them responded with relative silence.

Could this behavioral inhibition affect self-inference? An affirmative prediction comes from one potential bias in the self-perception process: the tendency to draw weaker self-inferences from one's inaction than from one's logically equivalent action (Cioffi, 1994; Cioffi & Garner, 1996; Fazio, Sherman, & Herr, 1982). Thus, if a token in our above-described study wanted to speak in support of gender-relevant opinion X but was induced by her situation to express this opinion passively—that is, by what she didn't say rather than by what she did—she might have left that situation with a weakened personal commitment to X. However, we expected this sort of moderation in private opinions to occur mainly among token women who were most uncertain about their attitudes on these gender-relevant issues to begin with. This is because behavior-based inference of any sort is usually more likely when private, internal knowledge about one's values is relatively weak (Cioffi, 1995; Fazio, 1987; Jones, 1990; Rhodewalt, 1986; Schlenker & Trudeau, 1990; Tice, 1992). Indeed, 50% of the token women who were most uncertain about the gender-relevant topics before the start of the experiment became even more uncertain about them after the experiment (as compared to 15% of the more certain token subjects), and only for the uncertain women did their degree of behavioral inhibition while discussing that topic significantly correlate with increased uncertainty about it. Thus, although behavioral inhibition was induced in most female token subjects during gender-relevant discussions, only the previously uncertain women apparently viewed this socially induced silence as diagnostic of the "weakness" or instability of their private beliefs.

There are other reasons besides social anxiety why tokens may "do nothing" in certain interaction domains: Chronically grappling with perceived negative expectancies of others may produce exhaustion, frustration—and disengagement (Steele, 1997). Whether social passivity under such conditions can stimulate further disengagement through a route of behavior-based self-inference is an important question that awaits exploration.[2]

Compensatory Communication Goals

Of course, grappling with the stable expectancies of others sometimes elicits a rather more active response. A reflective expectancy is a presumption of bias in one's audience: in what they expect, in what they will "see," and in what they will "hear." Thus, if one's social motives include any particular self-presentational or communicative goal, the presumed biases of others must be taken into account if one is to succeed in meeting that goal (Cioffi, 1999). Just as the student who wants to convey a studious impression to a skeptical professor may try to compensate behaviorally for that skepticism, so the token who wants to communicate impression or opinion X to an audience biased to expect and to hear X minus 3 must boost her communication of X accordingly.

Will behavior that is altered in service of a social communication goal come to affect privately held views? Research on the "communication game" by McCann, Higgins, and colleagues speaks to precisely this question (McCann & Higgins, 1992). This work shows that under some conditions, people do "tune" their communications for their audience (i.e., compensate for the presumed biases of their listeners), and these altered communications in turn can affect the communicator's private beliefs. In this research, the actor's knowledge of audience bias is manipulated directly—by explicitly telling the communicator what his or her audience already believes. Preliminary studies in our lab (Cioffi & Hebl, 1994) explored whether reflective expectancies are sufficient to activate a presumption of listener bias, to produce communications tuned to correct for that bias, and to create subsequent alterations in private self-views (e.g., Darley, Fleming, Hilton, & Swann, 1988). Subjects were asked to convey a precise opinion (expressed as a numerical point on an opinion scale), and we varied whether the subjects thought that their audience would or would not know their sex when estimating the opinion conveyed in each script. Thus writers who thought that readers would know their sex were "unshielded" or "exposed" to any presumed gender-based assumptions of their audience, whereas writers who thought their sex would be unspecified were "shielded" from these presumed audience expectations. The pattern of results suggested that subjects did adjust their communications as a function of this manipulation. In comparison to the shielded women, unshielded women "pulled their punches" on gender-relevant scripts in which their assigned opinion conveyed the stereotypic "women's opinion." That is, they moderated the extremity of that expressed opinion, presumably in order to "hit" the assigned impression target in a reader who might already presume "pro-woman" opinions from the writer. Similarly, communications of the un-shielded women who were instructed to convey an opinion disagreeing with the stereotypic "woman's opinion" were more extremely opposed to the statement than were those written by unshielded women given that same communication goal—again, a pattern that can be interpreted as a compensation in service of meeting the assigned communication goal, given an audience who might have a particular (directional) expectancy about what a female writer would believe. Supplementary analyses provided some evidence for the self-perceptual impact of these tuned communications. Subjects who indicated an awareness of the relationship between their sex and their success at meeting the assigned communication goal (according to their responses on a final questionnaire) were somewhat less likely to alter the content of their gender-relevant scripts—and among these women, any tuning that did occur was less likely to predict subsequent shifts in private opinion on these topics. This suggests an attributional mediation for both behavioral alteration and subsequent self-perception: Clear cognizance that one may be swayed by the expectations of others may decrease the probability that one will in fact be so swayed (Neuberg, 1994), and for the same reason, any behavioral alterations that do occur may be internalized to a lesser degree (Fazio, 1987; Schlenker & Weigold,1992; Tice, 1992).

GENERAL SUMMARY AND CONCLUSIONS

Summary of the Literature Review

Research on self-presentation has grown in recent years, in part due to a revitalized interest in self-perception processes, with which it is both conceptually and functionally related. Much of this recent work illustrates how the self-presentation process is enmeshed with the self-perception process at the most fundamental levels. I have tried to unpack the implications of this theme by highlighting the degree to which both processes actually flow from the same perceptual construct: the actor's episodic construal. It is an integrated perception that will guide both social behavior and also behavior-based self-inference, because it describes the actor's understanding of the cause, function, and effect—indeed, the very meaning—of his or her social act.

The second major thesis advanced in this chapter is that token status often represents natural variations in one's episodic construal because of the same psychosocial parameters that create token status to begin with. A skewed distribution or biased accessibility of various situational scripts; multiple and potentially conflicting self-identifications and social identities; heightened social vigilance and self-awareness; greater perceived scrutiny of one's behavior and potentially more perceived pressure to be consistent; a sensitivity to social norms and to potential social sanctions or rewards; an enlarged set of attributional accounts for one's behavior—all these are different configurations of variables that will affect both the choice of public behavior and its subsequent effect on private self-views. Moreover, several potentially chronic features of token status relating to social anxiety and self-focus may sabotage various regulatory processes in particularly ironic and unkind ways, while the possibilities of particular attributions, behavioral inhibition, and corrective communications further complicate the social picture. The well-developed general literatures on self-presentation, self-inference, and social regulation are readily applicable to many questions of behavior choice and self-perception in the social token.

The Looking-Glass Self Revisited

"I feel I am what others tell me I am" is the simple looking-glass metaphor of an earlier time, in which we see ourselves as reflected in the appraisals of others (e.g., Cooley, 1902; Mead, 1934). Thia metaphor has since been modified by an awareness that this reflection is filtered through our own preexisting self-views (e.g., Felson, 1993; Kenny & DePaulo, 1993; Shrauger & Schoeneman, 1979; Stryker, 1981); we feel we are what others say we are, but we come to know what this is in part because of what we believe ourselves to be. The integration of the disparate literatures discussed in this chapter now suggests even more reflective pathways by which social interaction affects private self-views: The social milieu as apprehended by the actor shapes his or her public behavior, thereby plowing open two additional channels through which self-views may change. First, the actor may now have a different behavioral history upon which to draw in any process of behavior-based self-inference (path "d" of Figure 7.1). But just as often, the same psychosocial forces that have had a hand in shaping the public behavior have also simultaneously tinkered with the self-perceptual machine itself—by suggesting additional or alternate attributions for the behavior, by having activated different standards by which it is judged, or by increasing the accessibility of certain identities or social goals, to cite only a few examples (path "c" of Figure 7.1). Thus the looking-glass self stands not before a single social reflection, but in a veritable hall of mirrors.

Finally, although the central concepts of this chapter have been illustrated using the token as an example, there is nothing about the concepts themselves that would limit their application to this particular social phenomenon. This is because the dynamics of token status represent phenotypical examples of genotypical psychological processes—that is, particular configurations of larger psychosocial principles to which all social actors are subject. Moreover, any number of psychosocial phenomena might be illuminated by the notion that behavioral choice and self-perception are mediated by an actor's episodic construal. If the present ideas were to be applied to the study of behavioral choice and self-perception in the nontoken as well, this chapter would find its final reflective metaphor: In exploring the hall of mirrors that surrounds the social token, we may come to see ourselves more clearly.

ACKNOWLEDGMENTS

Thanks to Steven Neuberg, Barry Schlenker, and several anonymous grant reviewers for their engaged comments on earlier drafts of this chapter, and to Robert Cialdini, Martin Davidson, and Yolanda Niemann, whose conversations with me contributed to the ideas herein.

NOTES

1. Another exploration of this representative pressure might revolve around the theory of self-affirmation as advanced by Steele and colleagues (Steele, 1988; Steele, Spencer, & Lynch, 1993), especially in situations where one's behavior is substantially altered. Although the role constraint of representing one's group might normally induce a token to deflect some personal responsibility for strong public expression of group-related interests (Cioffi, 1995), and the extremity of one's behavior might also work against any change in self-views (Fazio, Zanna, & Cooper, 1977), the subsequent chance to affiliate with others of one's group may provide an opportunity to "reclaim" the spirit of these public utterances, thus mitigating any suspension of self-inference that might otherwise occur. The mediational role of ingroup interaction and affiliation on the self-perceptual effects of constrained public behavior is ripe for future research.

2. The ultimate irony is that any such silence or behavioral disengagement may actually exacerbate stereotypic perceptions rather than circumvent them. In a recent study (Cioffi, 1998), perceivers read what they were told were transcripts of discussions on various topics, purportedly among groups of different gender compositions (e.g., female minority vs. female majority). The *content* of the expressed opinions was held constant (all "discussants" expressed the same moderate opinion on each topic), but the *amount* of discussion by each individual was manipulated (relative verbosity vs. relative silence). When a lone woman in a group of men said relatively little during a discussion about sexism on campus, both male and female perceivers interpreted her relative silence as motivated by a desire to avoid "making trouble" as a token gender representative, and inferred from her nonbehavior a high involvement with and support of "women's issues."

REFERENCES

Abelson, R. (1981). Psychological status of the script concept. *American Psychologist, 36*, 715–729.

Allport, G. W. (1954). *The nature of prejudice.* Reading, MA: Addison-Wesley.

Archer, D. (1985). Social deviance. In G. Lindzey & E. Aronson (Eds.), *Handbook of social psychology: Vol. 2. Special fields and applications* (3rd ed., pp. 743–804). New York: Random House.

Baldwin, M. W. (1992). Relational schemas and the processing of social information. *Psychological Bulletin, 112*, 461–484.

Banaji, M. R., & Prentice, D. A. (1994). The self in social contexts. *Annual Review of Psychology, 45*, 297–332.

Baumeister, R. F. (1982). A self-presentational view of social phenomena. *Psychological Bulletin, 91*, 3–26.

Baumeister, R. F. (Ed.). (1986). *Public self and private self.* New York: Springer-Verlag.

Baumeister, R. F. (1990). Anxiety and deconstruction: On escaping the self. In J. M. Olson & M. P. Zanna (Eds.), *The Ontario symposium: Vol. 6. Self-inference processes* (pp. 259–291). Hillsdale, NJ: Erlbaum.

Baumeister, R. F. (1993). Understanding the inner nature of low self-esteem: Uncertain, fragile, protective, and conflicted. In R. F. Baumeister (Ed.), *Self-esteem: The puzzle of low self-regard* (pp. 201–218). New York: Plenum Press.

Baumeister, R. F., & Heatherton, T. F. (1996). Self-regulation failure: An overview. *Psychological Inquiry, 7,* 1–15.

Baumeister, R. F., & Kenneth, C. J. (1992). Repression and self-presentation: When audiences interfere with self-deceptive strategies. *Journal of Personality and Social Psychology, 62*, 851–862.

Bond, C. F. (1982). Social facilitation: A self-presentational view. *Journal of Personality and Social Psychology, 42*, 1042–1050.

Brewer, M. B. (1991). The social self: On being the same and different at the same time. *Personality and Social Psychology Bulletin, 17*, 475–482.

Brewer, M. B., Manzi, J. M., & Shaw, J. S. (1993). In-group identification as a function of depersonalization, disctinctiveness, and status. *Psychological Science, 4*, 88–92.

Brown, L. M. (1998). Ethnic stigma as a contextual experience: A possible selves perspective. *Personality and Social Psychology Bulletin, 24*, 163–172.

Chaiken, S., Liberman, A., & Eagly, A. H. (1989). Heuristic and systematic information processing within and beyond the persuasion context. In J. S. Uleman & J. A. Bargh (Eds.), *Unintended thought* (pp. 212–252). New York: Guilford Press.

Cheek, J. M. (1989). Identity orientations and self-interpretation. In D. M. Buss & N. Cantor (Eds.), *Personality psychology: Recent trends and emerging directions* (pp. 275–285). New York: Springer-Verlag.

Cialdini, R. B. (1993). *Influence: Science and practice.* New York: HarperCollins.

Cialdini, R. B., Green, B. L., & Rusch, A. J. (1992). When tactical pronouncements of change become real changes: The case of reciprocal persuasion. *Journal of Personality and Social Psychology, 63*, 30–41.

Cioffi, D. (1994). When good news is bad news: Medical wellness as a non-event. *Health Psychology, 13*, 63–72.

Cioffi, D. (1995). Who's opinion is this anyway?: Self-inferential affects of representing one's social group. *Social Cognition, 13*, 341–363.

Cioffi, D. (1998). *Expectancies and the perceived diagnosticity of nonbehavior.* Manuscript submitted for publication.

Cioffi, D. (1999). *Selective suspicion: Static and dynamic components of social stereotypes.* Manuscript submitted for publication.

Cioffi, D., & Garner, R. (1996). On doing the decision: The effects of active versus passive choice on commitment and self-perception. *Personality and Social Psychology Bulletin, 22*, 133–147.

Cioffi, D., & Hebl, M. (1994). [Communicative corrections for the bias of others: Effects on self-perception]. Unpublished raw data, Dartmouth College.

Cioffi, D., & Jaffe, S. (1993). [The effects of discussion topic on tokens' group behavior]. Unpublished raw data, Dartmouth College.

Clark, H. H., & Brennan, S. E. (1991). Grounding in communication. In L. B. Resnick, J. M. Levine, & S. D. Teasley (Eds.), *Perspectives on socially shared cognition* (pp. 127–149). Washington, DC: American Psychological Association.

Cooley, C. H. (1902). *Human nature and the social order.* New York: Scribner.

Crocker, J., & Major, B. (1989). Social stigma and self-esteem: The self-protective properties of stigma. *Psychological Review, 96*, 608–630.

Crocker, J., Major, B., & Steele, C. (1998). Social stigma. In D. T. Gilbert, S. T. Fiske, & G. Lindzey (Eds.), *Handbook of social psychology* (4th ed., Vol. 2, pp. 504–553). Boston: McGraw-Hill.

Darley, J. M., Fleming, J. H., Hilton, J. L., & Swann, W. B., Jr. (1988). Dispelling negative expectancies: The impact of interaction goals and target characteristics on the expectancy confirmation process. *Journal of Experimental Social Psychology, 24*, 19–36.

Davidson, M., & Cioffi, D. (1993). [Structured interviews with Black students at Dartmouth]. Unpublished raw data, Dartmouth College.

DePaulo, B. M., Epstein, J. A., & Lemay, C. S. (1990). Responses of the socially anxious to the prospect of interpersonal evaluation. *Journal of Personality, 58*, 623–640.

Doherty, K., & Schlenker, B. R. (1991). Self-consciousness and strategic self-presentation. *Journal of Personality, 59*, 1–18.

Dovidio, J. F., Brigham, J. C., Johnson, B. T., & Gaertner, S. L. (1996). Stereotyping, prejudice, and discrimination: Another look. In N. Macrae, C. Stangor, & M. Hewstone (Eds.), *Stereotypes and stereotyping* (pp. 276–319). New York: Guilford Press.

Emmons, R. A., King, L. A., & Sheldon, K. (1993). Goal conflict and the self-regulation of action. In D. M. Wegner & J. W. Pennebaker (Eds.), *Handbook of mental control* (pp. 528–551). Englewood Cliffs, NJ: Prentice-Hall.

Fazio, R. H. (1987). Self-perception theory: A current perspective. In M. P. Zanna, J. M. Olson, & C. P. Herman (Eds.), *The Ontario Symposium: Vol. 5. Social influence* (pp. 129–149). Hillsdale NJ: Erlbaum.

Fazio, R. H., Sherman, S. J., & Herr, P. M. (1982). The feature-positive effect in the self-perception process: Does not doing matter as much as doing? *Journal of Personality and Social Psychology, 42*, 404–411.

Fazio, R. H., Zanna, M. P., & Cooper, J. (1977). Dissonance and self-perception: An integrative view of each theory's domain of application. *Journal of Experimental Social Psychology, 13*, 464–479.

Felson, R. B. (1993). The (somewhat) social self: How others affect self-appraisals. In J. Suls (Ed.), *Psychological perspectives on the self* (Vol. 4, pp. 1–26). Hillsdale, NJ: Erlbaum.

Fleming, J. H., & Rudman, L. A. (1993). Between a rock and a hard place: Self-concept regulating and communicative properties of distancing behaviors. *Journal of Personality and Social Psychology, 64*, 44–59.

Frable, D. E. S. (1993). Dimensions of marginality: Distinctions among those who are different. *Personality and Social Psychology Bulletin, 19*, 370–380.

Frable, D. E. S., Blackstone, T., & Scherbaum, C. (1990). Marginal and mindful: Deviants in social interactions. *Journal of Personality and Social Psychology, 59*, 140–149.

Gardner, R. C. (1994). Stereotypes as consensual beliefs. In M. P. Zanna & J. M. Olson (Eds.), *The Ontario Symposium: Vol. 7. The psychology of prejudice* (pp. 1–31). Hillsdale, NJ: Erlbaum.

Gibbons, F. X. (1990). Self-attention and behavior: A review and theoretical update. In M. P. Zanna (Ed.), *Advances in experimental social psychology* (Vol. 23, pp. 249–303). San Diego, CA: Academic Press.

Gilbert, D. T., Pelham, B. W., & Krull, D. S. (1988). On cognitive busyness: When person perceivers meet persons perceived. *Journal of Personality and Social Psychology, 54*, 733–740.

Goffman, E. (1963). *Stigma: Notes on the management of spoiled identity.* Englewood Cliffs, NJ: Prentice-Hall.

Higgins, E. T. (1987). Self-discrepancy: A theory relating self and affect. *Psychological Review, 94*, 319–340.

Higgins, E. T. (1990). Personality, social psychology, and person–situation relations: Standards and knowledge activation as a common language. In L. A. Pervin (Ed.), *Handbook of personality: Theory and research* (pp. 301–338). New York: Guilford Press.

Jones, E. E. (1990). Constrained behavior and self-concept change. In J. M. Olson & M. P. Zanna (Ed.), *The Ontario symposium: Vol. 6. Self-inference processes* (pp. 69–86). Hillsdale, NJ: Erlbaum.

Jones, E. E., & Davis, K. E. (1965). From acts to dispositions: The attribution process in person perception. In L. Berkowitz (Ed.), *Advances in experimental social psychology* (Vol. 2, pp. 219–266). New York: Academic Press.

Jones, E. E., Farina, A., Hastorf, A. H., Markus, H., Miller, D. T., & Scott, R. A. (1984). *Social stigma: The psychology of marked relationships.* New York: Freeman.

Jones, E. E., & Pittman, T. S. (1982). Toward a general theory of strategic self-presentation. In J. Suls (Ed.), *Psychological perspectives on the self* (Vol. 1, pp. 231–262). Hillsdale, NJ: Erlbaum.

Josephs, R. A., Larrick, R. P., Steele, C. M., & Nisbett, R. E. (1992). Protecting the self from the negative consequences of risky decisions. *Journal of Personality and Social Psychology, 62,* 26–37.

Kenny, D. A., & DePaulo, B. M. (1993). Do people know how others view them?: An empirical and theoretical account. *Psychological Bulletin, 114,* 145–161.

LaRonde, C., & Swann, W. B. (1993). Caught in the crossfire: Positivity and self-verification strivings among people with low self-esteem. In R. F. Baumeister (Ed.), *Self-esteem: The puzzle of low self-regard* (pp. 147–166). New York: Plenum Press.

Leary, M. R. (1993). The interplay of private self-processes and interpersonal factors in self-presentation. In J. Suls (Ed.), *Psychological perspectives on the self* (Vol. 4, pp. 127–155). Hillsdale, NJ: Erlbaum.

Leary, M. R., & Kowalski, R. M. (1990). Impression management: A literature review and two-component model. *Psychological Bulletin, 107,* 34–47.

Lepper, M. R. (1983). Social-control processes and the internalization of social values: an attributional perspective. In E. T. Higgins, D. N. Ruble, & W. W. Hartup (Eds.), *Social cognition and social development* (pp. 294–330). New York: Cambridge University Press.

Levine, J. M., Resnik, L. B., & Higgins, E. T. (1993). Social foundations of cognition. *Annual Review of Psychology, 44,* 585–612.

Lord, C. G., Saenz, D. S., & Godfrey, D. K. (1987). Effects of perceived scrutiny on participant memory for social interactions. *Journal of Experimental Social Psychology, 23,* 498–517.

Major, B., & Crocker, J. (1993). Social stigma: The affective consequences of attributional ambiguity. In D. M. Mackie & D. L. Hamilton (Eds.), *Affect, cognition, and stereotyping* (pp. 345–370). San Diego, CA: Academic Press.

Markus, H., & Cross, S. (1990). The interpersonal self. In L. A. Pervin (Ed.), *Handbook of personality: Theory and research* (pp. 576–608). New York: Guilford Press.

Markus, H. R., & Kitayama, S. (1991). Culture and the self: Implications for cognition, emotion, and motivation. *Psychological Review, 98,* 224–253.

Martin, L. L., Tesser, A., & McIntosh, W. D. (1993). Wanting but not having: The effects of unattained goals on thoughts and feelings. In D. M. Wegner & J. W. Pennebaker (Eds.), *Handbook of mental control* (pp. 552–572). Englewood Cliffs, NJ: Prentice-Hall.

McArthur, L. Z., & Baron, R. M. (1983). Toward an ecological theory of social perception. *Psychological Review, 90,* 215–247.

McCann, C. D., & Higgins, E. T. (1992). Personal and contextual factors in communication: A review of "the communication game." In G. R. Semin & V. Fiedler (Eds.), *Language, interaction, and social cognition* (pp. 144–172). London: Sage.

McGuire, W. J., & McGuire, C. V. (1981). The spontaneous self-concept as affected by personal distinctiveness. In M. D. Lynch, A. Norem-Hebeisen, & K. Gergen (Eds.), *The self-concept* (pp. 147–171). Cambridge, MA: Ballinger.

Mead, G. H. (1934). *Mind, self, and society.* Chicago: University of Chicago Press.

Mullen, B. (1991). Group composition, salience, and cognitive representations: The phenomenology of being in a group. *Journal of Experimental Social Psychology, 27,* 297–323.

Neuberg, S. L. (1994). Expectancy-confirmation processes in stereotype-tinged social encounters: The moderating role of social goals. In M. P. Zanna & J. M.
Olson (Ed.), *The Ontario symposium: Vol. 7. The psychology of prejudice*
(pp. 103–130). Hillsdale, NJ: Erlbaum.

Niemann, Y. F., & Secord, P. F. (1995). The social ecology of stereotyping. *Journal
of the Theory of Social Behavior, 25,* 1–13.

Olson, J. M., & Zanna, M. P. (Eds.). (1990). *The Ontario Symposium: Vol. 6. Self-
inference processes.* Hillsdale, NJ: Erlbaum.

Oyserman, D., & Markus, H. R. (1993). The sociocultural self. In J. Suls (Ed.),
Psychological perspectives on the self (Vol. 4, pp. 187–220). Hillsdale, NJ:
Erlbaum.

Pendry, L. F., & Macrae, C. N. (1994). Stereotypes and mental life: The case of the
motivated but thwarted tactician. *Journal of Experimental Social Psychology, 30,* 303–325.

Pittman, T. S., & Heller, J. F. (1987). Social motivation. *Annual Review of Psychology, 38,* 461–489.

Rhodewalt, F. T. (1986). Self-presentation and the phenomenal self: On the stability and malleability of self-conceptions. In R. F. Baumeister (Ed.), *Public self
and private self* (pp. 117–142). New York: Springer-Verlag.

Rhodewalt, F., & Agustsdottir, S. (1986). Effects of self-presentation on the phenomenal self. *Journal of Personality and Social Psychology, 50,* 47–55.

Ross, L. (1990). Recognizing the role of construal processes. In I. Rock (Ed.), *The
legacy of Solomon Asch: Essays in cognition and social psychology* (pp. 77–
96). Hillsdale, NJ: Erlbaum.

Saenz, D. S. (1994). Token status and problem-solving deficits: Detrimental effects
of distinctiveness and performance monitoring. *Social Cognition, 12,* 61–74.

Scheier, M. F., & Carver, C. S. (1988). A model of behavioral self-regulation:
Translating intention into action. In L. Berkowitz (Ed.), *Advances in experi-
mental social psychology* (Vol. 21, pp. 303–346). New York: Academic
Press.

Schlenker, B. R. (1986). Self-identification: Toward an integration of the private
and public self. In R. F. Baumeister (Ed.), *Public self and private self* (pp. 21–
62). New York: Springer-Verlag.

Schlenker, B. R., Dlugolecki, D. W., & Doherty, K. (1994). The impact of self-presentations on self-appraisals and behavior: The power of public commitment.
Personality and Social Psychology Bulletin, 20, 20–33.

Schlenker, B. R., & Leary, M. R. (1982). Social anxiety and self-presentation: A
conceptualization and model. *Psychological Bulletin, 92,* 641–669.

Schlenker, B. R., & Trudeau, J. V. (1990). Impact of self-presentations on private
self-beliefs: Effects of prior self-beliefs and misattribution. *Journal of Personality and Social Psychology, 58,* 22–32.

Schlenker, B. R., & Weigold, M. F. (1992). Interpersonal processes involving impression regulation and management. *Annual Review of Psychology, 43,*
133–168.

Shilts, R. (1993). *Conduct unbecoming: Gays and lesbians in the U.S. military.*
New York: St. Martin's Press.

Shoda, Y., Mischel, W., & Wright, J. C. (1993). Links between personality judgments and contextualized behavior patterns: Situation–behavior profiles of personality prototypes. *Social Cognition, 11*, 399–429.

Shrauger, J. S., & Schoeneman, T. J. (1979). Symbolic interactionist view of self-concept: Through the looking glass darkly. *Psychological Bulletin, 86*, 549–573.

Smith, E. R. (1990). Content and process specificity in the effects of prior experiences. In T. K. Srull & R. S. Wyer (Eds.), *Advances in social cognition* (Vol. 3, pp. 1–59). Hillsdale, NJ: Erlbaum.

Steele, C. M. (1988). The psychology of self-affirmation: Sustaining the integrity of the self. In L. Berkowitz (Ed.), *Advances in experimental social psychology* (Vol. 21, pp. 261–302). New York: Academic Press.

Steele, C. M. (1997). A threat in the air: How stereotypes shape intellectual identity and performance. *American Psychologist, 52,* 613–629.

Steele, C. M., Spencer, S. J., & Lynch, M. (1993). Self-image resilience and dissonance: The role of affirmational resources. *Journal of Personality and Social Psychology, 64*, 885–896.

Stewart, A. (Producer). (1993, September 13). *MTV News.* New York: Music Television.

Stryker, S. (1981). Symbolic interactionism: Themes and variations. In M. Rosenberg & R. H. Turner (Ed.), *Social psychology: Sociological perspectives* (pp. 3–29). New York: Basic Books.

Swann, W. B., & Ely, R. J. (1984). A battle of wills: Self-verification versus behavioral confirmation. *Journal of Personality and Social Psychology, 46*, 1287–1302.

Tajfel, H., & Turner, J. C. (1986). The social identity theory of intergroup behavior. In S. Worchel & W. G. Austin (Eds.), *Psychology of intergroup relations* (pp. 7–24). Chicago: Nelson-Hall.

Tedeschi, J. T. (1986). Private and public experiences and the self. In R. F. Baumeister (Ed.), *Public self and private self* (pp. 1–20). New York: Springer-Verlag.

Tedeschi, J. T., & Norman, N. (1985). Social power, self-presentation, and the self. In B. R. Schlenker (Ed.), *The self and social life* (pp. 293–322). New York: McGraw-Hill.

Tice, D. M. (1992). Self-concept change and self-presentation: The looking glass self is also a magnifying glass. *Journal of Personality and Social Psychology, 63,* 435–451.

Tice, D. M. (1993). The social motivations of people with low self-esteem. In R. F. Baumeister (Ed.), *Self-esteem: The puzzle of low self-regard* (pp. 37–53). New York: Plenum Press.

Turner, J. C., Hogg, M., Oakes, P., Reicher, S., & Wetherell, M. (1987). *Rediscovering the social group: A self-categorization theory.* Oxford: Blackwell.

Vallacher, R. R., Wegner, D. M., McMahan, S. C., & Cotter, J. (1992). On winning friends and influencing people: Action identification and self-presentation success. *Social Cognition, 10*, 335–355.

Vorauer, J. D., & Miller, D. T. (1997). Failure to recognize the effect of implicit social influence on the presentation of self. *Journal of Personality and Social Psychology, 73*, 281–295.

Wegner, D. M., & Vallacher, R. R. (1986). Action identification. In R. M. Sorrentino & E. T. Higgins (Eds.), *Handbook of motivation and cognition: Foundations of social behavior* (Vol. 1, pp. 550–582). New York: Guilford Press.

Wicklund, R., & Gollwitzer, P. (1987). The fallacy of the private–public self-focus distinction. *Journal of Personality, 55*, 491–523.

Wilson, T. D. (1990). Self-persuasion via self-reflection. In J. M. Olson & M. P. Zanna (Ed.), *The Ontario symposium: Vol. 6. Self-inference processes* (pp. 43–68). Hillsdale, NJ: Erlbaum.

8

The Hidden Costs
of Hidden Stigma

LAURA SMART
DANIEL M. WEGNER

Given the choice, most of us would probably prefer that our stigmas were secret. The various social albatrosses we all carry with us would seem to be less weighty and might even fly away, perhaps, if no one else could see them. Social stigmas seem particularly likely to induce discrimination, maltreatment, and ostracism, after all—not to mention personal embarrassment and shame—when they are immediately perceptible to everyone. The ability to hide stigmas in a closet would seem to be a fine option, if we had that choice.

For some people, such a choice is available. As Goffman (1963) observed, people with stigmas that are not clearly visible to others—what we refer to as "concealable stigmas"—have the option of not telling. They can deliberately try to "pass" as "normal," unstigmatized individuals. In this way, it may be possible to exert some control over the prejudiced impressions that others may have. Under some circumstances, concealing one's stigma may be not only advantageous, but crucial to the ability to participate in social life. There are many kinds of stigmas, such as being gay or having certain mental or physical illnesses, for which concealment can prevent devastating personal consequences—including social rejection, loss of job, and even persecution (see Herek, 1996).

Even a concealable stigma can be costly, though, as aptly documented by Goffman (1963). In his book *Stigma: Notes on the Manage-*

ment of Spoiled Identity, he described how people encounter psychological strain in the process of concealing their true identity. Through several examples, he illustrated how attempts to pass may lead to feelings of isolation, fraud, and fear of discovery. These difficulties may be compounded by the reactions of interaction partners, who may become suspicious of a relative lack of disclosure (Herek, 1996). Withholding personal information about oneself from others can impede the development and maintenance of social relationships, insofar as self-disclosure is considered one of the essential ingredients to having meaningful relationships (Derlega & Berg, 1987). There is more than this, however. Concealing a stigma leads to an inner turmoil that is remarkable for its intensity and its capacity for absorbing an individual's mental life.

A telling example of this struggle with a concealable stigma is offered by the former Olympic diver Greg Louganis. In a 1996 autobiography, *Breaking the Surface,* he describes the torment that he experienced in hiding both his homosexuality and his status as an HIV-positive person. A turning point occurred in the 1988 Olympics in Seoul, Korea, when he struck his head on the diving board during one of his dives. As he bled into the water and as doctors came to his aid, Louganis was overwhelmed with terror—not so much by his being hurt or by possibly losing his position in the competition, but instead by the fact that he was perhaps jeopardizing the lives of everyone who was coming into contact with his blood. This experience eventually prompted Louganis to abandon the secrecy of his dual stigmas:

> I also want to set the record straight about who I am, because my secrets have become overwhelming. I want to start living my life the way normal people do, without having to watch every word, without having to remember what I've shared with whom. I want never again to feel compelled to hide out in my house in the California hills, avoiding situations in which I have to edit what I say and lie about my life. (1996, p. xiii)

Much of what has been written about concealable stigmas has focused on the interpersonal costs for those who try to conceal their stigmas (Crocker, Major, & Steele, 1998; Gibbons, 1986). Less theoretical and research attention has addressed the intrapersonal, cognitive consequences of concealing a stigma. As Louganis states, trying to manage what is said (and what is kept from being said) in social interaction demands a great deal of mental control (see Wegner & Erber, 1993). In the effort to hide their true identities, those with concealable stigmas must face an internal struggle that leads to anguish and perhaps even to psychopathology. In what follows, we present evidence that as stigmatized people try to maintain secrecy about their stigmas, they become obsessively preoccupied with thoughts of their stigmas. Such effects have important implications for daily functioning, and for the psychological—and even physical—well-being of stigmatized persons.

SECRECY AND SUPPRESSION

A college professor we know once announced in a statistics class that a case of cheating had been detected from a pattern of unusual answers on the previous exam, and that the perpetrator could escape possible expulsion from college by confessing. Several days went by until, late on a Friday night, a student appeared unannounced on the professor's front porch. She was in tears, and explained as she stood under the porch light that she had been wracked with guilt all week. Even worse, she revealed, was that she hadn't been able to get the incident off her mind for a moment. She mentioned that just looking at the textbook on the shelf was enough to remind her of her offense, and that images of what she had done and what might happen to her kept intruding on her thoughts no matter what else she was doing. She said that she kept thinking about telling someone but could not, and that she had not slept for days. All this went away in minutes when she confessed, and it was really a shame that she was not the perpetrator the professor had been expecting to catch.

The point here is that a secret, guilty or not, can be a tremendous burden. This appears to be the case because keeping a secret becomes a preoccupation. In the "preoccupation model of secrecy," Lane and Wegner (1995; see also Wegner & Lane, 1995) propose that attempts at secrecy typically activate a set of cognitive processes that lead to obsessive thinking about the secret. This happens because when people try to keep a secret, they try to suppress their thoughts of the secret. Thought suppression can be an effective secret-keeping strategy at first, because temporarily pushing the secret thoughts out of mind may allow for more attention to be focused on attempting to appear as sincere and truthful as possible, or on redirecting the conversation away from the taboo topic. Such suppression is particularly important when the person is interacting with those from whom the secret must be kept, as there is the danger that these thoughts might bubble up into conversation. The tendency for secrecy to promote suppression has been observed in several studies (e.g., Lane & Wegner, 1995; Wegner, Lane, & Dimitri, 1994).

The next step in the preoccupation model is that attempts at thought suppression lead to intrusive thoughts of the very thing that the person with the secret is trying to keep out of mind. This effect has been documented in research as well (e.g., Wegner & Erber, 1992; Wegner, Erber, & Zanakos, 1993) and can be accounted for by the theory of "ironic processes of mental control" (Wegner, 1994). This theory suggests that when people try not to think about something (e.g., a personal, concealable stigma), two mental processes are initiated: an intentional operating process and an ironic monitoring process. The intentional operating process is conscious and effortful; it serves to keep the unwanted thoughts out of mind by searching for distractors or topics other than the suppressed thoughts. The ironic monitoring process is unconscious and requires little cognitive effort. It functions to search for exactly those unwanted thoughts that are under suppression, thus ironically making the unwanted thoughts accessible and making it likely that they will return to conscious awareness. This increased thought accessibility during suppression is especially likely that when a person is under some sort of cognitive load, because the operating process is not able to function as effectively and the monitoring process takes over. Someone with a concealable stigma, then, may not have thoughts of the stigma in consciousness all of the time, but rather as periodic intrusions that result from the ironic monitoring process.

These thought intrusions result in renewed attempts to try to keep the secret thoughts out of consciousness. The motivation for the suppression may again be to try to keep the thoughts out of mind in the service of trying to maintain the secret, or it might also be to try to reduce the distress and anxiety provoked by having the intrusive thoughts (see Wegner & Gold, 1995). Such motivated suppression completes the last stage of the model: a constant preoccupation with the secret thoughts, in which thought suppression and thought intrusion occur cyclically in response to each other. The thoughts pop into mind as attempts to suppress them increase, which fuels further attempts at suppression, which yields more intrusion, and so on. The secret becomes a fixed idea of sorts—a constant companion that becomes particularly unruly when audiences are encountered from whom the secret is to be kept.

The preoccupation model of secrecy provides some insight into why it is important to focus on the concealability dimension (Jones et al., 1984) in trying to understand the experience of being stigmatized. People with visible stigmas have to contend with the everyday negative reactions of others to their stigmas, and must deal with the assortment of prejudices that others hold about them. They have what Goffman (1963) referred to as a "discredited identity." Their challenges arise, then, in dealing with already "spoiled" social interactions. Although they may be thinking quite a bit about how their interaction partners perceive them, their thoughts are directed toward using this information to manage and repair the interactions. In addition, both people in such interactions know about the stigma—so while fears or prejudices may need to be hidden, at least the topic itself can be addressed directly in the conversation.

When people try to conceal their stigmas, however, their struggles are different. The preoccupation model suggests that when one has a concealable stigma and actively tries to hide it, this secret can become highly accessible just when one is trying hardest not to think about it. Those with concealable stigmas need to grapple with the assortment of negative feelings that are evoked when they hide important information about themselves—but they must also contend with their own obsessive preoccupation with their stigmas. This preoccupation may itself become a problem, as it can permeate judgments and behaviors. Therefore, people with concealable stigmas are psychologically burdened in different ways than those with visible stigmas, which may lead to unique kinds of consequences.

There are many circumstances that may necessitate the concealment of a stigma, including formal settings (such as a job interview) or a variety of more informal settings (such as casual conversation with friends or acquaintances, the early stages of a romantic relationship, or family interactions). There are also situations that may not *require* hiding a stigma, but that may motivate a person to conceal it nonetheless. These situations often occur when the revelation of a stigma promises to disrupt a relationship; the alienation of a potentially understanding friend or family member through stigma disclosure may be especially undesirable. For people with concealable stigmas, a wide variety of "active concealment" situations will set into motion the cognitive processes of the preoccupation model.

DEEP COGNITIVE ACTIVATION

How could preoccupation with a stigma be a problem? It might seem that a person who thinks a lot about a secret stigma might simply be a bit withdrawn or inattentive, as the preoccupation might be no more debilitating than a pain in the neck or an annoying worry about a problem at work. As it happens, such mere inattention is only the simplest and least costly of the consequences of preoccupation. We suspect that a variety of further complications arise because the preoccupation has continued insidious effects. It is useful to describe these in terms of the state of "deep cognitive activation" (Wegner & Smart, 1997).

In deep cognitive activation, stigma-related thoughts are accessible and influential over behavior and judgment, although they are not currently conscious. Such a state may occur because of the initial suppression of thoughts about the stigma, and may be maintained by repeated attempts to suppress the thoughts during the course of preoccupation. The state of deep activation differs from one in which a thought is both conscious and accessible ("full activation"), such as times when people become strongly absorbed with a thought—both thinking of it in consciousness and tending to have it come into consciousness again. Deep activation is also different from a state when a thought is conscious but not currently accessible. Such surface activation occurs when people attempt to distract themselves with a conscious thought in order to avoid thinking about another, more accessible and perhaps unpleasant thought. Elsewhere, we (Wegner & Smart, 1997) describe deep activation as a motivated state of mind, in which a person is typically trying to keep something out of consciousness even while that object is made highly accessible by the suppression and so is inclined to pop into consciousness periodically.

The potential for deep cognitive activation to occur for those with concealable stigmas has far-reaching consequences. It suggests that this process of concealing a stigmatized identity may lead to behavioral and judgmental effects that are indirect—that is, not connected to the activated thought in a way that may be logical or obvious. Such indirect effects can be profound for the very reason that their origins are unclear to individuals. In the process of trying to hide stigmas, people may be cognitively affected in ways that are subtle and seem only loosely linked to the activated thoughts of the stigmas themselves, but that may still cause a great deal of distress. Furthermore, there may be times when such people are not even consciously aware that they are preoccupied with their stigmas. They may consider their attempts to suppress thoughts of their stigmas to be successful, although these thoughts may still be influencing their behaviors and judgments.

Deep activation is a useful way of conceptualizing how people respond to any thought that is unpleasant to think. So, for instance, we (Wegner & Smart, 1997) have proposed that thoughts of death are often deeply activated, as are thoughts of one's susceptibility to illness and thoughts of personal losses. Consistent with this first idea, Arndt, Greenberg, Solomon, Pyszczynski, and Simon (1997) have found that people who have been reminded of their own death exhibit increased accessibility of death-related thoughts (as measured by techniques that do not depend on self-reported thinking), while at the same time reporting no conscious thought of the topic. And consistent with the second idea, Swann, Morris, and Blumberg (1996) found that sexually active college students who had seen a film on AIDS experienced higher accessibility of AIDS-related thoughts on a Stroop-type interference task. People whose thoughts of AIDS were deeply activated in this way were slow to name the colors in which these words appeared on a computer monitor, particularly when they were under cognitive load. In other research, Morris and Swann (1996) found that sexually active people reminded of AIDS by such a film did not express much conscious thought about AIDS.

The deep activation of thoughts of personal losses, in turn, was gauged in research by Wegner and Gold (1995). In these studies, people who had followed instructions to suppress thoughts of a past relationship that they still valued were given the opportunity to express their thoughts about it aloud after the suppression period was over. As compared to those who were not asked to suppress the thought beforehand, these individuals showed increased psychophysiological arousal (as indexed by skin conductance level)—all the while showing a marked tendency *not* to talk about the past relationship. They kept it out of consciousness, even though their bodies simultaneously revealed a deep concern with this loss. The state of deep cognitive activation appears to be prompted by circumstances that force people to think about what they would rather avoid. Under these conditions, people may show little conscious awareness of the unwanted thoughts, even while these are measurably present in the cognitive and psychophysiological responses over which they have less control.

Although there is as yet little research attempting to extend this analysis to the case of concealable stigmas, there is one promising line of inquiry. In a series of studies, Steele and Aronson (1995) found that when African American students focused their attention on the significance of their test performance in light of negative stereotypes about their racial group, their performance suffered considerably. The intriguing finding here, from our perspective, was that these students also showed evidence of increased cognitive accessibility for the negative stereotype. This is a hint that suppression was present (see Wegner, 1994). Although the degree to which the African American students could report these thoughts consciously was not assessed in this work, our guess is that such stigmatizing thoughts might well be ushered out of awareness by suppression in many cases. A full examination of the role of deep activation in this "stereotype threat" effect would be interesting indeed, as it might also uncover the degree to which visible stigmas such as race might suddenly come to behave like concealable ones when people are in situations (such as test taking) when previously visible stigmas are less evident.

The most interesting feature of deep activation is that people might, as a result of it, show predictable cognitive and behavioral effects of which they are oddly unaware. One such phenomenon has already been observed: the occurrence of the projection of suppressed personal characteristics onto others. A series of studies by Newman, Baumeister, and

Duff (1997) indicated support for a suppression model of "defensive projection." Their model departs markedly from a Freudian formulation by focusing on the implications of conscious suppression. It suggests that when people are faced with threatening information about themselves (e.g., negative feedback about their personalities), they will respond to this ego threat by denying the possibility and suppressing thoughts about it. These defensive processes should then result in both a belief that they do not possess the unwanted traits and chronic accessibility of the trait concepts that are being suppressed. Such enhanced accessibility, in turn, makes it likely that evidence of exactly these traits will be picked up in perceptions of *others*. The result of this defensive process is that the threatening traits are projected onto others. The lack of conscious awareness of the trait in themselves that comes from the denial and disbelief, in turn, makes it unlikely that those who are projecting will become aware of their own contribution to the perception.

The consequences of deep activation could very well be played out in the lives of those who conceal their stigmas. Deep activation could yield both a diminished capacity to process social information, and a pervasive tendency for such a person to interpret the social world in terms of the stigma and process stigma-relevant information quite readily. We would expect, too, that a person hiding a stigma might notice suppressing it, and so should report exerting this effort. It also makes sense that such a person would experience intrusive thoughts of the stigma and could report these. Measures tapping the degree of accessibility of thoughts of the stigma should be strongly affected for an individual hiding a stigma and indirect indications of preoccupation, such as defensive projection of the stigma, might be observed as well.

PAST RESEARCH ON COGNITIVE EFFECTS

Past research has yielded some evidence relevant to our predictions. First of all, possessing a stigma may lead to an impairment of cognitive abilities for the stigmatized person. Being a token member of a group (e.g., being the only female in an all-male discussion group) has been found to lead to memory deficits for the content of a group discussion (Lord & Saenz, 1985). This impairment effect has not been observed or even explored, however, for people who have concealable stigmas. There is evidence that deception takes cognitive capacity (cf. Gilbert, Krull, & Pelham, 1988; Lane & Wegner, 1995), but it is not clear that this effect extends to the case of simply remaining silent about a personal stigma.

Few studies have examined the dimension of visibility in determining the cognitive effects of stigmatization. This dimension was consid-

ered, however, in a study on "master status conditions" (Frable, Blackstone, & Scherbaum, 1990). A master status condition is related to
stigma, in that it is something about a person that is statistically unusual
and central to the understanding of his or her character—but, unlike
stigma, it can be either positive or negative. For example, being gay is
considered a master status condition, but so is having extremely wealthy
parents. In the study by Frable et al. (1990), pairs of people (one with a
master status condition and one without) sat in a room together for 5
minutes. Inevitably, the participants would begin to talk during this time
period. Unbeknownst to them, each interaction was videotaped. When
the participants were then separated and asked to recall everything that
they could about the interaction, the researchers discovered that people
who possessed master status conditions were more "mindful" in social
interactions than those without such conditions. "Mindfulness" in this
case was defined as paying greater attention to aspects of the situation.

When the master status people were further divided according to
the visibility of their conditions, it was found that visible deviants tended
to focus more on the environment (details of the experimental room)
and on their partners' physical appearance than on the conversations
that took place. Those with concealed master status characteristics
tended to focus more on the conversation by often taking their partners'
perspective, making frequent references to the conversations, and spontaneously remembering what their partners said. This difference reflects
the shifts in attention depending upon the visibility of the master status.
Frable et al. (1990) speculated that "visibles" need to focus on an already spoiled interaction and need to be alert for signs of true attitudes
and feelings, while "invisibles," those with concealed master statuses,
need to manage the conversation and pay close attention to what is being said. Perhaps, too, a person with a concealable stigma concentrates
on what his or her partner is thinking in order to steer the interaction in
ways that will allow the continued concealment of the stigma. This
study, then, does not indicate that concealed stigma produces any general deficit in cognitive function; instead, it suggests that people in this
circumstance may actually be focusing quite effectively on the interaction.

These past studies have not explored at all what we believe to be the
most interesting and intense circumstance for a person with a concealable stigma: an interaction *about the concealable stigma*. This is the
predicament in which the most flagrant consequences of preoccupation
and deep activation should be observed. Interactions in a waiting room,
after all, need not bring to mind a concealable stigma, or motivate much
in the way of concealment. However, being asked direct questions relevant to the stigma should prompt several of the predicted effects. A for-

mer psychiatric patient being asked about mental stability, for example, or a closeted gay person being asked about sexual preferences, is pressed to begin an active form of concealment and so must engage in mental control. This condition was examined in the research we now describe.

THE "PRIVATE HELL" STUDIES

The preoccupation model of secrecy, and the notion of deep cognitive activation, provide some new ideas about the effects of concealable stigmatization. We (Smart & Wegner, 1999) conducted two studies to examine whether keeping a stigma hidden may lead to an obsessive preoccupation with the stigma. The studies also explored some of the cognitive and interpersonal effects that may accrue from such obsessive preoccupation, and focused in particular on the possibility that projection of the stigma onto others might occur as a result of deep cognitive activation. We call these "private hell" studies as a way of emphasizing what we believe to be the inner experience of the person who is hiding a concealable stigma.

Arranging a Concealed Stigma

In both of our studies, undergraduate women who had characteristics of anorexia nervosa and/or bulimia nervosa (referred to hereafter as eating disorders or EDs), or who did not have EDs, were recruited based on their responses in a mass pretesting session. Women in the first group endorsed items in a pretesting measure that captured thoughts and behaviors typical of EDs (e.g., "I am terrified of being overweight," "There have been times when I have vomited or taken laxatives after eating in order to purge," "I am always concerned with a desire to be thinner"). The women with EDs also indicated that no one or very few people in their lives knew this information about them, and that they would be moderately to extremely reluctant to disclose this information to another student chosen at random.

EDs were chosen as the concealable stigma in these studies because of the high prevalence of women in the mass pretesting session at the University of Virginia (approximately 5–7%) who admitted to having these thoughts and engaging in behaviors characteristic of EDs. The abnormal patterns of behavior and thought processes that are common to people with EDs often necessitate attempts to keep information about themselves hidden from others to avoid arousing concern and possible unwanted intervention. Persons with bulimia nervosa, for instance, frequently report preparing secretively for a binge or planning for it privately by hoarding food beforehand (Abraham & Llewellyn-Jones, 1992). Those who purge their food by vomiting or taking laxatives typically cloak these behaviors in secrecy as well.

When each participant arrived at the experimental session, she found another female "participant" also waiting; in actuality, the latter was a confederate of the experiment. Both were greeted by an experimenter, who told them that they were about to take part in an interview. For each experimental session, each participant was led to believe that she was randomly assigned to be either the interviewer or the interviewee. The situation in fact was prearranged so that the participant was always the one who was interviewed and the confederate was always the interviewer.

The experimenter then explained that during the interview, the interviewee would be asked to role-play someone either with an ED or without one. These roles were used to operationalize visibility of the stigma. The participants who were assigned to play the role of having an ED and who actually did have one were considered to have their stigma "visible." Those who actually had an ED and were instructed to play the role of not having one were considered to have their stigma "concealed." The purpose of this role-playing approach was to allow the participants to have the psychological experience of hiding or revealing details about their ED, but also to avoid having them feel as if they were forced to disclose information about themselves that they would have preferred to have kept hidden. In order to make it clear what exactly was meant by the term "eating disorder" in this context, the experimenter read two short paragraphs aloud that described someone with an ED and someone without one. The "ED profile" read:

> People with the eating disorders of anorexia nervosa or bulimia nervosa are generally characterized by obsessive–compulsive behaviors in relation to food and their bodies. Some behaviors that they typically may engage in are exercising for several hours a day, regulating their caloric intake daily, refusing to eat food even when they are hungry or eating excessively and then purging by vomiting, laxatives, or excessive exercise.

The "non-ED profile" read:

> People who do not have eating disorders generally eat for nourishment, enjoy eating, and if they exercise, they do so to maintain a healthy lifestyle.

Participants were told that the interviewer was not aware at this time whether or not they were playing a role. The participants were therefore under the impression that the interviewer would believe that they did or did not have an ED, depending on which role they were assigned to play. In fact, the confederate who played the interviewer was naive during the interview about each participant's ED status and role-playing assignment—although the role-playing assignment soon became clear as the participant began to answer the questions.

The interview began with several neutral questions (e.g., "Tell me about your morning routine, from when you wake up to when you go to class," "What do you like most so far about being in college?"). As the interview progressed, the questions became increasingly relevant to the participant's stigma. Examples of these items were as follows: "Does anyone [e.g., friends, roommates, family] ever tell you that you exercise too much?" "[If yes,] how do you typically respond?" "Does anyone [e.g., friends, roommates, family] ever tell you that you have strange eating habits?"

Following the role play, participants were asked to respond this time truthfully (i.e., no longer in their roles) to several self-report measures of their thought processes during the interview. After each participant had completed these measures, she was questioned for suspiciousness about the study and then was thoroughly debriefed. Those who experienced any distress about the topic or their current ED problem (and these were only a few) were given special attention and information, and, if they so desired, a referral for counseling and ED treatment.

The procedure was the same for both Studies 1 and 2, except that in Study 2, following the interview, participants completed a computerized Stroop-type measure (Stroop, 1935). It was adapted so that it was a measure of the accessibility of stigma-related thoughts (see Wegner & Erber, 1992; Wegner et al., 1993). At the start of the Stroop task, participants sat at a computer monitor, where they read the instructions: to respond quickly and accurately to a series of words, indicating whether each word was shown in red or blue by pressing one of the keys on the keyboard. Some of the words they saw were related to EDs (e.g., "flabby," "thighs," "diet"), but most were neutral words (e.g., "bird," "car," "radio"). Before each word appeared, either a two-digit number (low cognitive load) or a seven-digit number (high cognitive load) appeared on the screen. Participants were instructed to hold this number in mind while they were identifying the color of the word that followed. After identifying the color, they were asked to state the number into a tape recorder.

The results from these two studies provide some insight into the consequences of having a concealable stigma. Taken together, the results suggest that when people try to hide their stigmas from others, there is a lot more going on in their minds than we may suspect. To begin with, in both studies, the women whose stigma was concealed (having an ED but playing the role of not having one) reported the highest amount of thought suppression about their ED. So, at a basic self-report level, participants verified the use of thought suppression as a strategy during the concealment of a stigma. Those with a concealed stigma also reported, in both studies, higher levels of intrusive thoughts about EDs than did participants in the other conditions. Thus we observed evidence for the notion that the same conditions that prompt suppression also prompt intrusion. It is interesting to note that the participants who concealed their stigma showed more suppression and intrusions than did those participants who were actively playing the role of someone with the stigma and professing to have this stigma. The results support the appropriateness of conceptualizing the processes of maintaining a concealable stigma as similar to those of keeping a secret (Lane & Wegner, 1995). It would appear that persons with concealable stigmas are plagued by mental control problems.

The Stroop task administered in Study 2 corroborated this idea. Recall that this task was used in the expectation that it would allow for the detection of uncontrollable expressions of the deep activation of ED-related thoughts—those (ED-related) thoughts that might be influencing behavior or judgment but were not currently conscious. Under high cognitive load, the women who had an ED and were role-playing not having one had a slower mean reaction time for naming colors of words that were body-relevant (e.g., "fat," "flabby," "thighs") than for naming colors of neutral words (e.g., "bird," "letter," "shelf"). This effect was not obtained for participants who had an ED but were not keeping it a secret (i.e., were role-playing having an ED) or for participants who did not have an ED. This indicates that people who were keeping their ED a secret had increased cognitive accessibility of thoughts related to their stigma. These results are consistent with evidence of the hyperaccessibility of unwanted thoughts following suppression. Using a similar Stroop paradigm, Wegner and Erber (1992) found that participants had slower reaction times for naming colors of words when they were asked to suppress thinking of the words and under conditions of high cognitive load than when there was not a cognitive load or when participants were instructed to concentrate on the words. Lane and Wegner (1995) observed a similar accessibility effect for participants who were specifically instructed to keep a particular thought secret from an inquisitive experimenter. In the current studies, it is interesting to note that the participants were not specifically instructed to suppress thoughts of their stigma or to keep it secret. In merely trying to play the role of someone without the stigma, participants suffered the same hyperaccessibility of the unwanted thoughts. This provides further evidence for the idea that people with concealable stigmas may suffer from a preoccupation with their stigmas, and indicates, too, that this preoccupation introduces automatic and uncontrollable interference effects.

Although these various indications of preoccupation were measured at different points in the studies, and in different ways, it is worth taking a moment to recall the theoretical sequence of events. According to the preoccupation model, the need to conceal a stigma in an interview yields thought suppression. This, in turn, produces the accessibility of the thought. And finally, the intrusions experienced in this circumstance occur because the high levels of accessibility repeatedly thrust stigma-relevant thoughts into consciousness even when the conscious flow of thought is on topics quite unrelated to the stigma. One further effect of such accessibility was also observed in these studies—the projection we anticipated on the basis of the research by Newman et al. (1997).

The Projection of Stigma

In a novel called *The Dwarf*, Pär Lagerkvist (1953) provided an example of projection of stigma:

> I have noticed that sometimes I frighten people; what they really fear is themselves. They think it is I who scare them, but it is the dwarf within them, the ape-faced man-like being who sticks its head from the depths of their souls. They are afraid because they do not know that they have another being inside. And they are deformed though it does not show on the outside. (p. 20)

We see that the protagonist, the dwarf, rather than defining himself as deformed, projects onto those around him by stating that they are the ones who are physically or morally deviant. This way of viewing the world may be one of the unconscious byproducts of concealing a stigma (although in the case of the dwarf, his stigma is clearly visible), and it may be one of the indirect effects of the state of deep cognitive activation.

In our (Smart & Wegner, 1999) studies, this possibility was measured. Participants with EDs were provided with the opportunity to project their thoughts and behaviors concerning their EDs onto the interviewer, as their perceptions of the confederate were collected following the interaction; in particular, their perception that she might also have an ED was specifically assessed. And as it happened, women who were concealing their stigma projected their concerns onto the interviewer by rating her higher on a set of questions about her likelihood of having an ED (her perfectionism, concern with her body image, and control of eating) than did those with EDs who were playing the disordered role. This suggests that the process of concealment and the resulting preoccupation with the secret are what stimulate this type of projective effect.

The desire to keep a stigma a secret may be coupled with a motivation for those with a concealable stigma to deny the stigma in themselves. Women with EDs seem to have relatively little insight into their distorted thinking and pathological behaviors. Since the women in our studies were self-identified as having thoughts and behaviors characteristic of EDs, their projection may have been motivated by a desire to deny the severity or abnormality of their thoughts and behaviors rather than the existence of them. The implications of the link between keeping secret a concealable stigma and distortions in how these people perceive others are intriguing. People with such stigmas may be constructing a world in which their stigmas are perceived as more common than they actually are. Perhaps this even ends up being useful. This way of thinking may serve a coping function and may temporarily relieve some of the stress that may arise from the unwanted thoughts (see Sherwood, 1981).

Interpersonal Skills

The possibility that the preoccupation with a concealable stigma would produce uneasy and stilted interactions was also examined in our (Smart & Wegner, 1999) studies. It would make sense, after all, that the burden of trying to keep information about themselves hidden, as well as the anticipation of the judgment of the interviewer if the stigma was revealed, might interfere with normative social behavior. As Goffman (1963, p. 88) put it, "He who passes will have to be alive to aspects of the social situation which others treat as uncalculated and unattended. What are unthinking routines for normals can become management problems for the discreditable." Jones et al. (1984) similarly suggested that social interactions between a person with a concealed stigma and a nonstigmatized person would be negatively altered (compared to an interaction between two nonstigmatized people), with the normal flow of conversation being hampered: "The effects of asymmetrical knowledge may show themselves in the awkward reticence of the markable, as he closes off entire areas of conversation to avoid revealing the nature of his mark" (p. 186).

We did not observe such effects. Although the participants in the "private hell" studies who had EDs and were concealing their stigma were indeed demonstrating stigma-related thought accessibility, thought intrusion, and projection, they appeared to be generally socially adept to independent judges who rated the taped interviews on many interpersonal dimensions. The results from the judges' ratings of the interviews showed that across both of the studies, people who were keeping their

EDs a secret did not appear to be interpersonally awkward or lacking in social skills in any way. Their inner struggles were not evident in their outward appearances. For example, the women with a concealed stigma were actually rated by the judges as being more likeable and less anxious than the women who had a visible stigma.

There are several possible explanations for this discrepancy between the inability to keep stigma-related thoughts out of mind and apparent ease in social interaction. The one we favor involves a practice effect. Perhaps those women with a concealable stigma had integrated secrecy into their lives for so long that they had become very skilled at hiding their stigma so as not to disrupt their social functioning. The participants with EDs in the study were generally viewed as socially skilled, and it is quite possible that individuals who develop EDs are unusually sensitive to others and even more socially motivated and adept than the usual research participants. The moments of concealment we engineered in the laboratory may have been no great challenge for women who had been doing this for a long time, and may instead have merely engaged their usual social coping skills. This interpretation is consistent with the notion of deep cognitive activation, in that the surface and conscious indications of stigmatization were not present.

It is also possible that the judges were responding to the heightened sense of arousal that those with a concealable stigma may have been experiencing in this type of interview situation. If this were the case, then these participants may have appeared more sociable and more expressive to the judges, which may have led to more positive ratings of their interpersonal functioning (e.g., Friedman, Riggio, & Casella, 1988; Sabatelli & Rubin, 1986). The key comparison for this research was between women with EDs who were revealing their stigma and those who were concealing it, of course, and perhaps revealing it was so disturbing that it disrupted these otherwise highly composed participants. Thus the participants who were concealing EDs may not have appeared particularly nonplussed by the situation because they were perhaps less flustered than those who were revealing.

Perhaps concealing a stigma affects long-term social relationships more than it does short-term interactions with strangers. Having a concealable stigma may affect the types of social relationships in which stigmatized people choose to become involved; for example, they may opt for shallow relationships in which hiding is relatively easy. Hiding their stigma may allow them to assimilate into the mainstream community life. At the same time, one of the consequences may be that they avoid associating with other similarly stigmatized people. In doing so, they deny themselves many of the benefits—the social support, social services, and social relationships—that come with being open about a stigma (Gibbons, 1986). In addition, they are unable to engage in downward social comparison because they are likely to want to avoid others who may be more clearly stigmatized than they are, in an effort to avoid being associated with the stigma and possibly implicated in also possessing it (Crocker et al., 1998).

The tendency to employ defensive projection raises an interesting issue regarding the social relationships of those with concealable stigmas. As suggested earlier, the increased use of projection by people with concealable stigmas may be evaluated on different levels in terms of effectiveness. With regard to initial interactions, projection may serve an adaptive function. It may allow people to rationalize their behaviors to themselves and reduce the negative affect that may be associated with repeated intrusive thoughts about their stigmas. In longer and perhaps more meaningful relationships, however, this kind of projection could well be disconfirmed repeatedly and serve as a barrier to relationship development.

Our studies shed some light on the consequences of leading a double life—presenting an "unmarked" image to those with whom one interacts, while keeping an important part of oneself hidden. The data suggest that while people with concealable stigmas may appear at ease in an interaction, they experience deep cognitive activation of their stigmas. Thus the preoccupation model, although developed to account for the cognitive consequences of secrecy in general, has much to offer in terms of insights pertaining to the specific effects of keeping a stigma secret from others.

HEALTH IMPLICATIONS AND CONCEALABLE STIGMAS

There is some evidence that keeping a stigma hidden may also take its toll on physical health. HIV infection, for example, has been found to advance more rapidly in HIV-positive men who conceal their homosexual identity than in men who are more open about their identity (Cole, Kemeny, Taylor, Visscher, & Fahey, 1996). Similarly, Crandall and Coleman (1992) have found that HIV-positive people who do not disclose their status to significant others are likely to become more isolated, more depressed, and more anxious than those who selectively confide in people whom they feel they can trust.

It has been argued that it may be beneficial to keep a secret concealed (Kelly & McKillop, 1996; Vangelisti, 1994). Of course, people do not usually keep secrets for imaginary or unimportant reasons, and it makes sense that there are often good reasons to hide a stigma. The reasons for secrecy may include the possibilities of receiving nonsupportive responses, for example, or disrupting personal boundaries that may be desired by the listener. Indeed, fear of a poor reception if concealed stigmas are revealed is likely to be what motivates the majority of people who are able to conceal their stigmas to perpetuate their assimilated status. Someone admits a stigma, for example, but the person to whom he or she has revealed this information is not able to handle this revelation and closes off future discussion of it. In this kind of situation, the person with the concealable stigma is still required to hide the stigma, but now his or her worst fear has been confirmed: People really do not understand. Secrecy attempts may then be renewed with even more zeal.

Under certain conditions, as in the presence of a safe and supportive audience or when one is able to preserve anonymity, making a concealed stigma visible may be highly beneficial. The health benefits of disclosing traumatic experiences have been researched extensively by Pennebaker and his colleagues (see Pennebaker, 1990). In one such study (Pennebaker, Kiecolt-Glaser, & Glaser, 1988), participants wrote in detail about events (many of which were potentially stigmatizing—e.g., incest victimization, perpetrating violence, having a spouse commit suicide) that they had not talked about with others. People who wrote more about concealed events (high disclosers) showed an improved immunological response relative to low disclosers and to controls. Pennebaker and his colleagues argue that the mechanism underlying this effect is that emotional expression involves confronting thoughts and feelings about stressful events. Through this process, people may be able to cognitively restructure the events and better understand them. It is also possible that the act of expression works its magic by allowing people to relax their pursuit of mental control, and so eliminates the costs of continuous deep activation.

Lepore (1997) also found health benefits for disclosing to a supportive audience in response to a stressful event. Participants in his experimental group who were instructed to write their deepest thoughts and feelings about an upcoming graduate exam had a decline in depressive symptoms from 1 month (Time 1) to 3 days (Time 2) before the exam. Those in the control group wrote about a trivial topic maintained a relatively high level of depressive symptoms over this same period of time. Like Pennebaker, Lepore maintains that being able to express one's thoughts and feelings about a particular stressor promotes emotional adaptation to the stressor by lessening the emotional impact of the intrusive thoughts. Our interpretation is that expression diminishes the deep cognitive activation of the stressor, and so eliminates the cognitive preoccupation and its costs.

Advancing technology may provide additional ways to reveal stigmas. There is some evidence that the Internet may be a valuable resource for "identity demarginalization" for people with concealable stigmas. McKenna and Bargh (1998) found that becoming a member of a newsgroup related to a marginalized aspect of one's identity led to greater self-acceptance, as well as an increased likelihood to reveal the concealable stigma to family and friends.

CONCEALABLE STIGMAS AND MENTAL CONTROL

Is there any way that concealable stigmas can be erased in the mind? Perhaps the greatest wish a person with a concealable stigma might have is not for the stigma to go away, but for the thought of it to go away. One wonders whether there might be conditions under which thoughts actually could be wished into oblivion—when personal stigmas could be forgotten and life could go on without the mental turmoil that regularly surrounds preoccupation. We can envision several ways in which this might happen.

One possibility is "automatization of suppression." If a person becomes highly practiced at mental control, it may come to be done expertly and efficiently. An individual with a sordid past that he or she wants to hide, for instance, may find that after many years of hiding it, the hiding gets easier. Just as riding a bicycle is learned and then not forgotten, the person with effective suppression strategies that are well practiced may be quite able to control the expressions and consciously perceptible repercussions of preoccupation. There is almost no current research on this possibility, but the notion that conscious mental control may become automatic and thus more effective deserves investigation in the area of stigma (see Smart & Wegner, 1996; Wegner, 1994; Wegner & Bargh, 1998). A person often has a stigma for life, after all, and it seems reasonable to expect that the person who has to rehearse suppression may become good at it.

A second way in which stigma may be forgotten is through "situation management." An individual with a concealable stigma may keep from being put in the position of having to pursue secrecy and suppression by avoiding situations in which the stigma must be hidden. This may involve, on the one hand, an engagement in only the most superficial relationships—ones that require almost no interaction about oneself. This is perhaps what we think of most readily when we consider a person who is in the process of avoiding an unwanted aspect of self. On the other hand, a situation management strategy may also prompt just the opposite kind of behavior. Interactions and settings may be sought out that maximize the degree of explicit focus on the stigma, as such circumstances will also free the person from the needs for secrecy and suppression. Becoming immersed in a homosexual lifestyle, for example, may well provide significant relief from secrecy to someone who has been hiding this identity.

A third strategy that may often succeed in reducing the pain of constant secrecy involves "redefinition of the stigma." If one can interpret a stigma in such a way that it is no longer stigmatizing, or perhaps at least no longer relevant to questions that may arise about one's identity, then it can be forgotten because active secrecy will no longer be needed. The utility of this strategy will depend, of course, on the nature of the stigma. A person who formerly abused drugs, for example, may be able to identify the self as a "convert," as having come clean and adopted a new identity. With this conversion comes a partition of the person's autobiography into a "former self" and a "current self," and secrecy need no longer be focused on the current self. The former identity can be talked about freely, or for that matter it can be kept secret—but it is not seen as highly relevant to the current self. Interactions that focus on the concealable stigma may not yield the need for concealment when the stigma is understood to be applicable only to one's former self, the owner of a spoiled identity that is no longer present.

Ultimately, the methods people use to manage their concealable stigmas will be many. In this chapter, we have examined some key phenomena that motivate such management. We have seen that a concealable stigma is a constant source of psychic pain: It requires work to suppress; it returns to mind in the form of intrusive thoughts that derail one's preferred course of thinking; and it can metastasize in a way, promoting projection and other insidious expressions of its extremely high levels of cognitive activation.

In a very clever experiment, Kleck and Strenta (1980) once made people think that they were visibly stigmatized in an interaction, even though no such stigma was present. The researchers attached false scars to participants' faces before an interaction, and then surreptitiously removed the scars in a flourish just before the interaction began. Those who thought they were stigmatized in this way reported being uncomfortable, and even were seen as ill at ease by observers—none of whom, of course, saw any scar. In a way, a concealable stigma perpetrates a similar hoax on the person who hides it. Although the person may have no stigma at all in others' eyes, he or she becomes preoccupied and ultimately devastated by the chore of trying to cover up something that cannot be seen.

ACKNOWLEDGMENT

Research reported in this chapter was supported by a National Institute of Mental Health (NIMH) predoctoral National Research Service Award (No. MH 11443-01) and by NIMH Grant No. MH 49127.

REFERENCES

Abraham, S., & Llewellyn-Jones, D. (1992). *Eating disorders: The facts.* New York: Oxford University Press.

Arndt, J., Greenberg, J., Solomon, S., Pyszczynski, T., & Simon, L. (1997). Suppression, accessibility of death-related thoughts, and cultural worldview defense: Exploring the psychodynamics of terror management. *Journal of Personality and Social Psychology, 73,* 5–18.

Cole, S. W., Kemeny, M. E., Taylor, S. E., Visscher, B. R., & Fahey, J. L. (1996). Accelerated course of human immunodeficiency virus infection in gay men who conceal their homosexual identity. *Psychosomatic Medicine, 58,* 219–231.

Crandall, C. S., & Coleman, R. (1992). AIDS-related stigmatization and the disruption of social relationships. *Journal of Social and Personal Relationships, 9,* 163–177.

Crocker, J., Major, B., & Steele, C. (1998). Social stigma. In D. T. Gilbert, S. T. Fiske, & G. Lindzey (Eds.), *Handbook of social psychology* (4th ed., Vol. 2, pp. 504–553). Boston: McGraw-Hill.

Derlega, V. J., & Berg, J. H. (1987). *Self-disclosure: Theory, research, and therapy.* New York: Plenum Press.

Frable, D. E. S., Blackstone, T., & Scherbaum, C. (1990). Marginal and mindful: Deviants in social interactions. *Journal of Personality and Social Psychology, 59,* 140-149.

Friedman, H. S., Riggio, R. E., & Casella, D. F. (1988). Nonverbal skill, personal charisma, and initial attraction. *Personality and Social Psychology Bulletin, 14,* 203–211.

Gibbons, F. X. (1986). Stigma and interpersonal relationships. In S. C. Ainlay, G. Becker, & L. M. Coleman (Eds.), *The dilemma of difference* (pp. 123–156). New York: Plenum Press.

Gilbert, D. T., Krull, D. S., & Pelham, B. W. (1988). Of thoughts unspoken: Social inference and the self-regulation of behavior. *Journal of Personality and Social Psychology, 55,* 685–694.

Goffman, E. (1963). *Stigma: Notes on the management of spoiled identity.* Englewood Cliffs, NJ: Prentice-Hall.

Herek, G. M. (1996). Why tell if you're not asked?: Self-disclosure, intergroup contact, and heterosexuals' attitudes toward lesbians and gay men. In G. M. Herek, J. B. Jobe, & R. M. Carney (Eds.), *Out in force: Sexual orientation and the military* (pp. 197–225). Chicago: University of Chicago Press.

Jones, E. E., Farina, A., Hastorf, A. H., Markus, H., Miller, D. T., & Scott, R. A. (1984). *Social stigma: The psychology of marked relationships.* New York: Freeman.

Kelly, A. E., & McKillop, K. J. (1996). Consequences of revealing personal secrets. *Psychological Bulletin, 120,* 450–465.

Kleck, R. E., & Strenta, A. (1980). Perceptions of the impact of negatively valued physical characteristics on social interaction. *Journal of Personality and Social Psychology, 39,* 861–873.

Lagerkvist, P. (1953). *The dwarf.* London: Chatto & Windus.

Lane, J. D., & Wegner, D. M. (1995). The cognitive consequences of secrecy. *Journal of Personality and Social Psychology, 69,* 1-17.

Lepore, S. J. (1997). Expressive writing moderates the relation between intrusive thoughts and depressive symptoms. *Journal of Personality and Social Psychology, 73,* 1030–1037.

Lord, C. G., & Saenz, D. S. (1985). Memory deficits and memory surfeits: Differential cognitive consequences for tokens and observers. *Journal of Personality and Social Psychology, 49,* 918-926.

Louganis, G. (1996). *Breaking the surface.* New York: Plume.

McKenna, K. Y. A., & Bargh, J. A. (1998). Coming out in the age of the Internet: Identity "de-marginalization" through virtual group participation. *Journal of Personality and Social Psychology, 75,* 681–694.

Morris, K. A., & Swann, W. B., Jr. (1996). Denial of the AIDS crisis: On wishing away the threat of AIDS. In S. Oskamp & S. C. Thompson (Eds.), *Understanding and preventing HIV risk behavior* (pp. 57–79). Thousand Oaks, CA: Sage.

Newman, L. S., Baumeister, R. F., & Duff, K. J. (1997). A new look at defensive projection: Thought suppression, accessibility, and biased person perception. *Journal of Personality and Social Psychology, 72,* 980–1001.

Pennebaker, J. W. (1990). *Opening up: The healing power of confiding in others.* New York: Morrow.

Pennebaker, J. W., Kiecolt-Glaser, J. K., & Glaser, R. (1988). Disclosure of traumas and immune function: Health implications for psychotherapy. *Journal of Consulting and Clinical Psychology, 56,* 239–245.

Sabatelli, R. M., & Rubin, M. (1986). Nonverbal expressiveness and physical attractiveness as mediators of interpersonal perceptions. *Journal of Nonverbal Behavior, 10,* 120–133.

Sherwood, G. G. (1981). Self-serving bias in person perception: A reexamination of projection as a mechanism of defense. *Psychological Bulletin, 90,* 445–459.

Smart, L., & Wegner, D. M. (1996). Strength of will. *Psychological Inquiry, 7,* 79–83.

Smart, L., & Wegner, D. M. (1999). Covering up what can't be seen: Concealable stigma and mental control. *Journal of Personality and Social Psychology, 77,* 474–486.

Steele, C. M., & Aronson, J. (1995). Stereotype threat and the intellectual test performance of African Americans. *Journal of Personality and Social Psychology, 69,* 797-811.

Stroop, J. R. (1935). Studies of interference in serial verbal reactions. *Journal of Experimental Psychology, 18,* 643–662.

Swann, W. B., Jr., Morris, K., & Blumberg, S. J. (1996). *Thought suppression as an obstacle to AIDS prevention.* Manuscript in preparation.

Vangelisti, A. L. (1994). Family secrets: Forms, functions and correlates. *Journal of Social and Personal Relationships, 11,* 113-135.

Wegner, D. M. (1994). Ironic processes of mental control. *Psychological Review, 101,* 34–52.

Wegner, D. M., & Bargh, J. A. (1998). Control and automaticity in social life. In

D. T. Gilbert, S. T. Fiske, & G. Lindzey (Eds.), *Handbook of social psychology* (4th ed., Vol. 1, pp. 446–496). Boston: McGraw-Hill.

Wegner, D. M., & Erber, R. (1992). The hyperaccessibility of suppressed thoughts. *Journal of Personality and Social Psychology, 63,* 903–912.

Wegner, D. M., & Erber, R. (1993). Social foundations of mental control. In D. M. Wegner & J. W. Pennebaker (Eds.), *Handbook of mental control* (pp. 36–56). Englewood Cliffs, NJ: Prentice-Hall.

Wegner, D. M., Erber, R., & Zanakos, S. (1993). Ironic processes in the mental control of mood and mood-related thought. *Journal of Personality and Social Psychology, 65,* 1093–1104.

Wegner, D. M., & Gold, D. B. (1995). Fanning old flames: Emotional and cognitive effects of suppressing thoughts of a past relationship. *Journal of Personality and Social Psychology, 68,* 782–792.

Wegner, D. M., & Lane, J. D. (1995). From secrecy to psychopathology. In J. W. Pennebaker (Ed.), *Emotion, disclosure, and health* (pp. 25–46). Washington, DC: American Psychological Association.

Wegner, D. M., Lane, J. D., & Dimitri, S. (1994). The allure of secret relationships. *Journal of Personality and Social Psychology, 66,* 287–300.

Wegner, D. M., & Smart, L. (1997). Deep cognitive activation: A new approach to the unconscious. *Journal of Consulting and Clinical Psychology, 65,* 984–995.

9

Coping with Stigma
and Prejudice

CAROL T. MILLER
BRENDA MAJOR

This chapter applies a stress-and-coping framework to understanding the experiences and adaptive reactions of individuals who are
targets of prejudice because they possess a social stigma. Our analysis is
guided by several key assumptions. The first is that possessing a social
stigma is a potentially stressful life event. Second, we assume that theoretical paradigms that have been used to understand how people cope
with and adapt to other types of stressful life events can be fruitfully applied to understanding how people cope with and adapt to being stigmatized. A central premise of a coping perspective is that there is not a simple direct relationship between exposure to stressors and adaptation
outcomes. Thus, although those who possess a stigma may experience
more stress, this does not necessarily translate into poorer outcomes,
such as poor mental health (e.g., Crocker & Major, 1989). Our third assumption is that although stigmas differ in a variety of important ways
that are likely to affect coping strategies (e.g., visibility, controllability),
there are also similarities across stigmas in how people cope with them
(Crocker, Major, & Steele, 1998). Finally, we assume that coping responses may focus on the problems associated with stigma or on the
emotions these problems cause (Major, Quinton, McCoy, & Schmader,
in press; Miller & Myers, 1998; Swim, Cohen, & Hyers, 1998).

STIGMA AS A STRESSOR

People who are stigmatized possess an attribute that conveys a devalued social identity in a particular context (Crocker et al., 1998). This devaluation, and the consequences that follow from it, can subject stigmatized people to stressors that are similar in many ways to other types of acute and/or chronic stressors. Although "stress" has been defined in a variety of ways, we adopt the definition of it as "any event in which environmental demands, internal demands, or both tax or exceed the adaptive resources of an individual, social system, or tissue system" (Monat & Lazarus, 1991, p. 3). Membership in a stigmatized group can pose a variety of environmental demands on an individual (Allison, 1998). Crocker and colleagues (1998) discuss several core features of the experience of stigma that are likely to tax or exceed the adaptive resources of an individual. One is the ever-present possibility that the person will be a target of prejudice or discrimination. There is substantial evidence that members of stigmatized groups are more likely to experience derision, exclusion, discrimination, and violence than are those who are not stigmatized. Hence, stigma increases the frequency and/or intensity of threats to the self. A second core aspect of stigma is awareness of the devalued quality of one's social identity. Stigmatized individuals' awareness that others do not like, value, or respect them is a major threat to self-esteem (Baumeister & Leary, 1995). A third key aspect of the experience of stigma is awareness that others hold specific negative stereotypes about one's social identity. Stigmatized persons are often threatened by these stereotypes even if they give no credence to them (Steele & Aronson, 1995; Steele, 1997). A fourth defining experience of stigma is uncertainty about whether one is being treated in a prejudicial manner on the basis of one's stigma. This uncertainty comes about in part because nonstigmatized people often try to hide or disguise their true attitudes toward stigmatized people, out of sympathy or concern about not appearing prejudiced (Carver, Glass, & Katz, 1977). Consequently, the behavior of nonstigmatized individuals toward stigmatized individuals may not be an accurate indicator of their true attitudes (Devine, 1989; Dovidio & Gaertner, 1986; Katz & Hass, 1988). The attributional ambiguity and uncertainty that this creates for stigmatized persons is likely to be a source of stress (Crocker & Major, 1989; Crocker, Voelkl, Testa, & Major, 1991; Major & Crocker, 1993).

Stigma also produces stress indirectly. Discrimination against stigmatized persons, for example, limits their access to resources such as health care, housing, education, and employment. The lives of stigmatized people are more subject to daily hassles and chronic strains than are those of more affluent and higher-status people (Allison, 1998).

Social rejection of stigmatized persons can lead to social isolation and lack of social support. All of these factors, in turn, can deplete or exceed an individual's adaptive resources (Dovidio & Gaertner, 1986).

Although stigma can be viewed as similar to other types of environmental demands that tax an individual's adaptive resources, there are ways in which stigma may pose unique demands on the individual. First, prejudice and discrimination are ever-present possibilities for a stigmatized person, whereas prejudice and discrimination are not defining features of other types of stressful experiences. Indeed, we would argue that if actual or anticipated prejudice and discrimination accompany a stressful experience (e.g., getting divorced or arrested), it is a stigmatizing experience. Second, awareness of social devaluation is at the heart of stigma. Stigmas that are chronic and visible features of the self, such as membership in devalued racial groups, disfigurements of the body, and physical disabilities, are likely to elicit actual or feared negative reactions from others across a broad range of contexts, making their impact on social interactions pervasive. Third, unlike most other types of stressors that researchers have studied, stigma is linked to a social identity. Hence, stigma and its accompanying threat are often experienced collectively as well as individually. Consider the controversy surrounding affirmative action. When others question whether particular individuals have achieved their status on their own merits or because of their membership in a protected group, their doubts pose a threat to the personal identity of the individuals involved. The assertion that otherwise unqualified minority individuals are advantaged over more qualified Whites also casts doubts, however, on the capabilities of minority group members as a whole. The fact that stigma threatens social identity as well as personal identity may make its implications more severe. But the social identity component of stigma may also provide a means by which the impact of stigma on personal identity can be buffered. In particular, a stigmatized person may be able to turn to other members of the stigmatized group for social support.

RESPONSES TO STIGMA

Many scholars assume that stress is an organismic response associated with negative physical and mental health outcomes (Allison, 1998). Consequently, a number of researchers have applied this approach to the domain of stigma by comparing the mental and/or physical health of members of stigmatized groups to that of members of nonstigmatized groups, on the assumption that group differences not attributed to culture are associated with prejudice. The often explicit assumption here is that stigma and prejudice leave various "marks of oppression" on their victims (e.g., personality flaws, neuroticism, self-hatred, increased aggressiveness, hypertension, etc.), which should show up when they are compared to those not so stigmatized (see Simpson & Yinger, 1985, for a review). For example, in his classic treatise *The Nature of Prejudice*, Allport (1954/1979) proposed that "since no one can be indifferent to the abuse and expectations of others we must anticipate that ego defensiveness will frequently be found among members of groups that are set off for ridicule, disparagement, and discrimination. It could not be otherwise" (p. 143).

Research taking this perspective has yielded mixed conclusions (see Allison, 1998, for a review). Few would argue that prejudice and discrimination against stigmatized persons do not have negative effects on their lives. Flacke and colleagues (1995), for example, report that African Americans have more physical health problems than European Americans, including shorter life expectancies, higher heart disease, and higher infant mortality. The evidence of poorer mental health outcomes among stigmatized than among nonstigmatized individuals, however, is less consistent (Rosenberg & Simmons, 1972; Simpson & Yinger, 1985). Crocker and Major (1989), for example, reviewed more than 20 years of research on stigma and self-esteem, and concluded that members of stigmatized groups frequently have self-esteem equal to or higher than that of nonstigmatized groups. Similar conclusions have been reached by other scholars (e.g., Feingold, 1992; Porter & Washington, 1979). Members of some stigmatized groups (such as overweight individuals), however, typically do have lower self-esteem than nonstigmatized people (Miller & Downey, 1999). Furthermore, there is considerable variation within stigmatized groups, such that some members have low self-esteem whereas others do not (e.g., Major, Barr, Zubek, & Babey, 1999). These findings emphasize that there is not a one-to-one relationship between exposure to environmental stressors and adaptational outcomes. Some stigmatized groups fare well whereas others do not, and some individuals within a stigmatized group fare better than do others. It is inappropriate to assume that because a person possesses a stigmatizing attribute, he or she will necessarily suffer emotional distress or diminished well-being as a consequence.

A COPING PERSPECTIVE ON STIGMA

How can we explain the paradoxical finding that people who are exposed to more frequent and more intense environmental demands do not necessarily suffer reduced well-being? Psychological perspectives on stress provide a useful framework. According to psychological perspectives, two central mediators of how individuals respond to potentially stressful life events are cognitive appraisals and coping (Bandura, 1977, 1982; Lazarus & Folkman, 1984). Two types of cognitive appraisals are central in Lazarus and Folkman's (1984) influential theory of coping. In "primary appraisal," an individual evaluates whether he or she has anything personally at stake in an encounter—for example, whether there is potential for harm, benefit, or loss. In "secondary appraisal," an individual evaluates existing coping resources and options to determine what (if anything) can be done to overcome or prevent harm, or to improve the prospects for benefit. An event is appraised as stressful when primary appraisals of threat exceed secondary appraisals of coping abilities (Folkman, Lazarus, Gruen, & DeLongis, 1986). Likewise, Bandura (1982) postulates that "self-efficacy beliefs"—beliefs about whether the individual can achieve mastery or control over the environment—are critical determinants of how individuals will respond in potentially stressful encounters.

A second key mediator of stressful person–environment relations and adaptational outcomes is coping. "Coping" is defined in Lazarus and Folkman's (1984) model as a person's "constantly changing cognitive and behavioral efforts to manage specific external and/or internal demands that are appraised as taxing or exceeding the person's resources" (p. 141). Coping occurs when an event or situation is appraised as stressful (or potentially stressful). Coping efforts are process-oriented and context-specific, and are distinguished both from more stable dispositions that can serve as coping resources (e.g., self-esteem, locus of control) and from the outcomes of coping efforts (whether or not they are successful). Thus people may engage in a variety of coping efforts, only some of which (or none of which) may be successful.

In short, a psychological stress-and-coping perspective implies that a stigma (e.g., obesity) or a stigma-related event (e.g., social rejection due to prejudice) will be appraised as stressful only if the stigmatized condition or the stigma-related event poses a personally relevant threat outstripping the individual's coping resources. Furthermore, this perspective implies that stigmatized individuals who do appraise their stigma or a stigma-related event as stressful will not necessarily suffer from reduced well-being if they use coping strategies that are effective at managing the internal or external demands posed by the appraised threat.

Appraisals of Stigma-Related Threat

One issue this perspective raises is to what extent stigmatized people appraise their stigma as a source of stress. As noted above, most analyses of stigma assume that stigmatized individuals are aware of the potential their stigma has to lead to prejudice and discrimination. They also assume that such individuals are aware of the social devaluation, negative stereotypes, and attributional ambiguity that accompany their stigma (e.g., Crocker et al., 1998; Goffman, 1963; Jones et al., 1984). Wright (1960) asserted that stigmatized persons interpret all of their interactions through the lens of their stigma. Several scholars have also suggested that the chronically stigmatized are vigilant to signs of prejudice and discrimination in others (e.g., Allport, 1954/1979; Goffman, 1963). For example, in his discussion of "traits" due to victimization, Allport wrote that "both vigilance and hypersensitiveness may be among the ego defenses of the minority group" (1954/1979, p. 144). Some evidence suggests that temporarily stigmatized people do interpret their social interactions through the lens of their stigma even when it in fact has no effect on the treatment that they receive (Kleck & Strenta, 1980), and that members of chronically stigmatized groups (e.g., African Americans, homosexuals) are more conscious of the impact their group membership has on their interactions than are members of nonstigmatized groups (e.g., European Americans, heterosexuals; Pinel, 1999). Members of stigmatized groups (e.g., ethnic minority groups, women) are also far more likely than members of nonstigmatized groups (European Americans, men) to report that both they personally and members of their group have more frequently been victims of discrimination (e.g., Crosby, 1984; Major, Levin, Schmader, & Sidanius, 1999).

Other theory and research, however, suggest that stigmatized people sometimes do not appraise their stigma as stressful and/or do not recognize the role their stigma plays in stigma-related events (Feldman-Barrett & Swim, 1998; Major, 1994). Members of oppressed social groups often fail to see the injustice of their personal situations and are "paradoxically content" even when they are objectively disadvantaged by virtue of their group membership (e.g., Crosby, 1984; Jost & Banaji, 1994; Major, 1987, 1994; Sidanius & Pratto, 1993). Tendencies to compare oneself with similar others can result in a lesser sense of personal entitlement, because such comparisons often prevent disadvantaged people from discovering that dissimilar others are more advantaged than they are (Major, 1987). Even when they become aware that they and/or their group are disadvantaged, endorsement of ideologies that justify the social hierarchy may preclude stigmatized individuals from seeing their treatment as unfair (see Major, 1994, for a review).

Stigmatized people also may not perceive themselves as victims of discrimination because of the costs such a perception may entail, such as relinquishing control over their outcomes and acknowledging that they are victims (Crocker & Major, 1994; Crosby, 1984; Crosby,

Pufall, Snyder, O'Connell, & Whalen, 1989; Major, 1987; Swim et al., 1998). It may be more psychologically adaptive for stigmatized individuals to deny that they are discriminated against than to abandon their belief in control, which would follow from an acknowledgment that they are victims of injustice (e.g., Crosby et al., 1989; Major, 1987, 1994). Indeed, self-blame rather than blaming others often is more adaptive for victims of misfortune (e.g., Wortman, 1983). Ruggiero and Taylor (1995, 1997) demonstrated experimentally that members of stigmatized groups (women, African Americans, and Asian Americans) tend to minimize discrimination as a cause of negative performance feedback relative to objective probabilities of discrimination. Perceiving oneself as a victim of others also may have social costs for stigmatized individuals (see Swim et al., 1998). People who claim that they have been discriminated against often experience significant interpersonal difficulties and social rejection.

To summarize, there is some evidence to suggest that under some circumstances stigmatized people do not appraise their stigma as a stressor. Furthermore, there is evidence to suggest that they sometimes minimize the causal association between their stigma and their outcomes. There is also substantial evidence to indicate, however, that they are highly aware of and attuned to their stigma's potential negative implications for their lives. Consequently, we assume that stigmatized individuals frequently appraise their stigma as a stressor and realize its potential negative impact on their outcomes.

Coping with Stigma-Related Threat

How do individuals who appraise their stigma or stigma-related events as stressful (or potentially stressful) respond to their predicament? A number of authors have tackled this question, often by listing the variety of victims' responses to prejudice or unfair treatment. For example, Allport (1954/1979) listed 14 different types of "ego defenses" that he believed victims of prejudice might adopt. Likewise, Goffman (1963) generated a number of ways in which people who are stigmatized may respond to their situation, as did Jones and colleagues (1984) and Crocker and Major (1989). The ways in which members of minority groups (e.g., Simpson & Yinger, 1985), members of groups characterized by a negative social identity (e.g., Branscombe & Ellemers, 1998; Tajfel & Turner, 1986), people who are relatively deprived (e.g., Crosby, 1982), or people who are inequitably treated (e.g., Walster, Walster, & Berscheid, 1978) respond to their situations have also been considered. Several different types of responses have been identified. For example, Allport identified two general types of ego defenses used by victims of prejudice: "extropunitive" or "intropunitive." Extropunitive defenses attack the source of the difficulty; victims who adopt these strategies blame outside causes for their handicaps. By contrast, victims employing intropunitive strategies take the responsibility upon themselves for adjusting to the situation. Other distinctions include behavioral versus psychological responses to inequity (e.g., Adams, 1965; Walster et al., 1978); individual versus collective or group-level reactions (Ellemers & Van Rijswijk, 1997); social mobility, social creativity, or social change responses to a negative social identity (Tajfel & Turner, 1986); and assertive versus nonassertive responses to prejudice (Swim, Cohen, & Hyers, 1998).

We believe that the various responses of stigmatized individuals to their predicament can be fruitfully conceptualized within a stress-and-coping framework. Within such a framework, people are described as active agents who attempt to manage stressors and/or emotions associated with those stressors. The empirical literature illustrates that people report using a wide variety of strategies to cope with life situations they appraise as stressful, and that they often use more than one strategy at a time (e.g., Amirkhan, 1990; Carver, Scheier, & Weintraub, 1989; Major, Richards, Cooper, Cozzarelli, & Zubek, 1998). One widely used coping inventory (the COPE scale; Carver et al., 1989), for example, identified 13 different ways people say they cope with events they appraise as stressful, including avoidance, denial, mental disengagement, behavioral disengagement, acceptance, positive reframing, venting negative emotions, seeking emotional support, seeking instrumental social support, religious coping, suppressing activities, active coping, and planful coping. We assume that the responses of stigmatized persons to prejudice and discrimination are similar to the types of coping strategies people use in attempting to manage other types of stressful life events.

A key assumption of stress-and-coping frameworks is that no one "best" coping strategy is effective for all people in all situations. Rather, different coping strategies are effective for different people in different situations. Forsythe and Compas (1987), for example, found that the perceived controllability of a stressful event moderated the association between coping strategy and psychological adjustment. Students who were coping with events they perceived as uncontrollable were less distressed if they used coping efforts targeted at managing their negative emotions. Students who were coping with events they perceived as controllable, in contrast, were less distressed if they used coping efforts that were targeted at solving the problem causing the stress.

How effective a particular strategy is also depends upon the person's goals. Coping is typically conceptualized as having two major goals. The first is altering the troubled person–environment relationship that is causing the perceived stress; the type of coping used to meet this goal is sometimes called "active" or "problem-focused" coping (Folkman et al., 1986). Examples of problem-focused coping efforts include trying to lose weight, filing a grievance about a prejudicial boss, or studying extra hard for an upcoming exam on a topic area in which one's group is stereotyped as being incapable. Each of these strategies has as its goal changing the nature of the relationship between the person and the environment, and hence eliminating the source of stress. The second major goal of coping is generally considered to be regulating stressful emotions; the type of coping employed to achieve this goal is often referred to as "emotion-focused" coping (Folkman et al., 1986). Examples of emotion-focused efforts to cope with stigma include attributing a failure to external factors rather than to one's own limitations, devaluing the importance of a domain in which one has experienced a failure, or engaging in downward social comparisons. Each of these strategies can help an individual reduce negative affect and/or maintain a sense of self-worth. Although both goals can sometimes be served by the same coping strategy, these goals often lead to incompatible coping strategies. For example, attributing a job rejection to prejudice rather than to personal deficiencies can potentially protect the self-esteem of a stigmatized individual (Major & Crocker, 1993); it may also be a means by which the employer could be forced to reconsider the decision not to hire the individual. However, if the job was denied because of genuine shortcomings in the interview performance of the stigmatized person, an attribution to prejudice could prevent the person from improving performance in an interview setting, and hence prevent the person from ultimately obtaining the desired outcome.

In addition to the problem-focused versus emotion-focused distinction among coping strategies described above, coping strategies can be distinguished in other ways. For example, coping efforts may be distinguished by their timing relative to the occurrence of the stressful event. Coping has typically been viewed as something that people do in reaction to events or circumstances that have already occurred and that have been appraised as problematical or stress-provoking. Coping can also be proactive, however (Aspinwall & Taylor, 1997). Proactive strategies are undertaken in anticipation of potentially stressful events. These strategies have as their goal decreasing the probability that the anticipated problem will ensue from the interaction or increasing the likelihood that the person's self-regard or affective state will emerge from the interaction unscathed. It may be harder to recognize proactive than reactive coping efforts, because if the former are successful, they will reduce the likelihood that stressful situations will eventuate. The line between proactive and reactive coping is sometimes blurred. For example, a

heavyweight person who in the past has encountered prejudicial comments at the beach may avoid going to the beach in the future so as to
reduce the likelihood of encountering prejudice again. This avoidance
strategy is both a problem-focused reaction to past pain, and a proactive
strategy to avoid future pain.

We believe that a stress-and-coping framework provides a useful
way of organizing the accumulated body of knowledge on how stigmatized people respond to and attempt to manage the stress posed by their
predicament. In the following discussion, we overview a variety of ways
in which stigmatized persons cope with their predicament. We organize
our discussion around the distinction between problem-focused and
emotion-focused strategies, although we recognize that there is considerable overlap between these types of strategies and that people typically
engage in both emotion-focused and problem-focused strategies simultaneously. We also recognize that coping strategies are interrelated. The
outcome of one strategy serves as feedback to other strategies, and has
implications for future coping efforts.

Problem-Focused Coping with Stigma

Problem-focused strategies can be targeted toward the self, toward others, or toward the situation in which the self and others interact. Coping
efforts that target the self involve changing some aspect of the self to reduce the likelihood that stigma will have a negative impact on interactions with others. Coping efforts that target others involve attempts to
change others so that they either will be prevented from devaluing the
stigmatized person or will be prevented from acting on their perception
of the stigmatized person's devalued social status. Coping efforts that
target the interaction are aimed at structuring situations so that the
stigma does not produce negative consequences for the stigmatized individual. Stigmatized individuals may target any number of these interaction elements (self, others, interaction) in coping with stigma, and may
target them simultaneously. The element they focus on at any particular
time will depend upon their assessment of self, others, and the specific
interaction situation.

Target of Coping Efforts: Self

Most coping efforts that target the self involve reducing the applicability
of the stigma to the self. One obvious way to do this is to eliminate the
stigmatizing condition. The popularity of dieting to achieve weight loss,
of cosmetic surgery to eliminate the signs of aging or to alter body parts
deemed less than perfect, and of therapy to overcome mental illness and

addictions suggests that elimination of one's stigmatized status is a common coping response. Another way to reduce the applicability of the stigmatizing condition to the self is to conceal or disguise it (Goffman, 1963). People conceal a wide variety of conditions, including homosexuality, mental disorders, physical illnesses, and abortion (e.g., Cole, Kemeny, & Taylor, 1997; Major & Gramzow, 1999). Members of stigmatized racial and ethnic minority groups can also sometimes "pass" as nonstigmatized persons (Goffman, 1963).

Stigmatized people also may try to compensate for the problems stigma creates in social interactions (Miller & Myers, 1998; Miller, Rothblum, Felicio, & Brand, 1995). Compensation is a coping response in which stigmatized persons alter their behavior so that they achieve their interaction goals despite the fact that the people with whom they are interacting may be prejudiced against them. Interaction goals may include gaining access to resources that another person controls (e.g., getting a raise from a prejudiced boss), being accepted by another, or expressing one's identity. Compensation can include exerting more effort or developing and refining interaction skills (Miller & Myers, 1998). Stigmatized people often express the belief that they have to work harder to receive the same evaluations that nonstigmatized persons would get (Jackson, Thoits, & Taylor, 1995). They may try harder and be more persistent than their nonstigmatized counterparts in social situations (Dion & Stein, 1978). Stigmatized people may behave in a more socially skilled manner when faced with the threat of prejudice (Miller et al., 1995). Other skills that may enable stigmatized people to achieve their goals despite prejudice include assertiveness (Dion & Stein, 1978; Miller & Myers, 1998), the ability to decipher subtle cues about the interaction partners' affect and motivation (Hall, 1978), and careful attention to situational cues (Frable, Blackstone, & Scherbaum, 1990). Stigmatized individuals may also develop bicultural skills, so that they can effectively function in the dominant culture as well as in the culture of their stigmatized group. African Americans, for example, often become adept at "code switching," which is using the dialect (Standard or Black English) used by the people with whom they are speaking at any given time (Agerton & Moran, 1995; Townsend, 1998).

One decision stigmatized people face when they compensate for others' prejudice is whether to try to confirm or disconfirm stereotyped expectations. Disconfirmation of stereotypes distances a stigmatized person from the stigma: The stigmatized person displays attitudes, behaviors, symbols, and signs that he or she is not like other people in the stigmatized group. In contrast, confirmation invites others to perceive the stigmatized person as a member of the stigmatized group. Although at first glance disconfirmation would seem to be the more adaptive coping response, research indicates that the stigmatized use both strategies. For example, Steele and Aronson (2000) found that when African American college students were faced with a test of academic ability under conditions in which the stereotype that African Americans do poorly in academic domains was salient, they disavowed having interests and preferences consistent with stereotypes about their group (e.g., liking rap music). Similarly, Kaiser and Miller (1999) found that women who thought a self-descriptive essay might be evaluated by a sexist judge described themselves in more masculine and less feminine terms than did women who did not anticipate sexism. These studies suggest that when faced with the threat of being stereotyped, stigmatized people may be motivated to disconfirm stereotypes about their group.

Sometimes, however, it may be more beneficial for stigmatized people to confirm a stereotype in order to achieve their goals. When others have power over stigmatized people, and expect stigmatized people to assume certain identities and behave in certain ways, it may behoove a stigmatized person to fulfill those expectations to obtain what he or she wants (Deaux & Major, 1987). Von Baeyer, Sherk, and Zanna (1981) showed this coping response in a study in which college women were interviewed for a job by a male interviewer who supposedly had either liberal or traditional views about the role of women. The women tailored their appearance and performance during the interview to fit the interviewer's expectations.

Although the experimental situations in the studies described above differed in several respects, one key difference was whether others' expectations and desires were clearly communicated to the stigmatized person. In the study in which stereotype confirmation occurred (Von Baeyer et al., 1981), the women knew the interviewers' preferences. In the other studies (Kaiser & Miller, 2000; Steele & Aronson, 1995), stereotypes were salient, but it was not clear whether the others would prefer a confirming or disconfirming response.

We would not wish to leave the impression that stigmatized people are always, or even usually, preoccupied with the question of whether they will be perceived in stereotype-consistent or stereotype-inconsistent fashion. Sometimes they may simply want to convey certain images—for example, that they are competent, moral, powerful, or likable (Jones & Pittman, 1982; Leary & Kowalski, 1990)—regardless of whether these images are consistent, inconsistent, or even relevant to stereotypes about their group. In other words, stigmatized people may bypass the issue of stereotype confirmation completely and focus their attention on general self-presentation strategies that anyone might use in a situation. They may recognize that more effort or skill may be required for them to create desired images, gain acceptance, or get access to resources that others control than would be the case if they were not stigmatized. But this recognition of the barrier posed by prejudice to achieving their interaction goals does not dictate that their only choice is to confirm or disconfirm a stereotype.

Target of Efforts: Situations

People can also cope with stigma by structuring situations in ways that avoid the problems of prejudice. One way to do this is to avoid situations that expose them to the prejudice of others (see Swim et al., 1998, for a review). Heavyweight people may avoid places such as fast-food restaurants or the beach, which are especially likely to expose them to censure (Myers, 1998). Ethnic minorities may develop their own communities or relocate to areas where prejudice is less prevalent, and deaf students may restrict their school attendance to deaf-only schools. Stigmatized people may also try to avoid nonstigmatized individuals who they know, suspect, or predict will exhibit prejudice against them. For example, women avoid interactions with men who are reputed to be sexist (Fitzgerald, Swan, & Fischer, 1995).

Total avoidance of nonstigmatized others may not be possible or desired, however. For this reason, stigmatized people may evaluate specific situations for the likelihood that prejudice may have negative consequences. They may then avoid especially those situations in which the possibility of prejudice-based responses is high. These may include situations in which stigmatized people occupy roles of relatively low status. Unequal status serves to perpetuate stereotypes and conflict between stigmatized and nonstigmatized people (Pettigrew, 1986). Professional women at business meetings, for example, may decline the opportunity to take minutes for the group, to avoid any suggestion that they are content to fulfill the stereotypic role of assistant rather than that of policy maker. A stigmatized person may also avoid being the solo or token representative of his or her group in a situation (Cohen & Swim, 1995). Tokens believe that others judge them harshly and view their behavior in dispositional terms (Imamura, 1990)—a perception that accurately reflects the demonstrated effects of solo status (Cohen & Swim, 1995; Fiske, 1998).

The flip side of avoiding nonstigmatized others is to affiliate oneself selectively with members of the stigmatized group. A large body of research shows that people are attracted to and seek affiliation with similar others (see Berscheid & Reis, 1998, for a review). The benefits of interactions with similar others include validation of beliefs and attitudes (Byrne, 1971), mutual need gratification (Condon & Crano, 1988), mutual understanding (Levenger & Breedlove, 1966), and interaction compatibility (Ickes, 1985; Ickes & Barnes, 1978), as well as provision of emotional and instrumental social support. By affiliating with similarly stigmatized others, stigmatized people gain a respite from prejudice, in addition to all of the benefits that may ordinarily occur as a consequence of affiliation with similar others. Separatist movements, in which groups such as African Americans and deaf people segregate themselves from society at large and focus on developing their own culture, are one form of selective affiliation. More commonly, stigmatized people may gravitate toward members of their own group for voluntary contacts such as socializing, without seeking to withdraw completely from interactions with nonstigmatized people.

Target of Efforts: Others

There would be no need to target coping efforts at changing either the self or the interaction if the stigmatized group's social devaluation could be eliminated. There have indeed been many efforts to eliminate the prejudice of others. Usually these efforts take the form of education and persuasion campaigns. The "Black is beautiful" movement, the National Association for the Advancement of Fat Acceptance, and the "gay pride" movement represent just a few of the many efforts that have been made to advocate greater acceptance of stigmatized people. One way to gain acceptance can involve increased emphasis on biological or medical models to explain the origins of stigmatized conditions. People are held less responsible for stigmas caused by genetic endowment or illness, and others generally have more sympathy for people whose stigmatizing condition is perceived as outside their control than for people who are perceived as being responsible for their stigmatizing condition (Crocker & Major, 1994; Weiner, Perry, & Magnusson, 1988).

If prejudice cannot be eliminated, coexistence may be possible if others can be prevented from acting on their prejudice. Stigmatized people may strive to influence the political process to obtain enforcement of their civil rights. Laws that prohibit gender, ethnic, and religious discrimination and that require reasonable accommodations for people with disabilities are examples. Affirmative action represents another attempt to provide a more level playing field for stigmatized people. In addition, stigmatized individuals may strive to create social norms that make it socially undesirable to express prejudice. For example, researchers are increasingly turning to unobtrusive measures of prejudice toward African Americans, because people are not willing to answer questionnaire or survey questions in ways that make them appear to be prejudiced (Crosby, Bromley, & Saxe, 1980; Fazio, Jackson, Dunton, & Williams, 1995; McConahay, 1986). Efforts to make expressions of prejudice socially unacceptable have been more successful for some stigmatized groups than for others. In the United States, for example, expressions of prejudice toward African Americans, Hispanics, and people with disabilities are likely to bring censure in many social circles. People with other types of stigmas have had less success in creating norms against prejudice. Prejudice against fat persons continues to be overt and socially acceptable, for instance (Crandall, 1994). During the effort to impeach President Clinton for his relationship with Monica Lewinsky, many derisive public comments were made about her weight. Linda Tripp, who secretly recorded and then made public her phone conversations with Monica Lewinsky, stood accused of being ugly as well as fat, and it sometimes seemed that these stigmatizing conditions were perceived as more offensive than was her betrayal of the young woman who thought she was her friend.

Coping efforts that target others for change can also become collective efforts (Tajfel & Turner, 1986; Wright, Taylor, & Moghaddam, 1990). Although a single person can exert pressure on the majority if that individual's arguments are powerful and consistent, more sources of influence increase social pressure (Latané & Wolf, 1981; Nemeth, 1986). Collective actions by the stigmatized individuals, however, are surprisingly rare (e.g., Wright et al., 1990). One reason such actions are rare is that they are likely to be met with resistance from nonstigmatized people. Collective efforts to create social change endanger nonstigmatized persons' control over power and resources, challenge the legitimacy of the current status situation, and threaten nonstigmatized individuals' self-esteem (Crocker et al., 1998; Major, 1994; Sidanius & Pratto, 1993). Consequently, stigmatized individuals who engage in collective actions are likely to incur significant personal costs. Nonetheless, collective coping efforts may be most likely to produce long-term social change.

Emotion-Focused Coping with Stigma

The problem-focused strategies described above attempt, either directly or indirectly, to change the relationship between a person and the environment so as to reduce the extent to which the person will experience stigma-related problems. Emotion-focused coping strategies, in contrast, are used to regulate emotions associated with stressors. In the domain of stigma, emotion-focused strategies seek especially to minimize negative affect and protect self-esteem from stigma-related stressors such as prejudice. A wide variety of strategies can be used to regulate negative emotion and to protect self-esteem from threats to the self. Because emotion-focused strategies have been the focus of a recent review (e.g., Crocker et al., 1998), our consideration of these strategies here is brief and selective.

Social comparisons constitute one way in which the stigmatized may protect their self-esteem and regulate stressful emotions related to stigma (Crocker & Major, 1989). Comparisons with others provide a reference, or standard, against which the self and one's outcomes are evaluated. By restricting their social comparisons to others who are like them—who share their stigmatized status—stigmatized persons can protect themselves from exposure to, and the potentially painful emotional consequences of, upward comparisons with nonstigmatized others (see Crocker et al., 1998, and Major, 1994, for reviews). Downward social comparisons with others who are worse off can also regulate negative emotion following threat (Wills, 1981). The emotional benefits of comparisons with others who share a stigmatizing attribute account, in part, for the prevalence of support groups for individuals with various disabilities, and for the popularity of ethnically and religiously oriented clubs on campuses.

Stigmatized people can also protect their self-esteem and emotional well-being through selective construals of available comparison information. Upward comparisons with others who are dissimilar to the self in some way, even a minor way, may be dismissed as not self-relevant, thereby protecting affect and self-esteem (e.g., Major, Sciacchitano, & Crocker, 1993). Furthermore, upward comparisons with advantaged others may be inspiring rather than demoralizing, if they are accompanied by the belief that one's own situation may improve (Major, Testa, & Bylsma, 1991; Testa & Major, 1990). Comparison strategies can also be used to protect collective self-esteem in the face of threats to one's social group. Tajfel and Turner (1986), for example, note that stigmatized persons may compare their ingroup to the outgroup on some new dimension on which the ingroup is not relatively disadvantaged; may change the values assigned to the attributes of the ingroup, so that comparisons that were previously negative are now seen as positive; or may change the outgroup with which the ingroup is compared, so that a higher-status outgroup is no longer used as a comparative frame of reference. In short, various comparison strategies may help the stigmatized to regulate emotion and protect personal and collective self-esteem in the face of stigma-related stressors.

Attributions can also help stigmatized individuals to protect self-esteem and regulate emotional reactions in the face of stigma-related stressors. According to attributional models of emotion, negative outcomes attributed to external factors are less likely to lead to negative emotion than are negative outcomes attributed to internal factors (e.g., Weiner, 1985). Following from this premise, Crocker and Major (1989) hypothesized that one way in which stigmatized persons may protect their self-esteem from stigma-related threats is by attributing negative outcomes to prejudice and discrimination rather than to their own personal deservingness. Consistent with this hypothesis, when prejudice is blatant and/or is seen as unjustified, attributions to prejudice do protect self-esteem from negative outcomes (Crocker et al., 1991; Major & Quinton, 1999). Likewise, when tests are seen as biased against one's group, failures on those tests have less negative impact on self-esteem than do failures on tests are seen as unbiased (Major, Spencer, Schmader, Wolfe, & Crocker, 1998).

Attributions to prejudice, however, are not always protective of self-esteem. When prejudice is seen as potentially justifiable, such as when it is believed to be due to lesser ability or is believed to be based on potentially controllable factors such as weight, attributions to prejudice do not protect self-esteem (Crocker & Major, 1994; Crocker, Cornwell, & Major, 1993). Furthermore, a tendency to attribute negative outcomes to prejudice in the absence of clear situational cues that prejudice is a plausible cause of outcomes is not self-protective. Major and Quinton (1999) found that the more women attributed a rejection to sex discrimination when situational cues indicative of prejudice were absent, the lower was their self-esteem. In contrast, the more women attributed a rejection to sex discrimination when clear situational cues indicative of prejudice were present, the higher was their subsequent self-esteem. These findings illustrate that blaming misfortune on prejudice is not always an effective strategy for regulating negative emotion in response to stigma-related stressors.

Indeed, one way stigmatized people may cope with emotions due to stigma-related stress is by denying or minimizing the extent to which they are targets of prejudice. As noted earlier, denial of discrimination can sometimes be an adaptive strategy, at least in the short run, compared to acknowledging oneself as a victim and relinquishing a sense of control over one's own outcomes. Branscombe, Schmitt, and Harvey (1999) recently found that the less African American students saw themselves as targets of racial prejudice in general, the higher their self-esteem was. This finding is consistent with earlier studies indicating that self-blame for misfortune is often more adaptive than is blaming others (e.g., Wortman, 1983). Much research within the literature on stress and coping, however, has found that using denial as a coping strategy is associated with poorer physical and mental health outcomes over time (e.g., Aldwin & Levenson, 1994). Whether denying or acknowledging prejudice as a potential cause of one's outcomes is adaptive or not is likely to depend on a variety of factors, such as the extent to which prejudice is flagrant, the extent to which others agree with one's own interpretation of events, and the degree of control one perceives oneself to have over the situation.

Stigmatized people may also cope emotionally with stigma-related stressors by restructuring their self-concept in such a way that stigma-related stressors have less damaging implications for the self (see Crocker et al., 1998, for a review). For example, they may selectively devalue, or reduce the importance to the self, of domains in which they or others like them are disadvantaged, and selectively value domains in which they or others like them are advantaged (Crocker & Major, 1989; Major & Schmader, 1998). The impact of evaluative feedback in a particular domain on self-esteem and affect is moderated in an important way by the psychological centrality of that domain to the self (e.g., Tesser, 1988). By diminishing the importance of domains in the self-concept, stigmatized persons lessen the extent to which they will suffer emotionally as a consequence of doing poorly in a domain. This process can lead them to disengage or unlink their self-esteem from their performance or outcomes in certain domains, either temporarily or chronically (Major & Schmader, 1998; Steele, 1997). Major and Schmader (1998) and Steele (1997) have argued that disidentification from school may account in part for how African American students maintain high self-esteem in the face of poor school performance.

MODERATORS OF COPING STRATEGIES

Various factors are likely to moderate the strategies that the stigmatized use to cope with stigma-related stress (Jones et al., 1984). We believe that three are especially important: the extent to which a stigma is associated with a group identity, the extent to which the stigma is concealable, and the extent to which a stigmatized person perceives control over the stigma or responses to it.

Group Identity

Some stigmas, such as stigmas based on race or religion, are associated with a recognizable group identity, whereas other stigmas, such as those based on physical deformities or obesity, are not. People who possess stigmas that are more collective in nature (i.e., that have a recognizable group identity) are more likely to identify with that group than are those whose stigmas are more individual. People with strong group identities, in turn, may be more likely to recognize the role that their stigmatized status plays in causing their outcomes (Branscombe & Ellemers, 1998; Major, 1994). They therefore may be more likely to attribute outcomes to prejudice (Major, Levin, Schmader, & Sidanius, 1999; Major & Quinton, 1999) than those who are less group-identified. Individuals who are highly group-identified may also be more likely to compare themselves to other members of their ingroup, selectively affiliate with members of their ingroup, seek social support from stigmatized others, and engage in collective efforts on behalf of their ingroup.

Stigma Concealability

The extent to which a stigma is visible or concealable is also likely to be important in how individuals cope. People with visible stigmas should be more likely to attribute their outcomes to prejudice, because their stigmatizing condition is immediately apparent to others. Although they may often question about whether stigma or some other factor was responsible for a particular outcome, they are rarely in doubt about whether their stigmatized status was known to the other. People with invisible stigmas, in contrast, are often in doubt about both questions. People with invisible stigmas may be more likely to conceal them. In fact, for people with stigmas that are associated with relatively few overt behaviors or other indicators, such as women who have had abortions, the default condition may be that others do not know about the stigma unless a stigmatized person reveals it. People with invisible stigmas also may be less likely to seek social support or engage in collective coping strategies, because these responses would expose their previously concealed stigmatizing condition. Other strategies may be relatively ineffective for people with invisible stigmas. For example, making self-protective attributions of poor outcomes to prejudice may be counterproductive for people with invisible stigmas, because the point of concealing the stigma is that others' prejudice will not be a cause of the outcomes received by the stigmatized person.

Perceived Control

Perceived control is a multifaceted variable as it relates to coping with stigma. In the coping literature, perceived control over the problem is a major determinant of problem-focused and emotion-focused coping efforts. Individuals who believe that they have some control over the problem are more likely to engage in problem-focused coping, whereas those who perceive little control are more likely to focus on emotion regulation (Folkman et al., 1986). Likewise, stigmatized people who perceive some control over the problems of stigma should be more likely to take a problem-focused approach than those who perceive that they have less control.

One important element of perceived control as it relates to stigma involves control over the stigmatizing condition itself. People who believe that their stigmatizing condition is controllable are more likely to use coping strategies that focus on changing the self (e.g., losing weight). High perceived control over a stigmatizing condition can diminish the effectiveness of other coping responses. For example, heavyweight college women who were rejected by a male partner attributed his rejection to their weight, but did not blame him for this rejection because they blamed themselves for being heavyweight (Crocker et al., 1993). This may explain why people with heavy body weight have low self-esteem, whereas people with stigmas that are perceived as less controllable do not (Miller & Downey, 1999). The perceptions of others about the controllability of the stigma are also important. As we have previously described, stigmatized people may attempt to change others' perceptions about the controllability of their stigmatizing condition as a way to reduce others' proclivity to devalue them for having the condition.

Perceived control also includes perceptions about the controllability of prejudice and prejudice-based responses. Stigmatized individuals who believe that others' prejudice can be reduced may be more likely to cope by attempting to persuade or educate others about prejudice. Those who believe that expressions of prejudice can be controlled may try to create and enforce norms that discourage the expression of prejudice. The belief that others can be prevented from expressing prejudiced responses should also promote the use of compensatory strategies. Stigmatized people are not likely to use greater skill or effort to achieve interaction goals unless they have some hope that these coping responses can control others' prejudiced responses. Stigma affects how much control over important outcomes people actually have. Social systems that tolerate overt or implicit prejudice and discrimination can limit the opportunities of stigmatized people, thereby rendering them relatively powerless to achieve mastery over their environment (Fiske, 1993; Sidanius & Pratto, 1993). This powerlessness may encourage the use of coping strategies that focus on managing the emotions and threats to self-esteem that stigma creates, rather than on how situations might be changed to reduce the stress.

COSTS OF COPING

Every response made to cope with stigma exacts costs from a stigmatized person. Accordingly, the costs of a coping response must be weighed against its likely value in reducing stigma-related stress. The costs and benefits will vary, depending on the nature of the stigmatizing condition, the resources of the stigmatized person, his or her goals in a particular situation, the characteristics of the people with whom the stigmatized person interacts, and the nature of the situation in which the interaction occurs. Stigmatized people may anticipate the costs of a coping response and decide that, all things considered, this response is still the most adaptive strategy at this time. In other cases the costs may not be foreseen (see Baumeister & Scher, 1988, for a similar discussion of costs). For example, when stigmatized people compare their outcomes with members of their own group, they may not foresee that a consequence of this strategy is that they may deprive themselves of information that would enable them to evaluate the fairness of their outcomes (Major, 1987, 1994). Costs associated with a particular coping response also may not be recognized as such when they occur. For example, when stigmatized people compensate for prejudice by using increased skills or effort, they may experience physical symptoms or other problems as a result of the stress involved in making these efforts. These consequences may not be identified as a direct result of the compensatory effort. Finally, it is critical to keep in mind that both problem-focused and emotion-focused strategies can be costly for a stigmatized person.

Consider the costs of problem-focused coping efforts targeted at the self. Eliminating a stigmatizing condition usually involves physical, emotional, and financial costs. A failed effort to remove a stigmatizing condition may be stressful, because the stigmatized person may consider the inability to change as a personal shortcoming. Stigmatized people who conceal their stigmatizing condition face the constant risk of discovery. Avoiding discovery may require vigilance to avoid giving the secret away. This can create a host of problems, including intrusive thoughts about the stigma and reduced resistance to physical ills (Cole et al., 1997; Major & Gramzow, 1999; Smart & Wegner, Chapter 8, this volume). Social identity can also become problematic for people who conceal a stigmatizing condition. They may lose the opportunity for social comparison, social support, and validation that would be provided by affiliation with other stigmatized individuals. Even if a stigmatized person is not attempting to hide a concealable stigmatizing condition, each new encounter raises the question of when and how the stigmatized person should reveal the stigma to the other. Compensation for prejudice also carries risks. Unskilled application of compensatory skills can lead to overcompensation, in which the stigmatized person's efforts to compensate backfire and make the situation worse (Kaiser & Miller, 1999; Miller & Myers, 1998). Moreover, compensation may drain the individual's resources and increase vulnerability to stress-related problems. For example, in a sample of working-class Southern African American men, an orientation toward active coping efforts coupled with the belief that hard work and determination can achieve one's goals ("John Henry-ism") was associated with hypertension (James, Hartnett, & Kalsbeek, 1983).

Coping efforts aimed at reducing prejudice in others can also de-mand commitments of time, money, energy, and other resources. Unfor-tunately, they are likely to have a low probability of success as well. Re-duction of prejudice is not simply a matter of convincing people that it is not acceptable to devalue some groups of people (see Crocker et al., 1998, for a review). Even well-meaning people with egalitarian values may harbor ambivalent feelings toward stigmatized people (Katz, 1981; Katz, Wackenhut, & Hass, 1986). Individualism may vie with egalitari-anism for the upper hand in nonstigmatized people's response to stigma-tized people. Perhaps most important is the fact that expressions of prejudice may not be completely controllable (Devine, 1989). When nonstigmatized people are stressed, preoccupied, or experiencing emo-tional arousal, prejudice-based responses that they ordinarily suppress may elude their control efforts (Dovidio & Gaertner, 1986). Conse-quently, being motivated not to be prejudiced is not sufficient to elimi-nate expressions of prejudice (Devine, Monteith, Zuwerink, & Elliot, 1991). For this reason, stigmatized people may become discouraged at the intractable nature of others' prejudice against their group. Stigma-tized people who attempt to create social norms that discourage the ex-pression of prejudice are often accused of creating a climate of "political correctness," in which innocent or careless expressions are severely cen-sured. Moreover, some efforts to eliminate prejudice as a determinant of outcomes received by stigmatized people can create other costs. Affirma-tive action provides educational and employment opportunities to stig-matized people that they otherwise would not have had, but are costly in terms of the attributions others make about stigmatized people who en-joy these opportunities (Heilman, Block, & Stathatos, 1997).

Avoiding situations in which prejudice may be encountered may limit stigmatized individuals' access to resources controlled by nonstig-matized people. Avoidance may also preclude the possibility that stigma-tized individuals can dispel stereotypes and prejudice through their inter-actions with nonstigmatized others. Avoiding situations that might expose one to stigma-based harassment severely circumscribes one's freedom. Women who travel alone are well aware of how constraining this can be.

One damaging consequence of the emotion-focused coping re-sponses reviewed above can be reduction of motivation to succeed in a domain. For example, devaluing academics may protect stigmatized stu-dents from negative stereotypes about their group in the school domain, but may do so at the cost of reducing their motivation and interest in academic pursuits. Severing the link between academic performance and self-esteem can lead to decreased persistence in schoolwork and/or withdrawal from school, thereby increasing the likelihood of experiencing academic setbacks (Major & Schmader, 1998; Steele, 1997). Similarly, regularly perceiving prejudice as the cause for negative outcomes may prevent a stigmatized person from recognizing instances in which he or she played a role in producing these outcomes. In situations in which greater effort or ability would have produced a better outcome, the attribution to prejudice may lead the stigmatized person to give up prematurely or unnecessarily (Major & Crocker, 1993). The strategy of avoiding comparisons with nonstigmatized people can prevent stigmatized people from recognizing the injustice of the outcomes they receive (Major, 1987).

SUMMARY AND CONCLUSIONS

In this chapter, we have used a stress-and-coping framework to understand the experiences and adaptive reactions of individuals who are targets of prejudice because they are stigmatized. We argue that possession of a stigma is a potentially stressful life experience, similar to other types of chronic and/or acute stressors. Furthermore, we argue that how stigmatized people appraise and cope with their situation is an important determinant of their adaptation. This framework allows us to understand both between-group and within-group variations in vulnerability and resilience to stigma.

An important message of this chapter is that there is nothing pathological or neurotic about the approaches taken by stigmatized individuals to cope with stigma-related stress. People use a variety of strategies to cope with stigma and stigma-related prejudice, just as they use a variety of strategies to cope with other types of life circumstances that are appraised as stressful. Both individual differences and situational factors determine the strategies that are used, as well as the effectiveness of those strategies. No one strategy is likely to be effective across all situations. Rather, the appropriate question is what strategy works best for which individual in what situation. The stigmatized person's goals are critically important in what type of strategy will best serve his or her needs. Both problem-focused and emotion-focused coping are likely to be employed to cope with stigma, and use of each strategy has multiple effects. Some of these effects are costly, as our brief review indicates. Thus successful adaptation of stigmatized persons is typically not achieved without a price.

Values inevitably enter into any discussion of how stigmatized people cope with stigma. Many assume that only coping efforts focused on changing the status quo are desirable. The implicit assumption of this view is that only direct challenges to prejudiced people will help stigmatized people achieve their goals. Although this view may be correct with respect to achieving long-term social change, one consequence of valuing some coping responses more than others is that stigmatized people can encounter criticism both from within and outside their stigmatized group for choosing the "wrong" coping response. This disapproval itself becomes yet another source of stigma-related stress. People differ in the goals they want to achieve, the resources they can draw on, their perception of the level and pervasiveness of prejudice they face, and the extent to which identification with the stigmatized group is important to them. This diversity must be respected as we seek to understand how people cope with the consequences of stigma.

REFERENCES

Adams, J. S. (1965). Inequity in social exchange. In L. Berkowitz (Ed.), *Advances in experimental social psychology* (Vol. 2, pp. 267–298). New York: Academic Press.

Agerton, E. P., & Moran, M. J. (1995). Effects of race and dialect of examiner on language samples elicited from southern African American preschoolers. *Journal of Childhood Communication Disorders, 16,* 25–30.

Aldwin, C. M., & Levenson, M. R. (1994). Aging and personality assessment. *Annual Review of Gerontology and Geriatrics, 14,* 182–209.

Allison, K. W. (1998). Stress and oppressed social category membership. In J. K. Swim & C. Stangor (Eds.), *Prejudice: The target's perspective* (pp. 145–170). San Diego, CA: Academic Press.

Allport, G. (1979). *The nature of prejudice.* New York: Doubleday/Anchor. (Original work published 1954)

Amirkhan, J. H. (1990). Applying attribution theory to the study of stress and coping. In S. Graham & S. Folkes (Eds.), *Attribution theory: Applications to achievement, mental health, and interpersonal conflict* (pp. 79–102). Hillsdale, NJ: Erlbaum.

Aspinwall, L. G., & Taylor, S. E. (1997). A stitch in time: Self-regulation and proactive coping. *Psychological Bulletin, 121,* 417–436.

Bandura, A. (1977). Self-efficacy: Toward a unifying theory of behavioral change. *Psychological Review, 84,* 191–215.

Bandura, A. (1982). Self-efficacy mechanism in human agency. *American Psychologist, 37,* 122–147.

Baumeister, R. F., & Leary, M. R. (1995). The need to belong: Desire for interpersonal attachments as a fundamental human motivation. *Psychological Bulletin, 117,* 497–529.

Baumeister, R. F., & Scher, S. J. (1988). Self-defeating behavior among normal individuals: Review and analysis of common self-destructive tendencies. *Psychological Bulletin, 104*, 3–22.

Berscheid, E., & Reis, H. T. (1998). Attraction and close relationships. In D. T. Gilbert, S. T. Fiske, & G. Lindzey (Eds.), *Handbook of social psychology* (4th ed., Vol. 2, pp. 193–281). Boston: McGraw-Hill.

Branscombe, N. R., & Ellemers, N. (1998). Coping with group-based discrimination: Individualistic versus group-level strategies. In J. K. Swim & C. Stangor (Eds.), *Prejudice: The target's perspective* (pp. 243–266). San Diego, CA: Academic Press.

Branscombe, N. R., Schmitt, M. T. & Harvey, R. D. (1999). Perceiving pervasive discrimination among African-Americans: Implications for group identification and well-being. *Journal of Personality and Social Psychology, 77*, 135–149.

Byrne, D. (1971). *The attraction paradigm*. New York: Academic Press.

Carver, C. S., Glass, D. C., & Katz, I. (1977). Favorable evaluations of Blacks and the handicapped: Positive prejudice, unconscious denial, or social desirability? *Journal of Applied Social Psychology, 8*, 97–106.

Carver, C. S., Scheier, M. F., & Weintraub, J. K. (1989). Assessing coping strategies: A theoretically based approach. *Journal of Personality and Social Psychology, 56*, 267–283.

Cohen, L. L., & Swim, J. K. (1995). The differential effect of gender ratios on women and men: Tokenism, self-confidence, and expectations. *Personality and Social Psychology Bulletin, 21*, 876–884.

Cole, S. W., Kemeny, M. E., & Taylor, S. E. (1997). Social identity and physical health: Accelerated HIV progression in rejection-sensitive gay men. *Journal of Personality and Social Psychology, 72*, 320–335.

Condon, J. W., & Crano, W. D. (1988). Inferred evaluation and the relation between attitude similarity and interpersonal attraction. *Journal of Personality and Social Psychology, 54*, 789–797.

Crandall, C. S. (1994). Prejudice against fat people: Ideology and self-interest. *Journal of Personality and Social Psychology, 66*, 882–894.

Crocker, J., Cornwell, B., & Major, B. (1993). The stigma of overweight: Affective consequences of attributional ambiguity. *Journal of Personality and Social Psychology, 64*, 60–70.

Crocker, J., & Major, B. (1989). Social stigma and self-esteem: The self-protective properties of stigma. *Psychological Bulletin, 96*, 608–630.

Crocker, J., & Major, B. (1994). Reactions to stigma: The moderating effect of justifications. In M. P. Zanna & J. M. Olson (Eds.), *The Ontario Symposium: Vol 7. The psychology of prejudice* (pp. 289–314). Hillsdale, NJ: Erlbaum.

Crocker, J., Major, B., & Steele, C. (1998). Social stigma. In D. T. Gilbert, S. T. Fiske, & G. Lindzey (Eds.), *Handbook of social psychology*, (4th ed., Vol. 2, pp. 504–553). Boston: McGraw-Hill.

Crocker, J., Voelkl, K., Testa, M., & Major, B. (1991). Social stigma: The affective consequences of attributional ambiguity. *Journal of Personality and Social Psychology, 60*, 218–228.

Crosby, F. (1982). *Relative deprivation and working women*. New York: Oxford University Press.

Crosby, F. (1984). The denial of personal discrimination. *American Behavioral Scientist, 27,* 371–386.

Crosby, F., Bromley, S., & Saxe, L. (1980). Recent unobtrusive studies of Black and White discrimination and prejudice: A literature review. *Psychological Bulletin, 87,* 546–563.

Crosby, F., Pufall, A., Snyder, R. C., O'Connell, M., & Whalen, P. (1989). The denial of personal disadvantage among you, me, and all the other ostriches. In M. Crawford & M. Gentry (Eds.), *Gender and thought: Psychological perspectives* (pp. 79–99). New York: Springer-Verlag.

Deaux, K., & Major, B. (1987). Putting gender into context: An integrative model of gender-related behavior. *Psychological Review, 94,* 369–389.

Devine, P. G. (1989). Stereotyping and prejudice: Their automatic and controlled components. *Journal of Personality and Social Psychology, 56,* 5–18.

Devine, P. G., Monteith, M. J., Zuwerink, J. R., & Elliot, A. J. (1991). Prejudice with and without compunction. *Journal of Personality and Social Psychology, 60,* 817–830.

Dion, K. K., & Stein, S. (1978). Physical attractiveness and interpersonal influence. *Journal of Experimental Social Psychology, 14,* 97–108.

Dovidio, J. F., & Gaertner, S. L. (Eds.). (1986). *Prejudice, discrimination, and racism.* Orlando, FL: Academic Press.

Ellemers, N., & Van Rijswijk, W. (1997). Identity versus social opportunities: The use of group level and individual level identity management strategies. *Social Psychology Quarterly, 60,* 52–65.

Fazio, R. H., Jackson, J. R., Dunton, B. C., & Williams, C. J. (1995). Variability in automatic activation as an unobtrusive measure of racial attitudes: A bona fide pipeline? *Journal of Personality and Social Psychology, 69,* 1013–1927.

Feingold, A. (1992). Good-looking people are not what we think. *Psychological Bulletin, 111,* 304–341.

Feldman-Barrett, L., & Swim, J. K. (1998). Appraisals of prejudice and discrimination. In J. K. Swim & C. Stangor (Eds.), *Prejudice: The target's perspective* (pp. 11–36). San Diego, CA: Academic Press.

Fiske, S. T. (1993). Controlling other people: The impact of power on stereotyping. *American Psychologist, 48,* 621–628.

Fiske, S. T. (1998). Stereotypes, prejudice, and discrimination. In D. T. Gilbert, S. T. Fiske, & G. Lindzey (Eds.) *Handbook of social psychology* (4th ed., Vol. 2, pp. 357–411). Boston: McGraw-Hill.

Fitzgerald, L. F., Swan, S., & Fischer, K. (1995). Why didn't she just report him? The psychological and legal implications of women's responses to sexual harassment. *Journal of Social Issues, 51,* 117–138.

Flacke, J. M., Amaro, H., Jenkin, S. W., Kunitz, S., Levy, J., Mikon, M., & Yu, E. (1995). Panel I: Epidemiology of minority health. *Health Psychology, 14,* 592–600.

Folkman, S., Lazarus, R. S., Gruen, J., & DeLongis, A. (1986). Appraisal, coping, health status, and psychological symptoms. *Journal of Personality and Social Psychology, 50,* 571–579.

Forsythe, C. J., & Compas, B. E. (1987). Interactions of coping and perceptions of control: Testing the goodness of fit hypothesis. *Cognitive Therapy and Research, 11*, 473–485.

Frable, D. E. E., Blackstone, T., & Scherbaum, C. (1990). Marginal and mindful: Deviants in social interaction. *Journal of Personality and Social Psychology, 59*, 140–149.

Goffman, E. (1963). *Stigma: Notes on the management of spoiled identity.* Englewood Cliffs, NJ: Prentice-Hall.

Hall, J. A. (1978). Gender effects in decoding nonverbal cues. *Psychological Bulletin, 85*, 845–887.

Heilman, M. E., Block, C. J., & Stathatos, P. (1997). The affirmative action stigma of incompetence: Effects of performance of information ambiguity. *Academy of Management Journal, 40*, 603–625.

Ickes, W. (Ed.). (1985). *Compatible and incompatible relationships.* New York: Springer.

Ickes, W., & Barnes, R. D. (1978). Boys and girls together and alienated: On enacting stereotyped sex roles in mixed sex dyads. *Journal of Personality and Social Psychology, 36*, 669–683.

Imamura, A. E. (1990). Strangers in a strange land: Coping with marginality in international marriage. *Journal of Comparative Family Studies, 21*, 171–191.

Jackson, P. B., Thoits, P. A., & Taylor, H. F. (1995). Composition of the workplace and psychological well-being: The effects of tokenism on America's Black elite. *Social Forces, 74*, 543–557.

James, S. A., Hartnett, S. A., & Kalsbeek, W. D. (1983). John Henryism and blood pressure differences among Black men. *Journal of Behavioral Medicine, 6*, 259–278.

Jones, E. E., Farina, A., Hastorf, A. H., Markus, H., Miller, D. T., & Scott, R. A. (1984). *Social stigma: The psychology of marked relationships.* New York: Freeman.

Jones, E. E., & Pittman, T. S. (1982). Toward a general theory of strategic self-presentation. In J. Suls (Ed.), *Psychological perspectives on the self* (Vol. 1, pp. 231–262). Hillsdale, NJ: Erlbaum.

Jost, J. T., & Banaji, M. R. (1994). The role of stereotyping in system justification and the production of false consciousness. *British Journal of Social Psychology, 33*, 1–27.

Kaiser, C., & Miller, C. T. (2000). *Reacting to impending discrimination: Compensation for prejudice and atrributions to discrimination.* Unpublished manuscript, University of Vermont.

Katz, I. (1981). *Stigma: A social-psychological perspective.* Hillsdale, NJ: Erlbaum.

Katz, I., & Hass, R. G. (1988). Racial ambivalence and value conflict: Correlational and priming studies of dual cognitive structures. *Journal of Personality and Social Psychology, 55*, 893–905.

Katz, I., Wackenhut, J., & Hass, R. G. (1986). Racial ambivalence, value duality, and behavior. In J. F. Dovidio & S. L. Gaertner (Eds.), *Prejudice, discrimination, and racism* (pp. 35–60). Orlando, FL: Academic Press.

Kleck, R. E., & Strenta, A. (1980). Perceptions of the impact of negatively valued physical characteristics on social interaction. *Journal of Personality and Social Psychology, 39*, 861–873.

Latané, B., & Wolf, S. (1981). The social impact of majorities and minorities. *Psychological Review, 88*, 438–453.

Lazarus, R. S., & Folkman, S. (1984). *Stress, appraisal, and coping*. New York: Springer.

Leary, M. R., & Kowalski, R. M. (1990). Impression management: A literature review and two-component model. *Psychological Bulletin, 107*, 34–47.

Levinger, G., & Breedlove, J. (1966). Interpersonal attraction and agreement. *Journal of Personality and Social Psychology, 3*, 367–372.

Major, B. (1987). Gender, justice, and the psychology of entitlement. In P. Shaver & C. Hendrick (Eds.), *Review of personality and social psychology* (Vol. 7, pp. 124–148). Beverly Hills, CA: Sage.

Major, B. (1994). From social inequality to personal entitlement: The role of social comparisons, legitimacy appraisals, and group membership. In L. Berkowitz (Ed.), *Advances in experimental social psychology* (Vol. 26, pp. 293–355). San Diego, CA: Academic Press.

Major, B., Barr, L., Zubek, J., & Babey, S. (1999). Gender and self-esteem: A meta-analysis. In W. B. Swann, Jr., J. H. Langlois, & L. A. Gilbert (Eds.), *Sexism and stereotypes in modern society: The gender science of Janet Taylor Spence* (pp. 223–253). Washington, DC: American Psychological Association.

Major, B., & Crocker, J. (1993). Social stigma: The affective consequences of attributional ambiguity. In D. M. Mackie & D. L. Hamilton (Eds.), *Affect, cognition, and stereotyping: Interactive processes in intergroup perception* (pp. 345–370). San Diego, CA: Academic Press.

Major, B., & Gramzow, R. (1999). Abortion as stigma: Cognitive and emotional implications of concealment. *Journal of Personality and Social Psychology, 77*, 735–745.

Major, B., Levin, S., Schmader, T., & Sidanius, J. (1999). *Implications of justice ideology, group identification, and ethnic group for perceptions of discrimination*. Manuscript in preparation.

Major, B., & Quinton, W. (1999). *Perceiving discrimination: Impact of group identification and illegitimacy*. Manuscript in preparation.

Major, B., Quinton, W., McCoy, S., & Schmader, T. (in press). Reducing prejudice: What can targets do? In S. Oskamp (Ed.), *Reducing prejudice: The Claremont Symposium*.

Major, B., Richards, M. C., Cooper, M. L., Cozzarelli, C., & Zubek, J. (1998). Personal resilience, cognitive appraisal, and coping: An integrative model of adjustment to abortion. *Journal of Personality and Social Psychology, 74*, 735–752.

Major, B., & Schmader, T. (1998). Coping with stigma through psychological disengagement. In J. K. Swim & C. Stangor (Eds.), *Prejudice: The target's perspective* (pp. 191–218). San Diego, CA: Academic Press.

Major, B., Sciacchitano, A. M., & Crocker, J. (1993). In-group versus out-group comparisons and self-esteem. *Personality and Social Psychology Bulletin, 19*, 711–721.

Major, B., Spencer, S., Schmader, T., Wolfe, C., & Crocker, J. (1998). Coping with negative stereotypes about intellectual performance: The role of psychological disengagement. *Personality and Social Psychology Bulletin, 24,* 34–50.

Major, B., Testa, M., & Bylsma, W. H. (1991). Responses to upward and downward social comparisons: The impact of esteem-relevance and perceived control. In J. Suls & T. A. Wills (Eds.), *Social comparison: Contemporary theory and research* (pp. 237–260). Hillsdale, NJ: Erlbaum.

McConahay, J. B. (1986). Modern racism, ambivalence, and the Modern Racism Scale. In J. F. Dovidio & S. L. Gaertner (Eds.), *Prejudice, discrimination, and racism* (pp. 91–125). Orlando, FL: Academic Press.

Miller, C. T., & Downey, K. T. (1999). A meta-analysis of heavyweight and self-esteem. *Personality and Social Psychology Review, 3,* 68–84.

Miller, C. T., & Myers, A. M. (1998). Compensating for prejudice: How heavyweight people (and others) control outcomes despite prejudice. In J. K. Swim & C. Stangor (Eds.), *Prejudice: The target's perspective* (pp. 191–218). San Diego, CA: Academic Press.

Miller, C. T., Rothblum, E. D., Felicio, D., & Brand, P. (1995). Compensating for stigma: Obese and nonobese women's reactions to being visible. *Personality and Social Psychology Bulletin, 21,* 1093–1106.

Monat, A., & Lazarus, R. S. (Eds.). (1991). *Stress and coping: An anthology* (3rd ed.). New York: Columbia University Press.

Myers, A. M. (1998). *Fat, stigma, and coping: Relation to mental health symptoms, body-image, and self-esteem.* Unpublished doctoral dissertation, University of Vermont.

Nemeth, C. J. (1986). Differential contributions of majority and minority influence. *Psychological Review, 93,* 23–32.

Pettigrew, T. F. (1986). The contact hypothesis revisited. In M. Hewstone & R. Brown (Eds.), *Contact and conflict in intergroup encounters* (pp. 169–195). Oxford: Blackwell.

Pinel, E. C. (1999). Stigma consciousness: The psychological legacy of social stereotypes. *Journal of Personality and Social Psychology, 76,* 114–128.

Porter, J. R., & Washington, R. E. (1979). Black identity and self-esteem: A few studies of Black self concept. *Annual Review of Sociology, 5,* 53–74.

Rosenberg, M., & Simmons, R. G. (1972). *Black and White self-esteem: The urban school child.* Washington, DC: American Sociological Association.

Ruggiero, K. M., & Taylor, D. M. (1995). Coping with discrimination: How disadvantaged group members perceive the discrimination that confronts them. *Journal of Personality and Social Psychology, 68,* 826–838.

Ruggiero, K. M., & Taylor, D. M. (1997). Why minority group members perceive or do not perceive the discrimination that confronts them: The role of self-esteem and perceived control. *Journal of Personality and Social Psychology, 72,* 373–389.

Sidanius, J., & Pratto, F. (1993). The inevitability of oppression and the dynamics of social dominance. In P. M. Sniderman, P. E. Tetlock, & E. G. Carmines (Eds.), *Prejudice, politics, and the American dilemma* (pp. 173–211). Stanford, CA: Stanford University Press.

Simpson, G. E., & Yinger, J. M. (1985). *Racial and cultural minorities: An analysis of prejudice and discrimination* (5th ed.). New York: Plenum Press.

Steele, C. M. (1997). A threat in the air: How stereotypes shape intellectual identity and performance. *American Psychologist, 52,* 613–629.

Steele, C. M., & Aronson, J. (1995). Stereotype threat and intellectual performance of African Americans. *Journal of Personality and Social Psychology, 69,* 797–811.

Swim, J. K., Cohen, L. L., & Hyers, L. L. (1998). Experiencing everyday prejudice and discrimination. In J. K. Swim & C. Stangor (Eds.), *Prejudice: The target's perspective* (pp. 37–60). San Diego, CA: Academic Press.

Tajfel, H., & Turner, J. C. (1986). The social identity theory of intergroup behavior. In S. Worchel & W. G. Austin (Eds.), *Psychology of intergroup relations* (pp. 7–24). Chicago: Nelson-Hall.

Tesser, A. (1988). Toward a self-evaluation maintenance model of social behavior. In L. Berkowitz (Ed.), *Advances in experimental social psychology* (Vol. 21, pp. 181–227). San Diego, CA: Academic Press.

Testa, M., & Major, B. (1990). The impact of social comparisons after failure: The moderating effects of perceived control. *Basic and Applied Social Psychology, 11,* 205–218.

Townsend, B. L. (1998). Social friendships and networks among African American children and youth. In L. H. Meyer, H. Park, M. Grenot-Scheyer, I. S. Schwartz, & B. Harry (Eds.), *Making friends: The influence of culture and development* (pp. 225–241). Baltimore: Brookes.

Von Baeyer, C. L., Sherk, D. L., & Zanna, M. P. (1981). Impression management on the job interview: When the female applicant meets the male (chauvinist) interviewer. *Personality and Social Psychology Bulletin, 7,* 45–51.

Walster, E., Walster, G. W., & Berscheid, E. (1978). *Equity: Theory and research.* Boston: Allyn & Bacon.

Weiner, B. (1985). An attributional theory of achievement motivation. *Psychological Review, 92,* 548–573.

Weiner, B., Perry, R. P., & Magnusson, J. (1988). An attributional analysis of reactions to stigma. *Journal of Personality and Social Psychology, 55,* 738–748.

Wills, T. A. (1981). Downward comparison principles in social psychology. *Psychological Bulletin, 90,* 245–271.

Wortman, C. B. (1983). Coping with victimization: Conclusions and implications for future research. *Journal of Social Issues, 39,* 195–221.

Wright, B. (1960). *Physical disability: A psychological approach.* New York: Harper & Row.

Wright, S. C., Taylor, D. M., & Moghaddam, F. M. (1990). Responding to membership in a disadvantaged group: From acceptance to collective protest. *Journal of Personality and Social Psychology, 58,* 994–1003.

III

THE SOCIAL INTERFACE

10

Awkward Moments in Interactions between Nonstigmatized and Stigmatized Individuals

MICHELLE R. HEBL
JENNIFER TICKLE
TODD F. HEATHERTON

Most people can call to mind some interaction they have had with a stigmatized individual during which they said or did something that created some anxiety, discomfort, tension, or embarrassment to themselves and/or their stigmatized interactant. Recent descriptions of such transactions from our students have revealed a plethora of such examples. For instance, one student asked a paraplegic stranger who had fallen from his wheelchair how his legs felt. Another student told her facially scarred friend that the young man they were looking at would be attractive if only it weren't for his facial scar—a mark she realized immediately thereafter was almost identical to her friend's scar. One student recalled asking a blind person whether he had seen a hot-air balloon lift-off. Several White students recalled stuttering noticeably in deliberating whether to use the term "Blacks" or "African Americans" in conversations with Black individuals. Another student described staring at her interactant's stump of an arm that was slightly protruding from the sleeve. And one student stated that she remembered deliberately backing away from shaking hands with a person she knew was HIV-positive. Although these particular examples of undesirable social exchanges may not be universal experiences, most people have experienced the overarching discomfort that accompanies such marred interactions. We call these feelings "awkward moments," and what seems to be a commonality across diverse experiences of these moments is the precursor or presence of interaction anxiety that directly or indirectly arises from the stigma.

In this chapter, we explore awkward moments that occur in "mixed interactions," or interactions that involve stigmatized and nonstigmatized interactants (Goffman, 1963). We begin by describing some features of stigma that influence the production of awkward moments. We then present a number of firsthand accounts of awkward moments from the perspectives of both types of interactants, together with empirical research that reveals the hesitation both sides have in pursuing social interactions with each other. Next, we gain insight into awkward moments by considering a number of reasons why tensions and anxieties are likely to occur; we present readers with a comprehensive, although not exhaustive, list of potential factors that may lead to or maintain awkwardness in both nonstigmatized and stigmatized individuals. Finally, we discuss strategies for alleviating awkward moments, which we believe will not only benefit social interactions but also lead to a more general mainstreaming of stigmatized individuals into our society. Such remediation strategies have been shown to immunize stigmatized individuals from threats and to enhance mixed interactions and dialogue, as well as to attenuate experiences of awkwardness. Our belief is that some very straightforward cognitive and behavioral interventions, targeted at both the dyadic and societal levels, can work to reduce anxiety and the presence of awkward moments in nonoptimal mixed interactions.

FEATURES OF STIGMAS INFLUENCING THE PRODUCTION OF AWKWARD MOMENTS

A general understanding of social stigma is helpful in understanding the dynamics of mixed interactions. As early as ancient Greek civilization, records indicate that individuals possessed "stigmas," defined as undesirable brands or marks connoting devalued differentness from others and from expectations (see Archer, 1985; Crocker, Major, & Steele, 1998; Goffman, 1963; Jones et al., 1984). In the last century, dozens of groups have been viewed as stigmatized, including individuals who are alcoholic (Dean & Poremba, 1983; Weinberg & Vogler, 1990), Black (Dovidio & Gaertner, 1986, 1993), blind (Albrecht, Walker, & Levy,

1982), diagnosed with cancer (Bloom & Kessler, 1994; Muzzin, Anderson, Figueredo, & Gudelis, 1994), facially scarred (Bull & Rumsey, 1988), homosexual (Dunbar, Brown, & Amoroso, 1973; Neuberg, 1994), obese (Allon, 1982; Crandall & Biernat, 1990; DeJong & Kleck, 1986), physically disabled (Kleck, Ono, & Hastorf, 1966; Perlman & Routh, 1980), stutterers (Woods & Williams, 1976), and female (Heilbrun, 1976). Because of the wide variation in stigmatized groups, researchers have attempted to classify stigmas into different typologies (see, e.g., Northcraft, 1980). Undoubtedly the most widely recognized classification is Goffman's (1963) conceptualization of three stigma categories: (1) "blemishes of individual character," such as alcoholism, homosexuality, unemployment, and addiction; (2) "abominations of the body," such as physical deformities and conspicuous disabilities; and (3) "tribal identities," such as race, nation, and religion.

An alternative way of conceptualizing stigmas is to consider specific features inherent in stigmas that may influence strongly how stigmatized individuals are perceived and treated. One such feature is the extent to which a stigma is perceived to be controllable (Weiner, 1995). Stigmas that society perceives to be largely controllable (e.g., obesity, alcoholism, homosexuality) tend to coincide with those viewed as character blemishes, and may be particularly aversive to nonstigmatized interactants because possessors tend to be held accountable for such conditions. In addition, most people believe that these conditions could be altered or prevented with some effort, but that this effort is not put forth. Thus these stigmatized individuals have been viewed as weak and undisciplined, and have been reacted to with greater hostility and less sympathy (Hebl, 1997; Farina, Holland, & Ring, 1966; Levine & McBurney, 1977; Weiner, Magnusson, & Perry, 1988). Perceptually, they are reduced from whole and "normal" people to contaminated, rejected ones (see, e.g., Herek, 1988; National Gay Task Force, 1988).

A second distinguishing feature of stigmas, particularly ones that might lead to increased awkward moments, is the extent to which stigmas are disruptive in a social interaction. Described as an important dimension by Jones et al. (1984), "disruptiveness" refers to the extent to which a stigma makes itself visible in an interaction. Disruptiveness is heightened, according to Jones et al., when a stigma is aesthetically unappealing, when a stigma is visible, and when the "peril" of a stigma (dangerousness of the stigma to the perceiver) is high. Disruptiveness, then, may be a direct gauge of the strain or difficulty characterizing interchanges between mixed interactants. Empirical evidence suggests that nonstigmatized individuals have strengthened stereotypes of individuals who possess disruptive stigmas (McGuire, 1998), which may directly lead to more aversive reactions in social interactions. In addition, those who have less disruptive stigmas may even be able to hide the evidence of being stigmatized (see also Goffman's [1963] "discredited vs. discreditable" categorization).

When we consider different categorizations of stigmas and some of their defining features, it becomes clear that many factors about a stigma itself can affect mixed interactions, aside from the more standard social-psychological effects of expectancies, situational factors, and individual differences. It is also important to note that while categorizations and lists of distinguishing features of stigmas may be helpful as a cognitive framework, they are simultaneously somewhat arbitrary and may be misleading in terms of making specific predictions about social interactions and their outcomes. That is, some stigmas may have less impact than others on the production of awkward moments. People's experiences with and perspectives concerning a given stigma are diverse, and what creates an awkward moment for one pair of interactants may not create the same anxiety in another pair. Given such variation in stigmas and their impact on interactions, we still find Goffman's (1963) categories and the delineation of certain features helpful in drawing comparisons and general trends across the broad range of stigmatizing conditions. By considering a number of personal accounts concerning diverse sets of stigmatizing conditions, we can observe some of these trends and can begin to better understand awkward moments.

FIRSTHAND ACCOUNTS OF AWKWARD MOMENTS

In indirect ways, awkward moments have been described throughout history by both nonstigmatized and stigmatized interactants, and by observers of these interactions. We begin this section by presenting some firsthand experiences of nonstigmatized individuals. In particular, we asked college students to describe their personal experiences, observations, and expectations regarding social interactions with stigmatized individuals. Consistently across our sample, the students reported interactions that involved experiences of awkward moments. The types of stigmas and specific comments included the following:

> *Albinism*: "In a conversation that I had with an albino, I was nervous because certain topics such as tanning, birthmarks, or color contacts seemed off limits, and I was so afraid I would accidentally bring them up."
> *Being Black*: "Sometimes when I'm talking to them [Black people], I just feel angry at them. I know I shouldn't, but I just do."
> *Blindness*: "In my experience, the seeing person is quite prone to ac-

cidentally referring to visual stimuli, such as 'What do you think of the decorations?' and 'Wow, that woman is wearing an ugly dress!' Also, the seeing person feels uncomfortable terminating the conversation, having to decide if they just walk away and leave them [the blind person] standing there or ask if they need help getting to their next destination."

Obesity: "I've noticed one usually has an immediate reaction of revulsion, almost as if what they see is grotesque. This repulsion, which one attempts to hide, can change to anger in the interaction if gluttonous behavior or lazy behavior is pursued by the obese individual."

Physical Disability: "I have felt nervous and apprehensive about offending or upsetting people in wheelchairs. I'm never sure whether to stand and look down upon the person, to kneel, or to sit. I never want to mention activities that I have done for fear that the handicapped person will envy me and wish to be able to do such activities. Often such conversations only reach surface issues. I avoid discussing anything about how the person ended up in a wheelchair."

Stuttering: "We had never met before, and I was thinking about his stutter the whole time. But at the same time, I was trying really hard to look like I did *not* notice the stutter."

Awkward moments are further illuminated by considering accounts from stigmatized individuals, who corroborate the occurrence of nonoptimal interactions. Perhaps the best-known accounts come from Goffman's 1963 book, *Stigma: Notes on the Management of Spoiled Identity*, which presents poignant descriptions, case studies, and autobiographical stories about the lives of stigmatized individuals and their mixed interaction difficulties. Such descriptions, however, can also be found in other published autobiographies and sources of nonfiction:

Being Black: "When you are harried by day and haunted by night by the fact that you are a Negro, living constantly at tiptoe stance, never quite knowing what to expect next, [you] are plagued with inner fears and outer resentments ... " (King, 1986, p. 52).

Facial Deformation: "I like best to be out of sight of strange people. I envy to be normal like the other fellow. Ridicule is plenty and always" (MacGregor, Abel, Bryt, Lauer, & Weissmann, 1953, p. 94).

Obesity: "As a fat child (and even later as a fat adult) I have always felt some degree of alienation from those around me" (Wiley, 1994, p. 96).

Obesity: "He was quiet for a moment, then said, 'This is embarrassing. I'm not attracted to you because of your weight.' His answer devastated me . . . . My worst fear had happened" (Wiley, 1994, p. 126).

Physical Disability: "Two contradictory themes in American life [are] sympathy and self-reliance. Outside rehab, self-reliance was a high-risk proposition. To people raised on telethons, it looks suspiciously like a chip on the shoulder" (Hockenberry, 1995, p. 33).

Physical Disability: "People in the apartment watched me come and go. I didn't know them. They didn't ask about me. I didn't ask about them. I was alone" (Hockenberry, 1995, p. 116).

Stuttering: "We who stutter speak only when we must. We hide our defect, often so successfully that our intimates are surprised when in an unguarded moment, a word suddenly runs away with our tongues and we blurt and blat and grimace and choke until finally the spasm is over and we open our eyes to view the wreckage" (van Riper, 1939, p. 601).

An examination of these accounts from both nonstigmatized and stigmatized individuals reveals two main themes. First, anxiety is present as a precursor or as a concomitant to each awkward moment. By "anxiety," we refer to Leary's (1983) definition of physiological arousal accompanied by uneasiness concerning an impending negative outcome that a person believes is unavoidable. Anxiety is directly associated with—either enveloping or initiating—additional feelings of discomfort, tension, and forced or strained interactions (e.g., Ickes, 1984). Such a description can readily be applied to an impending mixed interaction, in which a perceiver may have expectancies that the situation will be extremely difficult or negative simply because it involves interaction with a stigmatized person. Such an expectancy may serve to increase the anxiety and arousal, and may subsequently lead to the confirmation of this expectancy. The stigmatized individual may also experience this anxiety simultaneously. However, an awkward moment may also occur when only one member of the interaction experiences discomfort, and this need not be made public or obvious to the other interactant.

The empirical examination of anxiety per se in mixed interactions has not gained a great deal of attention. One exception to this is the examination of the phenomenon of "intergroup anxiety," which suggests that anxiety toward outgroups and outgroup members may be embodied in many different forms (Devine, Evett, & Vasquez-Suson, 1996). Furthermore, Stephan and Stephan (1985) suggest that prior intergroup relations, intergroup cognitions, and situational factors lead to intergroup anxiety that has behavioral, cognitive, and affective consequences for the self and for the ingroup or outgroup. Recent research suggests that such consequences may include self-esteem loss (Crocker, Cornwell, & Major, 1993; Steele, 1988). In the following section, we describe precursors that lead one to become anxious.

The second theme that emerges in the personal accounts is avoidance. The very possibility of encountering a mixed interaction may lead both nonstigmatized and stigmatized individuals to arrange their lives so as to minimize or altogether avoid them. Goffman (1963) proposed that many stigmatized individuals remain at home and rarely enter the public eye of the nonstigmatized world, because they anticipate and dread the reactions of nonstigmatized individuals. A sizable amount of empirical research, particularly in the physical disability literature, also documents this tendency toward avoidance. For instance, Snyder, Kleck, Strenta, and Mentzer (1979) found that nondisabled persons avoided social interaction with disabled persons, particularly when a socially acceptable excuse was present. These researchers gave participants a choice between watching a movie together with a person wearing a metal leg brace or watching a very similar movie alone. Participants strongly preferred viewing the movie alone. However, if the movie was identical, then participants chose to watch it with the person wearing a leg brace. These results were interpreted to reveal nonstigmatized individuals' desire to avoid disabled persons, but only when the reasons for this avoidance could not have been attributed directly to prejudice or rejection of the disabled individual. Similarly, Kleck et al. (1966) examined a forced interaction in which participants were asked to interview a confederate who appeared either disabled or physically normal through the use of a specially designed wheelchair. Nonstigmatized individuals again appeared to avoid interaction by terminating the interview much sooner and showing more behavioral inhibition when interacting with the disabled versus the nondisabled individual (see Kleck, 1968a, 1968b). Additional research confirms this avoidance motivation (see, e.g., Belgrave, 1984; Devine et al., 1996; Mills, Belgrave, & Boyer, 1984; Stephan & Stephan, 1985).

In sum, both stigmatized and nonstigmatized individuals report the presence of anxiety and avoidance in mixed interactions. We believe that this emotion is responsible for initiating and perpetuating awkward moments. In the following section, we explore a number of explanations for the anxiety that arises and the awkward moments that result. In describing these cognitions, we consider both the perspective of both the nonstigmatized and stigmatized interactants.

WHY DO AWKWARD MOMENTS OCCUR?

Reasons for Nonstigmatized Individuals' Anxiety

Fear of Danger

Nonstigmatized individuals may experience anxiety because of an underlying fear they possess of stigmatized individuals. This fear may arise from a number of sources, the first of which is a fear tied to Jones et al.'s (1984) dimension of "peril," or danger to the perceiver. Certain stigmas convey either an imagined or a real threat to one's physical health, and are thus perilous. For instance, stereotypes of Blacks and of persons with characterological stigmas (e.g., imprisonment or addiction) lead many to believe that these people are dangerous to one's well-being. Although such individuals are not necessarily dangerous, the associated stereotypes may consolidate a nonstigmatized individual's experience of discomfort and anxiety in a mixed interaction. Fear may also be aroused in response to stigmas that have aggression or unpredictability tied to their stereotypes. For instance, persons with mental illness are often feared because of the unpredictability of their actions.

Second, nonstigmatized individuals may fear social or interpersonal contagion (Haidt, McCauley, & Rozin, 1994; Rozin, Markwith, & McCauley, 1994). This anxiety may arise from a fear that a stigma might spread merely because of an association with a stigmatized individual (Hastorf, Wildfogel, & Cassman, 1979). Although most people wish to avoid the possible contagion of stigmas, certain people voluntarily take on "courtesy stigmas" (Goffman, 1963). Such individuals include relatives of stigmatized individuals, as well as those individuals who work in settings that cater to stigmatized individuals (i.e., a nurse working with disabled patients, a heterosexual bartender working in a gay bar). Fears of spreading may take a "physical" or a "social" form. Fear of physical spreading is a fear of actual physical contamination. For instance, some people fear that they will contract AIDS or cancer from physical contact with those who already have these conditions. In some cases, this fear may be accurate. Fear of social spreading, by comparison, has more to do with the feared loss of social status or contamination of one's attitudes through contact. For instance, dating an overweight partner can portray negative characteristics and attributions about the other partner. Recent investigations affirm the notion that social spreading actually does occur in the case of the homosexuality stigma; hence, nonstigmatized individuals may actually be justified in maintaining distance from some stigmatized individuals (Sigelman, Howell, Cornell, Cutright, & Dewy, 1990). In particular, Neuberg, Smith, Hoffman, and Russell (1994) demonstrated that male individuals were rated less positively by participants if they associated with a homosexual man than if they associated with a heterosexual man. The stigma-by-association phenomenon is a condition, then, that fosters avoidance of and awkwardness in mixed contacts (see Bull & Rumsey, 1988).

Not only is the contagion of stigmatizing conditions sometimes based on faulty knowledge about stigmatizing conditions, but it is also often based on a lack of experience in interacting with members of stigmatized groups. This lack of experience does not necessarily stem from active avoidance of mixed interactions; it may also result from the fact that some types of stigmas are statistically infrequent.

Statistical Infrequencies of Some Stigmas, and General Lack of Experience and Knowledge

Certain types of stigmas in our world are statistically infrequent. This infrequency not only makes individuals with such stigmas more salient (see Zebrowitz-McArthur, 1982), but also results in a lack of contact with such persons and an uncertainty in how exactly to respond and behave once contact with them is established. Consider that a substantial percentage of individuals in our country is obese (approximately one out of every four), but that the number of disabled handicapped individuals in our country is far less than this. For example, approximately 0.6% of Americans use wheelchairs (McNeil, 1993), and 0.6% of Americans have an absence of major extremities (Dorgan, 1995). According to the theoretical contributions of Zebrowitz-McArthur (1982), different interaction dynamics in mixed contacts should be expected in nonstigmatized individuals' interactions with obese persons versus physically disabled persons. The uncertainty is simply not there in mixed interactions with obese individuals; rather, their heightened prevalence in society reduces the uncertainty in interacting with them. Exceptions might include exposure to individuals who are grossly obese or who have disproportionate distributions of weight. But overall, people seem to have less uncertainty in interactions with obese individuals because they come in contact with obese individuals so frequently.

In interactions with physically disabled individuals, however, there may be much more uncertainty and lack of know-how. Most individuals have simply had very limited experience in interacting with these and certain other types of stigmatized individuals. One reaction to this limited interaction is for nonstigmatized individuals to proceed with a degree of hesitancy. Because nonstigmatized individuals have been in so few similar situations, they are uncertain as to how they should respond. For instance, should they offer to push a person in the wheelchair if this person is having trouble? Should they be sympathetic, ask questions, be overly optimistic? Should they guide a blind person across the street? Research on bystander intervention (Latané & Darley, 1970) suggests that people are less likely to help others or to take risks if the situation is ambiguous, if the others are deindividuated, or if the others may be embarrassed by their actions. In the same way, nonstigmatized individuals may refrain from action because the ambiguity is heightened.

Given that most nondisabled individuals (and many disabled individuals themselves) have little to no contact with physically disabled persons and are uncertain about how exactly to respond and behave once contact with such individuals is established, it is understandable that anxiety and awkwardness will emerge. Such uncertainty and lack of know-how have been labeled "interaction pathology" (Davis, 1961; Goffman, 1959, 1963).

Violation of Norms and Expectations

The lack of experience that many nonstigmatized individuals have in mixed interactions is compounded by the fact that such individuals bring prior expectations to mixed interactions and have schemas for how interactions should proceed. For instance, nonstigmatized individuals may expect their interactants to be likewise nonstigmatized and for interactions to proceed smoothly. When interactants meet expectations, the resulting behavior on the part of the nonstigmatized individuals may be routinized and predictable. However, when interactants are stigmatized and interactions become mixed, expectations are violated. Suddenly, nonstigmatized individuals may find themselves scriptless, their schemas having been disrupted. One result of such scriptlessness is a heightened attention to both their interactants' behavior and their own behavior. In the service of maintaining a posture of normality, nonstigmatized individuals may increase their self-monitoring, think more about their word choices and responses, and feel restrictions in their normal range of verbal and nonverbal behaviors. Given such violations in expectations and the possibility of a sudden focus on behaviors that are not normally considered, it is easy to understand how awkward moments might emerge.

Thought Suppression

In addition to simply not knowing how to act and being suddenly overly cognizant of what is typically routinized behavior, many nonstigmatized individuals try not to say the wrong thing, although they may simultaneously never be sure exactly what the right or wrong thing is. A nonstigmatized individual rarely introduces the subject of a stigma, as a societal norm governs that the topic of stigma should be introduced only by the stigmatized individual. The nonstigmatized individual may also attempt to suppress all thoughts concerning the stigma and may try to avoid referring to any topic even marginally related to it. He or she may avoid staring or showing any evidence of disruption potentially caused by the stigma. Although such behavior is intended in most cases to assist and smooth the interaction, research on thought suppression (Wegner, 1994) suggests that those who attempt to suppress unwanted thoughts often ultimately experience a "rebound" effect, whereby they experience a substantial number of such thoughts later. If a mixed interaction is still ongoing during this rebound phase, awkwardness seems unavoidable. Research by Macrae, Milne, and Bodenhausen (1994) found that individuals who were instructed not to think about stereotypes regarding one's devalued mark (e.g., being a "skinhead") were more likely to engage in increased stereotyping than were those who were given no suppression instructions. This finding was manifested in that those who suppressed, relative to those who did not, chose to sit farther away from an actual "skinhead" whom they later encountered. The researchers suggested that the thought suppression of the "skinhead" stereotype created tension in the form of a "bottling up" that later erupted.

Misinterpretations

In addition to thought suppression, nonstigmatized individuals possess some invalid assumptions about stigmatized individuals that may lead to awkward moments. For instance, nonstigmatized individuals may react with uncertainty and hesitation to stigmatized individuals because they believe that those possessing stigmas, particularly physically disabled individuals, are bitter, emotional, and morose about their stigmas (see Belgrave, 1985; Belgrave & Mills, 1981; Mills et al., 1984). In addition, nonstigmatized individuals avoid certain topics and sometimes interactions altogether because they believe that stigmatized individuals will be overly sensitive about their stigmas and readily offended on topics both related and unrelated to the stigmas. As Belgrave and Mills (1981) suggest, such expectations may arise from nonstigmatized individuals' trying to imagine themselves with similar stigmatizing conditions. But such misinterpretations may block interactants from getting to know each other and may have negative attributional consequences for interactions.

Hostility and Just-World Beliefs

Whereas some stigmatized individuals' awkward moments arise from the lack of experience, others' arise from deep-seated hostility and antipathy toward individuals who possess stigmas. In particular, nonstigmatized individuals report feeling the greatest amount of hostility toward persons who are alleged or known to abuse children or misuse drugs. This finding is probably due to the fact that such stigmas are perceived to be controllable in comparisons with other stigmas, such as AIDS, blindness, paraplegia, or obesity (Hebl, 1997; Weiner et al., 1988). In fact, increasing perceived responsibility for the onset of AIDS increases affective anger responses (and decreases sympathy) for those stigmatized with AIDS (causes ranked from least to most responsibility: blood transfusion, conventional sex, promiscuous sex, homosexuality, drug use) (Graham, Weiner, Giuliano, & Williams, 1993). Increasing one's hostility may lead directly to problematic mixed interactions, given that angry people have been shown to use stereotypes more than those who are not angry (Bodenhausen, Sheppard, & Kramer, 1994).

Nonstigmatized individuals may also express anxiety in mixed interactions because such interactions make them realize their own vulnerabilities. Individuals in the United States tend to ascribe to the belief that the world is just and that people not only get what they deserve but deserve what they get (see Crandall, 1994; Crandall & Martinez, 1996). Maintaining this ideology may be difficult for individuals who interact with stigmatized individuals and are forced to observe that many are innocent victims dealt a clearly undeserved fate (e.g., those with birth defects, those plagued with rare and unpreventable diseases) (see Lerner, 1980). For the most part, people do not want to have their values and beliefs challenged; in fact, individuals are likely to feel hostility toward minority groups that threaten their values (Haddock, Zanna, & Esses, 1993).

Fears associated with invulnerability are likewise embodied in the terror management theory of stigma (Greenberg et al., 1990; Rosenblatt, Greenberg, Solomon, Pyszczynski, & Lyon, 1989). This theory also proposes that people have a strong need to feel that the world is a just place. The derogation of stigmatized persons upholds a personal theory of the world that protects nonstigmatized persons against existential fear and anxiety. Nonstigmatized individuals alter their typical behaviors, then, because interactions with stigmatized individuals make them realize their own vulnerabilities. Empirical evidence supports this view by showing that individuals who have a great fear of someday becoming severely incapacitated elderly folks tend to blame currently elderly persons for problems associated with their age (Snyder & Miene, 1994).

Approach–Avoidance Mechanisms

Many nonstigmatized individuals report neither solely negative nor solely positive feelings, but rather the presence of competing sets of beliefs and experiences regarding stigmatized individuals. Such a phenomenon has been termed "ambivalence amplification" by Katz and his colleagues (Katz, 1981; Katz, Glass, Lucido, & Farber, 1979; Katz & Hass, 1988), and it describes how White individuals in a research context simultaneously offer more help and yet also deliver more shocks to Black than to White individuals. Feelings of hostility or disgust toward a stigmatized individual (e.g., a grossly obese individual, an AIDS patient) may be accompanied with a sincere interest in and desire to learn more about the condition. For instance, Langer, Fiske, Taylor, and Chanowitz (1976) proposed that discomfort toward stigmatized individuals arises because of the conflict between a desire to stare at a novel stimulus and the suppression of that desire for social acceptability's sake. They found that people stared at a photo of a disabled person longer when no observer was present with them. Other emotions also preside in creating awkwardness. Sympathy and guilt are two such emotions that nonstigmatized individuals commonly report (Scheier, Carver, Schulz, Glass, & Katz, 1978; Gibbons, Stephan, Stephenson, & Petty, 1980). Supporting this notion of ambivalence, Monteith (1993) found that guilt was more likely to be prevalent in people who were randomly told that they might possess subtle prejudice than in people who were not told they had such prejudice.

That ambivalence results in anxiety is not surprising. Among the earliest and most prominent social-psychological examinations was one revealing that anxiety may result when two dissonant emotions, cognitions, or behaviors are evoked (Festinger, 1957). More recently, Izard (1991) proposed that a combination of the emotions of fear and (to a lesser degree) sadness, shame and guilt may result in anxiety. When one considers the hesitancies that a nonstigmatized person may have about interacting with a stigmatized person, the guilt and shame that arise from not wanting to show negative affect that does exist, and the fear that this negative affect (or cognitions) will become known to the target or to others, it is no surprise that anxiety occurs and awkward moments arise.

In line with the idea of ambivalence, verbal and nonverbal behaviors emitted in mixed interactions often contradict each other. Nonstigmatized people's verbal behaviors directed toward stigmatized individuals tend to be positive and to credit the stigmatized individuals for the burdens they bear (Barker, Wright, Meyerson, & Gonick, 1953; Belgrave, 1985; Hastorf, Northcraft, & Picciotto, 1979). A study examining both verbal and nonverbal behaviors of nonstigmatized persons, however, revealed avoidant nonverbal behaviors, such as maintenance of a greater interaction distance and more rigidity in movement. The inconsistencies in behaviors directed toward stigmatized individuals support a two-factor phenomenon (Kleck et al., 1966; Kleck, 1969): Overt verbal behaviors directed toward stigmatized individuals (e.g., feedback, public attitudinal measures, the help they receive) seem to have an at least initially positive connotation, whereas covert, nonverbal behaviors (e.g., decreased spontaneity, less acceptance, increased social distance) seem to have an indisputable negative connotation.

Such conflicting behaviors may result in part from the fact that nonstigmatized individuals are able to regulate their verbal behaviors but are less skilled at regulating their nonverbal behaviors. This theory, however, does not by itself explain the observed discontinuity. Thus an approach–avoidance mechanism may be at work, and we observe this with the physical disability stigma. On the one hand, nonstigmatized individuals may be attuned to societal norms to be kind to disabled people (Kleck, 1969); on the other hand, they are motivated to avoid interacting with such people altogether. What results is inconsistency. A nonstigmatized individual can adeptly present a facade of acceptance for a stigmatized individual through very positive verbal behaviors, but negative nonverbal messages simultaneously resonate from the nonstigmatized interactant and create a mixed message.

Feelings of approach–avoidance may be very common to the experience of awkward moments. We should point out that if a nonstigmatized individual's feelings about or behaviors toward a stigmatized individual are entirely negative, awkwardness may still not result. Both interactants may be aware of and strongly disagree about each other's perspective, but this need not result in an awkward moment. What seems likely to instigate an awkward moment is the presence of this approach–avoidance, in which the nonstigmatized individual has very conflicting desires and beliefs.

Reasons for Stigmatized Individuals' Anxiety

Fear of Rejection

A stigmatized individual has a number of goals in any given interaction, and reducing the extent to which he or she is avoided seems to be foremost (e.g., Belgrave & Mills, 1981). In fact, stigmatized individuals define success in part by the extent to which they are successful at affiliating with and being accepted by nonstigmatized others (Wright, 1983). Recognizing this motivation, Goffman (1963) introduced the concept of "normalization" to refer to the extent to which a nonstigmatized individual treats a stigmatized person as if he or she does not have the stigma. Clearly, most stigmatized individuals aspire toward normalization. Such individuals often experience anxiety in interactions because each interaction is a potential threat to their self-esteem and happiness, since normalization may not occur. Rather, the smallest hint of rejection may create tension in stigmatized individuals, and lead to awkward moments in mixed interactions. As in a chain reaction, the initial sense of rejection may cause stigmatized individuals to act awkwardly, and ultimately reinforce and perpetuate nonstigmatized individuals' rejection behaviors.

Being "on Stage"

The fear of being rejected and viewed as flawed or abnormal (see Herek, 1988) is compounded by the fact that stigmatized individuals report being unable to avoid attentional focus once an interaction has been initiated. Stigmatized individuals report feeling that they are constantly "on stage" in conversations, meaning that they have heightened self-consciousness and continuously feel the need to create impressions of being normal despite their stigmas (Goffman, 1963; Wright, 1983). They report having less privacy and are treated as low-status individuals by nonstigmatized others (Wright, 1983). In addition, a stigmatized person is often reduced to the stigma itself (e.g., "the deaf-mute"), rather than conceptualized as a person who has a stigma ("Bob, who cannot hear"). Any difficulty observed by a nonstigmatized individual tends to be attributed to the presence of the stigma, even if the stigma is completely irrelevant. For instance, a disabled person who makes a bad decision is believed to make it because he or she has physical limitations, not because of the standard situational and personality influences that affected the decision. Similarly, a Black person who acts in a reserved manner may be interpreted as being "lazy" or "hostile." A nonstigmatized individual may also assume that because a person possesses a stigma, he or she simultaneously possesses other, additional problems. Hence, an interactant talks very loudly to a blind person or very slowly to a person who stutters. The sum of these behaviors places a great deal of emphasis on the verbal and nonverbal actions of stigmatized individuals. Such individuals are indeed "on stage," and an exaggerated attention to their behaviors may promote interaction awkwardness, confirm their feelings of rejection, and add to their insecurities and feelings of inferiority.

Self-Loathing

It may not be surprising, then, that stigmatized individuals themselves often view stigmas negatively, and that their interactions with other stigmatized individuals may also produce negative outcomes. For example, Comer and Piliavin (1972) found that physically disabled subjects terminated the interview sooner, were more inhibited in their gross motor movements, and engaged in less eye contact when they interacted with a disabled interviewer than with a nondisabled interviewer. Such negative reactions from members of their ingroup as well as from their outgroup may lead stigmatized individuals to experience decreases in mood and self-esteem, and increases in self-consciousness, social isolation, and discrimination (Bull & Rumsey, 1988; Crandall, 1994; Wright, 1983). Stigmatized individuals may enter interactions expecting to be treated badly, and thereby may engage in behavioral choices that are self-fulfilling and increase levels of anxiety.

Overinterpretation

The nonoptimal interaction dynamics and the self-loathing that stigmatized individuals experience may lead them to generalize and believe that all individuals are viewing them negatively. That is, not only do stigmatized individuals suffer at the hands of others, but stigmatized individuals may create a whole set of undesirable expectations themselves. Research confirms this, showing that stigmatized individuals sometimes interpret nondiscriminatory actions by nonstigmatized individuals as discriminatory actions against their stigmatized status. In particular, Kleck and Strenta (1980) found that subjects who believed that facial scars had been applied to their faces (with the help of cosmetics) prior to interactions with other individuals interpreted a number of neutral signs from their interactants as being signs of prejudice and antipathy against their deviant status. In reality, the facial scars could not explain interactants' behavior because the scars were removed, unbeknownst to the subjects, before the subjects ever interacted with the nonstigmatized individuals. Hence, subjects found evidence to confirm negative reactions to their stigma when no such reactions existed.

Although in many cases negative reactions do occur, this study showed that nonstigmatized individuals are not the only ones who exhibit biased behavior in mixed interactions. Rather, stigmatized individuals themselves share part of the responsibility for the negative reactions they accrue, particularly by overinterpreting or misinterpreting others' behaviors. Such conjectures may create a social reality of their own. It would be best if stigmatized individuals could realize that initial reactions against them are not necessarily signs of rejection, but represent either uncertainty as to how best to behave or some other not necessarily negative reaction. Instead, the sum of the interactional setbacks explains why stigmatized individuals often react by experiencing a great deal of anxiety within interactions and attempting to avoid such interactions altogether.

Summary

In sum, nonstigmatized individuals may experience fear, lack of knowledge, violations of expectations, a rebounding of suppressed thoughts, misinterpretations, prejudiced sets of beliefs, and ambivalence regarding stigmas and individuals who possess them. Furthermore, stigmatized individuals feel the pressures of rejection; feel that they cannot avoid being judged, at least in part, on the basis of their stigmatized status; have self-esteem issues; and sometimes react with hostility and/or misinterpretations toward their nonstigmatized interactants. In sum, many forces combine to create anxiety in mixed interactions, and the reasons behind the occurrence of awkward moments are manifold. Any given awkward moment may have a number of sources causing or maintaining it. The aforementioned factors do not constitute an exhaustive list, but are intended to provide readers with a general impression regarding some of the causes of interaction anxiety and awkward moments. Awkward moments, in turn, may perpetuate the negativity associated with mixed relations and lead to further misunderstandings between mixed interactants.

THE IMPORTANCE OF EXAMINING
AND ATTENUATING AWKWARD MOMENTS

The descriptions we have provided serve as guidelines for thought and provide an impetus for future research concerning awkward moments. Future research might carefully examine the emotional states of the interactants by attempting to describe and clarify their presence and influence in mixed interactions. Rather than naively believing that a single precursor leads to an awkward moment, we believe that many of these forces act together and reinforce each other, making interactions uniformly difficult. We hope that future research will continue to identify and analyze the building blocks of these awkward moments, and to determine their impact on interactants as well as on larger issues, such as intergroup attitudes and behaviors.

Each of the mechanisms we have described proposes some degree of anxiety, an emotional reaction to stigmatized persons. Yet almost no research has systematically examined the emotional responses of nonstigmatized people toward stigmatized people. Zajonc (1980) stated:

> There are practically no social phenomena that do not implicate affect in some important way. Affect dominates social interaction, and it is the major currency in which social intercourse is transacted. . . . One cannot be introduced to a person without experiencing some immediate

feeling of attraction or repulsion and without gauging such feelings on
the part of the other. We evaluate each other constantly, we evaluate
each other's behavior, and we evaluate the motives and the consequences of their behavior. (p. 153)

This perspective articulately reflects the notion that emotions play a central role in interactions with others, including stigmatized individuals.
Anecdotal reports of perceivers in interactions with stigmatized persons
suggest that in addition to anxiety, other emotions influence mixed interactions. Archer (1985) describes stigmas as affecting communication
mechanisms as well as producing strong effects in the perceiver such as
aversion, anxiety, fear, loathing, pity, and panic. Our review has
touched upon these emotions, but future research might further examine
how specific emotions intertwine with the experience of awkward moments.

It is also important to examine other aspects associated with mixed
interactions—those at the behavioral and cognitive levels—and to examine whether and how individual-difference variables influence the emotional manifestation of awkward moments. Monteith, Devine, and
Zuwerink (1993) discuss how highly prejudiced individuals may experience an outward-directed negative affect (including disgust, anger, and
irritation), as compared to low-prejudice individuals, who experience a
"diffuse discomfort." Clearly, emotional states color perceptions and the
way information is processed and interpreted, just as cognitions do—by
influencing encoding and subsequent recall, affecting the valence of
evaluative judgments, being used to infer judgments, or narrowing the
cognitive focus of the perceiver (see Clore, Schwarz, & Conway, 1994,
for a discussion; see also Mackie & Hamilton, 1993; Forgas, 1992).

In addition to providing research with a new direction, research on
awkward moments can work to attenuate the very nature and occurrence of interaction strain. Specific strategies that can be adopted by
both stigmatized and nonstigmatized individuals have gained recent research attention. These strategies can be categorized by their focus on a
dyadic interactional level or on a larger, societal level. The implementa-
tion of both interactional-level and societal-level strategies, we believe,
can serve to reduce the occurrence of anxiety and awkward moments in
mixed interactions.

Interactional-Level Strategies

Most of the strategies that work to reduce awkward moments attempt to
reduce avoidance and to increase contact and dialogue between mixed
interactants. Since the majority of the burden in possessing a stigma lies

with the bearer of this stigma (Goffman, 1963), we first focus on strategies that stigmatized persons might undertake. Because self-acceptance and openness have been found to be predictive of the well-being of stigmatized individuals, we believe that stigmatized individuals should work toward these goals not only for their own well-being, but also for the well-being of social interactions. Wright (1983) has proposed that the way for disabled individuals to gain self-acceptance is to retreat from the negative social images regarding disability and to accept differences as nondevaluating. In essence, there is a need to effect changes in stigmatized individuals' belief systems. With regard to physical disability, Wright believes that most individuals focus on the debilitating side of disability rather than the salient, unique status it offers and that for disabled individuals to do anything less than accept their situation would be disastrous to themselves and to their relationships with others. Disabled and other stigmatized individuals therefore should work to possess and maintain high levels of self-esteem as a buffer against interaction anxiety.

Self-acceptance also seems to predict other-acceptance. That is, the specific interpersonal manner (e.g., stereotyped, depressed style vs. socially appropriate and open, accepting style) that a physically disabled individual adopts in a given social interaction may influence the nondisabled individual's behaviors (Elliott & MacNair, 1991; Elliott, MacNair, Herrick, Yoder, & Byrne, 1991). A socially appropriate, nondepressed interpersonal style adopted by physically disabled individuals corresponds significantly with an enhanced amount of conversation, an increase in eye gazes, and greater positivity in social evaluations from nondisabled interactants. Thus it seems advantageous for some members of stigmatized groups to portray satisfaction to others.

Satisfaction may be garnered in part through a strategy referred to as "attributional ambiguity" (Crocker & Major, 1989, 1994; Snyder et al., 1979), which is one way individuals work to maintain and protect their self-esteem. Specifically, when stigmatized individuals are rejected or receive negative feedback from others and there is ambiguity about this feedback, one strategy is for them to attribute the negativity not to their own shortcomings but to the prejudice of others. Recent research has demonstrated that both women and Blacks who experience such ambiguity are able to attribute unfavorable feedback successfully to the other persons' reactions against them, rather than to their own lack of personal deservingness (Crocker & Major, 1994). Such a strategy not only alleviates a person's sense of being at fault, but it also transfers the feedback from the individual person to the stigmatized subgroup (i.e., women or Blacks) and creates a shift that can actually strengthen the self-concept of the individual (see Dion, 1986).

Another strategy that can maintain and even bolster a stigmatized person's sense of self-esteem is based on Steele's (1988) theory of "self-affirmation." This theory suggests that individuals can continue to view themselves positively when one aspect of their personhood is threatened by creating or focusing on another aspect of themselves that is positive. Self-affirmation processes are activated by information that threatens the perceived integrity of the self—for instance, when an obese individual is ridiculed by others for being overweight. The obese individual realizes that obese people in general are viewed as self-indulgent and undisciplined. Realizing that such views poses a threat to his or her perception of self-integrity, the individual is motivated to reduce the threat by engaging in some other affirmation of general self-integrity (i.e., joining a valued cause, spending more time with children, accomplishing more at the office). An article by Miller, Rothblum, Felicio, and Brand (1995) suggests the power of compensation as utilized by stigmatized individuals. Specifically, they found that obese women who were unaware that their partners could see them received low ratings of likability and social skills by such partners. Interestingly, however, such findings were not obtained when obese women were aware that their partners could see them. These results suggest that overweight women actively compensate when they know that other people can see them and discriminate against their size.

One way of compensating may involve a stigmatized individual's expressing some interests in common with a nonstigmatized individual. For example, walking a pet has been shown to provide a nonverbal statement of shared interest that can facilitate conversation between stigmatized and nonstigmatized individuals (Hart, Hart, & Bergin, 1987). Such increased conversation on a joint topic may be a gateway to uniting individuals in a superordinate interest, rather than pitting them against each other in a social interaction.

One strategy that seems particularly beneficial in fostering positive mixed-interaction dynamics is the "acknowledgment" strategy, or the tactic of disclosing a stigma to a nonstigmatized interactant. One of the earliest studies conducted on such a strategy revealed that a stigmatized individual's sensitivity about the stigma might reveal to nonstigmatized others whether the topic of the stigma was an open or closed one (Farina, Sherman, & Allen, 1968). If the stigmatized individual merely mentioned that his or her stigma caused some difficulties and then switched the topic, as in the Farina et al. (1968) article, the stigma topic was not clearly a safe one for nonstigmatized others to broach. Consequently, nonstigmatized individuals were left feeling that the topic was closed. However, if the stigmatized individual revealed information surrounding the possession of the stigma, recognized that others probably had questions about the stigma, and encouraged others to ask questions that they might have, the stigmatized individual was demonstrating less reactivity and a great deal of openness toward possessing the given stigma. Therefore, an acknowledgment devoid of defensiveness and hints of maladjustment leads to greater acceptance on the part of others.

Similarly, Hastorf, Wildfogel, and Cassman (1979) examined a physically disabled individual who either did not acknowledge being in a wheelchair, or acknowledged that being in the wheelchair was problematic but that he was learning to accept it and the difficulties associated with it. In addition, he acknowledged that he realized other people were afraid to talk about the handicap but that he encouraged others to ask questions, as he believed talking about it allowed others to set aside his handicap and eventually see him as a person. The experimenters found that 71% of the time the physically disabled individual who acknowledged his stigma was chosen as the preferred work partner by nonstigmatized others, whereas only 29% of the time the physically disabled individual who did not acknowledge his stigma was chosen as the preferred work partner.

Because the acknowledging partner might have been chosen as the preferred work partner simply on the basis that he made a personal disclosure, these investigators conducted a second study in which the acknowledgment condition was compared with another personal disclosure condition. Specifically, a male confederate either acknowledged his condition as in the first study, or described his relatively ordinary life (e.g., a girlfriend, some friends, parents). Again, the individual who acknowledged his stigma was preferred over the individual who personally disclosed other information.

In Hastorf, Wildfogel, and Cassman's (1979) third study, a "nervous mention" condition was compared with the personal disclosure condition. In this study, the confederate mentioned the stigma in a manner that conveyed tension by running his hand through his hair, avoiding eye contact, and clasping his hands tightly together. The results continued to reveal that mentioning the stigma was preferred over not mentioning it, despite the presence of tense behavior.

The acknowledgment strategy has been shown to be successful not only for physically disabled individuals, but also for individuals who have had laryngectomies and who stutter. In particular, 84% of subjects in one study indicated a strong preference for working with a laryngectomized individual who acknowledged the stigma over an individual who did not (Blood & Blood, 1982). Subjects rated the acknowledger as more pleasant, positive, calm, active, likeable, well-adjusted, hardworking, stronger, and tougher than the nonmentioning person. Similarly, 71% of subjects in another study indicated a strong preference for working with a stutterer who mentioned the condition over one who did not (Collins & Blood, 1990). Subjects described the acknowledger as having a greater ability to cope, overall ease in the speaking situation, [and] positive attitude and as being more of a "real person" than the nonmentioning person.

Before adopting the acknowledgment strategy as a way to reduce awkwardness, one must first consider the particular stigma. Recent research by Hebl (1997) suggests that acknowledgments may be beneficial for some stigmatized individuals but may actually be liabilities for others. Whereas acknowledging seems to yield positive outcomes (e.g., on person perception measures) for physically disabled individuals, stigmatized individuals who have more "controllable" stigmas (e.g., obesity) are not accorded more positivity and rather are denigrated for mentioning their stigmas. Thus acknowledgments may be limited in the benefits they provide in reducing awkward moments. Acknowledgments may be particularly beneficial for disruptive, visible stigmas such as disabilities, as they can provide a nonstigmatized interactant with information. In the absence of this information, the subject of an obvious stigma remains a subterranean topic. For instance, an individual with a missing arm may realize that the nonstigmatized individual is looking at and wondering what happened to the arm; in turn, the nonstigmatized individual may realize that he or she has been caught looking. This "I know that you know that I know" interplay serves to get the social interaction off to a weak start, because a focal point of the interaction has been passed over or omitted.

Additional research on the acknowledgment strategy suggests that more interactional success occurs when stigmatized individuals provide a context for the acknowledgment (Belgrave & Mills, 1981; Belgrave, 1984). That is, rather than the individual's mentioning the stigmatizing condition alone, requesting assistance and *then* mentioning the stigmatizing condition have been shown to facilitate acceptance of the stigmatized individual (Belgrave & Mills, 1981; Mills et al., 1984). For example, an individual in a wheelchair might be unable to utilize a pencil sharpener and thus ask a nonstigmatized interactant whether he or she would mind sharpening the pencil, because "there's just some things you can't do from a wheelchair" (Belgrave & Mills, 1981, p. 48). Asking for assistance prior to mentioning the stigma is hypothesized to work as a remediation strategy because acknowledgments of stigmas in the absence of requests are often perceived by nonstigmatized others as coming "out of the blue" (Belgrave & Mills, 1981, p. 46). Inappropriate acknowledgments may be deleterious if they indicate the presence, and not absence, of emotional duress associated with possession of a stigma. On the other hand, acknowledgments made after a request are thought to be perceived as being based less on emotions and more on the functional purpose (e.g., "I need to tell him why I can't open the door myself").

Societal-Level Strategies

Additional strategies, focused on a more global level, may also remediate the occurrence of awkward moments. These strategies tend to share the goals of making mixed contact more accessible and more likely, and reducing obstacles that restrict stigmatized individuals' access to resources. More societally focused strategies may at first seem like lofty goals in addressing remediation of problems at the dyadic level. However, we believe that interaction problems, such as awkwardness, cannot fully be attenuated without examining and addressing the larger, more complex societal influences and forces.

Perhaps the most widely examined strategy involves the "contact hypothesis," which is that simply increasing the contact between stigmatized and nonstigmatized individuals should facilitate ease of interaction. Early studies found a positive relationship between contact and acceptance of stigmatized individuals. For example, Deutsch and Collins (1951) found that amount of contact with Black women was positively correlated to the favorable attitudes that White women held toward Black women. While the contact hypothesis leads to favorable attitudes, many conditions (e.g., cooperative activities, personal interactions) are necessary (see Stephan, 1986). It may be especially important to increase nonstigmatized individuals' exposure to stigmatized individuals who are happy. This exposure allows others to learn that this oxymoron ("happy and stigmatized") can and does occur in many cases, and that the stereotype that stigmatized individuals are always morose and unhappy people is in many cases simply unfounded (Elliott & Frank, 1990; Elliott, Yoder, & Umlauf, 1990).

However, other early studies failed to find an increase in acceptance as a result of increased contact. In a classic study, Richardson, Goodman, Hastorf, and Dornbusch (1961) asked 10- and 11-year-old children from diverse backgrounds to view a standardized set of six pictures depicting a child who (1) had no physical disability, (2) had crutches and a leg brace on the left leg, (3) was sitting in a wheelchair with a blanket covering both legs, (4) was missing a left hand, (5) had a facial disfigurement on the left side of the mouth, or (6) was obese. Subjects were asked to rank-order the children according to whom they liked the most; not surprisingly, the child with no physical disability was consistently ranked first, indicating that this child was liked by others the most. What was surprising, however, was that this and other studies revealed that such rank orderings were not affected by increased contact with dis-

abled children (for a review, see DeJong, 1980). The continued possession of negative beliefs about other groups of stigmatized people (e.g.,
obese individuals) by medical professionals who must work with such
clients on a regular basis also suggests the lack of a positive relationship
between contact and acceptance (see Allon, 1982).

Some of the contradictory findings may be clarified by Kleck
(1968a), who suggested that the quality and not the quantity of contact
is the important determinant in ascertaining the impact of increased contact on acceptance. In particular, close social and personal contact may
result in greater acceptance than medical or rehabilitative contact (see
Kleck, 1968a, for a review). A sizable literature on the contact hypothesis reveals necessary conditions for contact to reduce hostile intergroup
relations. These conditions include groups having mutual goals (Sherif,
Harvey, White, Hood, & Sherif, 1961), having equal status (Aronson,
1984), and engaging in actual social interactions (Cook, 1978).

A second societal-level strategy is to increase legislation concerning
stigmas. In the past decade, awareness of the needs and rights of stigmatized individuals has grown tremendously. For example, laws mandate
that new buildings must be constructed to be accessible to those in
wheelchairs; nondiscriminatory policies on hiring are ubiquitous in cor-
porations and institutions; and the presence of individuals with stigmatizing conditions is at an all-time high on college campuses. The early
Civil Rights Act of 1964 was the first of these laws, and was expanded
in 1972. The Age Discrimination in Employment Act of 1967, and the
Americans with Disabilities Act of 1990, also paved the way for the removal of barriers faced by stigmatized individuals. State laws, too, are
changing in a way advantageous to stigmatized individuals. This currently may be happening most dramatically with the stigma of homosexuality: A growing number of states have repudiated laws restricting gay
rights, have increased civil rights protections for homosexuals, and are
even beginning to outlaw discrimination against gays and lesbians in
public schools. Such advances are resulting in much higher visibility for
stigmatized individuals in our society. As such trends proliferate, the
very nature of stigmas may be altered (see, e.g., Archer, 1985). For instance, being gay was once viewed as a psychiatric disorder and ridiculed; now being gay is not only more widely accepted, but is the basis
of a growing community and culture. Moreover, gay people are playing
recognized roles in politics, the media, and religion (for a review, see
Miller, 1995).

At the societal level, dispelling the myths surrounding stigmas will
also help to reduce problems at the interaction level. One arena in which
stereotypes seem to be accentuated is that of the mass media. People
tend to form attitudes and exhibit behaviors in line with media presenta-

tions. Studies spanning over the last several decades have revealed consistently negative depictions of stigmatized groups, including Blacks (Leab, 1975), Native Americans (Trimble, 1988), elderly people (Harris & Feinberg, 1977), physically disabled individuals (Hockenberry, 1995), and women (McArthur & Resko, 1975). Rather than presenting stereotypic portrayals of stigmatized individuals, the media have the power to normalize stigmatizing conditions. The media can inform and break down barriers by revealing and disproving many of our negative stereotypes concerning stigmas. Individuals who are quadriplegic are attending medical school; disabled individuals are driving taxis; individuals who are mentally retarded are holding down corporate jobs; and women are running for President. Stigmas can be "destigmatized," and the media are very powerful instruments for doing this.

Dispelling the myths also involves supplanting untruths with accuracies concerning stigmatizing conditions and the lives of those who are stigmatized. One attempt to give greater exposure to individuals who have had little exposure until now is the establishment of courses and, in some cases, even departments for the study of stigmatized groups within college and university settings (e.g., women's studies, African American studies, disability studies). Such courses and departments offer those who have little experience with or knowledge about such groups the opportunity to learn more; they give those who belong to such groups the opportunity not only to learn more, but to celebrate, respect, and destigmatize their groups. It is unclear what effects the development of such classes and departmental programs have had at either the societal or the interactional level, but we believe that providing some forum for learning about and gaining more exposure to stigmas can do much to alleviate the negativity experienced by stigmatized individuals, even at the level of awkwardness created in a dyadic social interaction.

CONCLUSION

This chapter has attempted to clarify the nature of "awkward moments" between stigmatized and nonstigmatized individuals. Such experiences are diverse; they are initiated by various factors, perpetuated by the same and other factors, and influenced by additional situational and personality variables. Stigmatized and nonstigmatized individuals have much in common in mixed interactions: They fear and are uncertain about each other, and they often experience anxiety. This anxiety, unfortunately, may perpetuate one of the main goals of the interactants, which is to avoid each other.

We believe that awkward moments are important experiences to understand. The affective, cognitive, and behavioral reasons for them, their impact on both individuals and groups, and the consequences of awkward moments are all areas that we hope will be illuminated by future research. We propose that an understanding of more global issues such as stereotyping, prejudice, and discrimination will be facilitated by a continued focus on understanding what transpires at the level of a single mixed interaction. Awkward moments have far-reaching consequences in the lives of both stigmatized and nonstigmatized individuals. But the research that is conducted and the strategies that are implemented in the future may reduce much of the anxiety and awkwardness that nonstigmatized and stigmatized individuals alike experience.

REFERENCES

Albrecht, G. L., Walker, V. G., & Levy, J. A. (1982). Social distance from the stigmatized: A test of two theories. *Social Science and Medicine, 16,* 1319–1327.

Allon, N. (1982). The stigma of overweight in everyday life. In B. B. Wolman (Ed.), *Psychological aspects of obesity: A handbook* (pp. 130–174). New York: Van Nostrand Reinhold.

Archer, D. (1985). Social deviance. In G. Lindzey & E. Aronson (Ed.), *Handbook of social psychology: Vol. 2. Special fields and applications* (3rd ed., pp. 413–483). New York: Random House.

Aronson, E. (1984). Modifying the environment of the desegregated classroom. In A. J. Stewart (Ed.), *Motivation and society.* San Francisco: Jossey-Bass.

Barker, R. G., Wright, B. A., Meyerson, L., & Gonick, M. R. (1953). *Adjustment to physical handicap and illness: A survey of the social psychology of physique and disability* (2nd ed.). New York: Social Science Research Council.

Belgrave, F. Z. (1984). The effectiveness of strategies for increasing social interaction with a physically disabled person. *Journal of Applied Social Psychology, 14,* 147–161.

Belgrave, F. Z. (1985). Reactions to a Black stimulus person under disabling and nondisabling conditions. *Journal of Rehabilitation, 2,* 53–57.

Belgrave, F. Z., & Mills, J. (1981). Effect upon desire for social interaction with a physically disabled person of mentioning the disability in different contexts. *Journal of Applied Social Psychology, 11,* 44–57.

Blood, G. W., & Blood, I. M. (1982). A tactic for facilitating social interaction with laryngectomees. *Journal of Speech and Hearing Disorders, 47,* 416–419.

Bloom, J. R., & Kessler, L. (1994). Emotional support following cancer: A test of the stigma and social activity hypotheses. *Journal of Health and Social Behavior, 35,* 118–133.

Bodenhausen, G. V., Sheppard, L. A., & Kramer, G. P. (1994). Negative affect and social judgment: The differential impact of anger and sadness. *European Journal of Social Psychology, 24,* 45–62.

Bull, R., & Rumsey, N. (1988). *The social psychology of facial appearance.* New York: Springer-Verlag.

Clore, G. L., Schwarz, N., & Conway, M. (1994). Affective causes and consequences of social information processing. In R. S. Wyer, Jr., & T. K. Srull (Eds.), *Handbook of social cognition: Vol. 2: Applications* (2nd ed., pp. 323–417). Hillsdale, NJ: Erlbaum.

Collins, C. R., & Blood, G. W. (1990). Acknowledgment and severity of stuttering as factors influencing nonstutterers' perceptions of stutterers. *Journal of Speech and Hearing Disorders, 55*(1), 75–81.

Comer, R. C., & Piliavin, J. A. (1972). The effects of physical deviance upon face-to-face interaction. The other side. *Journal of Personality and Social Psychology, 23*(1), 33–39.

Cook, S. W. (1978). Interpersonal and attitudinal outcomes in cooperating interracial groups. *Journal of Research and Development in Education, 12*, 97–113.

Crandall, C. (1994). Prejudice against fat people: Ideology and self-interest? *Journal of Personality and Social Psychology, 66*, 882–894.

Crandall, C., & Biernat, M. (1990). The ideology of anti-fat attitudes. *Journal of Applied Social Psychology, 20*, 227–243.

Crandall, C., & Martinez, R. (1996). Culture, ideology, and antifat attitudes. *Personality and Social Psychology Bulletin, 22*, 1165–1176.

Crocker, J., Cornwell, B., & Major, B. (1993). The stigma of overweight: Affective consequences of attributional ambiguity. *Journal of Personality and Social Psychology, 64*, 60–70.

Crocker, J., & Major, B. (1989). Social stigma and self-esteem: The self-protective properties of stigma. *Psychological Bulletin, 96*, 608–630.

Crocker, J., & Major, B. (1994). Reactions to stigma: The moderating role of justifications. In M. P. Zanna & J. M. Olson (Eds.), *The Ontario Symposium: Vol. 7. The psychology of prejudice* (pp. 289–314). Hillsdale, NJ: Erlbaum.

Crocker, J., Major, B., & Steele, C. (1998). Social stigma. In D. T. Gilbert, S. T. Fiske, & G. Lindzey (Eds.), *Handbook of social psychology* (4th ed., Vol. 2, pp. 504–553). Boston: McGraw-Hill.

Davis, F. (1961). Deviance disavowal: The management of strained interaction by the visibly handicapped. *Social Problems, 9*, 120–132.

Dean, J. C., & Poremba, G. A. (1983). The alcoholic stigma and the disease concept. *International Journal of the Addictions, 18*(5), 739–751.

DeJong, W. (1980). The stigma of obesity: The consequences of naive assumptions concerning the causes of physical deviance. *Journal of Health and Social Behavior, 21*, 75–87.

DeJong, W., & Kleck, R. E. (1986). The social psychological effects of overweight. In C. P. Herman, M. P. Zanna, & E. T. Higgins (Eds.), *The Ontario Symposium: Vol. 3. Physical appearance, stigma and social behavior* (pp. 65–87). Hillsdale, NJ: Erlbaum.

Deutsch, M., & Collins, M. E. (1951). *Interracial housing: A psychological evaluation of a social experiment.* Minneapolis: University of Minnesota Press.

Devine, P. G. (1989). Stereotypes and prejudice: Their automatic and controlled components. *Journal of Social and Personality Psychology, 56*(1), 5–18.

Devine, P. G., Evett, S. R., & Vasquez-Suson, K. A. (1996). Exploring the interpersonal dynamics of intergroup contact. In R. M. Sorrentino & E. T. Higgins

(Eds.), *Handbook of motivation and cognition: Vol. 3. The interpersonal context* (pp. 423–464). New York: Guilford Press.

Dion, K. L. (1986). Responses to perceived discrimination and relative deprivation. In J. M. Olson, C. P. Herman, & M. P. Zanna (Eds.), *The Ontario Symposium: Vol. 4. Relative deprivation and social comparison* (pp. 159–179). Hillsdale, NJ: Erlbaum.

Dorgan, C. A. (Ed.). (1995). *Statistical record of health and medicine.* New York: Gale Research.

Dovidio, J. F., & Gaertner, S. L. (Eds.). (1986). *Prejudice, discrimination, and racism.* Orlando, FL: Academic Press.

Dovidio, J. F., & Gaertner, S. L. (1993). Stereotypes and evaluative intergroup bias. In D. Mackie & D. Hamilton (Eds.), *Affect, cognition, and stereotyping: Interactive processes in intergroup perception* (pp. 167–193). San Diego, CA: Academic Press.

Dunbar, J., Brown, M., & Amoroso, D. M. (1973). Some correlates of attitudes toward homosexuality. *Journal of Social Psychology, 89*(2), 271–279.

Elliott, T. R., & Frank, R. G. (1990). Social and interpersonal reactions to depression and disability. *Rehabilitation Psychology, 35*(3), 135–147.

Elliott, T. R., & MacNair, R. R. (1991). Attributional processes in response to social displays of depression. *Journal of Social and Personal Relationships, 8,* 129–132.

Elliott, T. R., MacNair, R. R., Herrick, S. M., Yoder, B., & Byrne, C. A. (1991). Interpersonal reactions to depression and physical disability in dyadic interactions. *Journal of Applied Social Psychology, 21,* 1293–1302.

Elliott, T. R., Yoder, B., & Umlauf, R. (1990). Nurse and patient reactions to social displays of depression. *Rehabilitation Psychology, 35*(4), 195–204.

Farina, A., Holland, C. H., & Ring, K. (1966). The role of stigma and set in interpersonal interaction. *Journal of Abnormal Psychology, 71,* 421–428.

Farina, A., Sherman, M., & Allen, J. G. (1968). Role of physical abnormalities in interpersonal perception and behavior. *Journal of Abnormal Psychology, 73,* 590–595.

Festinger, L. (1957). *A theory of cognitive dissonance.* Stanford, CA: Stanford University Press.

Forgas, J. P. (1992). Affect in social judgments and decisions: A multiprocess model. In M. P. Zanna (Ed.), *Advances in experimental social psychology* (Vol. 25, pp. 227–275). San Diego, CA: Academic Press.

Gibbons, F. X., Stephan, W. G., Stephenson, B., & Petty, C. R. (1980). Reactions to stigmatized others: Response amplification vs. sympathy. *Journal of Experimental Social Psychology, 16,* 591–605.

Goffman, E. (1959). *The presentation of self in everyday life.* Garden City, NY: Doubleday.

Goffman, E. (1963). *Stigma: Notes on the management of spoiled identity.* Englewood Cliffs, NJ: Prentice-Hall.

Graham, S., Weiner, B., Giuliano, T., & Williams, E. (1993). An attributional analysis of reactions to Magic Johnson. *Journal of Applied Social Psychology, 23*(12), 996–1010.

Greenberg, J., Pyszczynski, T., Solomon, S., Rosenblatt, A., Veeder, M.,

Kirkland, S., & Lyon, D. (1990). Evidence for terror management theory: II. The effects of mortality salience on reactions to those who threaten or bolster the cultural worldview. *Journal of Personality and Social Psychology, 58*(2), 308–318.

Haddock, G., Zanna, M. P., & Esses, V. M. (1993). Assessing the structure of prejudicial attitudes: The case of attitudes toward homosexuals. *Journal of Personality and Social Psychology, 65,* 1105–1118.

Haidt, J., McCauley, C., & Rozin, P. (1994). Individual differences in sensitivity to disgust: A scale sampling seven domains of disgust elicitors. *Personality and Individual Differences, 16*(5), 701–713.

Harris, A., & Feinberg, J. (1977). Television and aging: Is what you see what you get? *Gerontologist, 18,* 464–468.

Hart, L. A., Hart, B. L., & Bergin, B. (1987). Socializing effects of service dogs for people with disabilities. *Anthrozooes, 1*(1), 41–44.

Hastorf, A. H., Northcraft, G. B., & Picciotto, S. R. (1979). Helping the handicapped: How realistic is the performance feedback received by the physically handicapped? *Personality and Social Psychology Bulletin, 5,* 373–376.

Hastorf, A. H., Wildfogel, J., & Cassman, T. (1979). Acknowledgment of handicap as a tactic in social interaction. *Journal of Personality and Social Psychology, 37,* 1790–1797.

Hebl, M. R. (1997). *Nonstigmatized individuals' reactions to the acknowledgment and valuation of a stigma by physically disabled and overweight individuals.* Unpublished doctoral dissertation, Dartmouth College.

Heilbrun, A. B. (1976). Measurement of masculine and feminine sex role identities as independent dimensions. *Journal of Consulting and Clinical Psychology, 44*(2), 183–190.

Heinemann, W., Pellander, F., Vogelbusch, A., & Wojtek, B. (1981). Meeting a deviant person: Subjective norms and affective reactions. *European Journal of Social Psychology, 11,* 1–25.

Herek, G. M. (1988). Heterosexuals' attitudes toward lesbians and gay men: Correlates and gender differences. *Journal of Sex Research, 25,* 451–477.

Hockenberry, J. (1995). *Moving violations: War zones, wheelchairs, and declarations of independence.* New York: Hyperion.

Ickes, W. (1984). Compositions in Black and White: Determinants of interaction in interracial dyads. *Journal of Personality and Social Psychology, 47*(2), 339–341.

Izard, C. E. (1991). *The psychology of emotions.* New York: Plenum Press.

Jones, E. E., Farina, A., Hastorf, A. H., Markus, H., Miller, D. T., & Scott, R. A. (1984). *Social stigma: The psychology of marked relationships.* New York: Freeman.

Katz, I. (1981). *Stigma: A social psychological analysis.* Hillsdale, NJ: Erlbaum.

Katz, I., Glass, D. C., Lucido, D. J., & Farber, J. (1979). Ambivalence, guilt, and the scapegoating of minority group victims. *Journal of Experimental Social Psychology, 9,* 423–436.

Katz, I., & Hass, R. G. (1988). Racial ambivalence and American value conflict: Correlational and prime studies of dual cognitive structures. *Journal of Personality and Social Psychology, 55,* 893–905.

King, M. L., Jr. (1986). Letter from Birmingham jail, April 16, 1963. *American Visions: The Magazine of Afro-American Culture, 1*(1), 52–59.

Kleck, R. (1966). Emotional arousal in interactions with stigmatized persons. *Psychological Reports, 19,* 1126.

Kleck, R. (1968a). The role of stigma as a factor in social interaction. In *Perspectives on human deprivation: Biological, psychological and sociological* (NICHD Task Force Report). Washington, DC: U.S. Department of Health, Education and Welfare.

Kleck, R. (1968b). Physical stigma and nonverbal cues emitted in face-to-face interaction. *Human Relations, 21,* 19–28.

Kleck, R. (1969). Physical stigma and task oriented interactions. *Human Relations, 22,* 53–60.

Kleck, R., Ono, H., & Hastorf, A. H. (1966). The effects of physical deviance upon face-to-face interaction. *Human Relations, 19*(4), 425–436.

Kleck, R., & Strenta, A. (1980). Perceptions of the impact of negatively valued physical characteristics on social interaction. *Journal of Personality and Social Psychology, 39,* 861–873.

Langer, E. J., Fiske, S., Taylor, S. E., & Chanowitz, B. (1976). Stigma, staring, and discomfort: A novel-stimulus hypothesis. *Journal of Experimental Social Psychology, 12,* 451–463.

Latané, B., & Darley, J. M. (1970). *The unresponsive bystander: Why doesn't he help?* New York: Appleton-Century-Crofts.

Leab, D. J. (1975). *From Sambo to Superspade: The Black experience in motion pictures.* Boston: Houghton Mifflin.

Leary, M. (1983). Social anxiousness: The construct and its measurement. *Journal of Personality Assessment, 47*(1), 66–75.

Lerner, M. J. (1980). *The belief in a just world: A fundamental delusion.* New York: Plenum Press.

Levine, J. M., & McBurney, D. H. (1977). Causes and consequences of effluvia: Body odor awareness and controllability as determinants of interpersonal evaluation. *Personality and Social Psychology Bulletin, 3,* 442–445.

MacGregor, F. C., Abel, T. M., Bryt, A., Lauer, E., & Weissmann, S. (1953). *Facial deformities and plastic surgery: A psychosocial study.* Springfield, IL: Thomas.

Mackie, D. M., & Hamilton, D. L. (Eds.). (1993). *Affect, cognition, and stereotyping: Interactive processes in intergroup perception.* San Diego, CA: Academic Press.

Macrae, C. N., Milne, A. B., & Bodenhausen, G. V. (1994). Stereotypes as energy-saving devices: A peek inside the cognitive toolbox. *Journal of Personality and Social Psychology, 66,* 37–47.

McArthur, L., & Resko, B. (1975). The portrayal of men and women in American television commercials. *Journal of Social Psychology, 97,* 209–220.

McGuire, J. A. (1998). *Tainted persons or tainted interactions: The effect of disruptive stigmas on the perceiver.* Honors thesis, Dartmouth College.

McNeil, J. M. (1993). *Americans with disabilities: 1991–1992* (Current Population Reports No. P-70-33). Washington, DC: U.S. Government Printing Office.

Miller, C. T., Rothblum, E. D., Felicio, D. M., & Brand, P. A. (1995). Compensating for stigma: Obese and nonobese women's reactions to being visible. *Personality and Social Psychology Bulletin, 21,* 1093–1106.

Miller, N. (1995). *Out of the past: Gay and lesbian history from 1869 to the present.* New York: Vintage Books.

Mills, J., Belgrave, F. Z., & Boyer, K. M. (1984). Reducing avoidance of social interaction with a physically disabled person by mentioning the disability following a request for aid. *Journal of Applied Social Psychology, 14,* 1–11.

Monteith, M. J. (1993). Self-regulation of prejudiced responses: Implications for progress in prejudice-reduction efforts. *Journal of Personality and Social Psychology, 65,* 469–485.

Monteith, M. J., Devine, P. G., & Zuwerink, J. R. (1993). Self-directed versus other-directed affect as a consequence of prejudice-related discrepancies. *Journal of Personality and Social Psychology, 64*(2), 198–210.

Muzzin, L. J., Anderson, N. J., Figueredo, A. T., & Gudelis, S. O. (1994). The experience of cancer. *Social Science and Medicine, 38*(9), 1201–1208.

National Gay Task Force. (1988). *Anti-gay violence, victimization, and defamation in 1987.* Washington, DC: Author.

Neuberg, S. L., Smith, D. M., Hoffman, J. C., & Russell, F. J. (1994). When we observe stigmatized and "normal" individuals interacting: Stigma by association. *Personality and Social Psychology Bulletin, 20,* 196–209.

Northcraft, G. B. (1980). *The perception of disability.* Unpublished manuscript, Stanford University.

Perlman, J. L., & Routh, D. K. (1980). Stigmatizing effects of a child's wheelchair in successive and simultaneous interactions. *Journal of Pediatric Psychology, 5*(1), 43–55.

Richardson, S. A., Goodman, N., Hastorf, A. H., & Dornbusch, S. M. (1961). Cultural uniformity in reaction to physical disabilities. *American Sociological Review, 26,* 241–247.

Rosenblatt, A., Greenberg, J., Solomon, S., Pyszczynski, T., & Lyon, D. (1989). Evidence for terror management theory: I. The effects of mortality salience on reactions to those who violate or uphold cultural values. *Journal of Personality and Social Psychology, 57*(4), 681–690.

Rozin, P., Markwith, M., & McCauley, C. (1994). Sensitivity to indirect contact with other persons: AIDS aversion as a composite of aversion to strangers, infection, moral taint, and misfortune. *Journal of Abnormal Psychology, 103*(3), 495–504.

Scheier, M. F., Carver, C. S., Schulz, R., Glass, D. C., & Katz, I. (1978). Sympathy, self-consciousness, and reactions to the stigmatized. *Journal of Applied Social Psychology, 8*(3), 270–282.

Sherif, M., Harvey, O. J., White, B. J., Hood, W. R., & Sherif, C. W. (1961). *Intergroup conflict and cooperation: The Robber's Cave experiment.* Norman, OK: University of Oklahoma Press.

Sigelman, C. K., Howell, J. L., Cornell, D. P., Cutright, J. D., & Dewey, J. C. (1991). Courtesy stigma: The social implications of associating with a gay person. *Journal of Social Psychology, 131,* 45–56.

Snyder, M. L., Kleck, R. E., Strenta, A., & Mentzer, S. J. (1979). Avoidance of the handicapped: An attributional ambiguity analysis. *Journal of Personality and Social Psychology, 37*(12), 2297–2306.

Snyder, M., & Miene, P. K. (1994). Stereotyping of the elderly: A functional approach. *British Journal of Social Psychology, 33*, 63–82.

Stephan, W. G. (1986). The effects of school desegregation: An evaluation 30 years after Brown. In M. J. Saks & L. Saxe (Eds.), *Advances in applied social psychology* (Vol. 3, pp. 181–206). Hillsdale, NJ: Erlbaum.

Steele, C. M. (1988). The psychology of self-affirmation: Sustaining the integrity of the self. In L. Berkowitz (Ed.), *Advances in experimental social psychology* (Vol. 21, pp. 261–302). San Diego, CA: Academic Press.

Stephan, W. G., & Stephan, C. W. (1985). Intergroup anxiety. *Journal of Social Issues, 41*(3), 157–175.

Trimble, J. E. (1988). Stereotypical images, American Indians, and prejudice. In P. A. Katz & D. A. Taylor (Eds.), *Eliminating racism: Profiles in controversy.* New York: Plenum Press.

Van Riper, C. (1939). *Do you stutter?* New York: Harper & Row.

Wegner, D. M. (1994). Ironic processes of mental control. *Psychological Review, 101*, 34–52.

Weinberg, T. S., & Vogler, C. C. (1990). Wives of alcoholics: Stigma management and adjustments to husband–wife interaction. *Deviant Behavior, 11*(4), 331–343.

Weiner, B. (1995). *Judgments of responsibility: A foundation for a theory of social conduct.* New York: Guilford Press.

Weiner, B., Perry, R. P., & Magnusson, J. (1988). An attributional analysis of reactions to stigma. *Journal of Personality and Social Psychology, 55*(5), 738–748.

Wiley, C. (1994). *Journeys to self-acceptance: Fat women speak.* Freedom, CA: Crossing Press.

Woods, C. L., & Williams, D. E. (1976). Traits attributed to stuttering and normally fluent males. *Journal of Speech and Hearing Research, 19*(2), 267–278.

Wright, B. (1983). *Physical disability: A psychological approach* (2nd ed.). New York: Harper.

Zajonc, R. B. (1980). Feeling and thinking: Preferences need no inferences. *American Psychologist, 35*(2), 151–175.

Zebrowitz-McArthur, L. (1982). Judging a book by its cover: A cognitive analysis of the relationship between physical appearance and stereotyping. In A. H. Hastorf & A. M. Isen (Eds.), *Cognitive social psychology* (pp. 149–211). New York: Elsevier.

11

Stigma, Threat, and Social Interactions

JIM BLASCOVICH
WENDY BERRY MENDES
SARAH B. HUNTER
BRIAN LICKEL

The chapters in this and many other volumes attest to the importance of stigma as a construct in psychology, sociology, and related disciplines. Not surprisingly, stigma has enjoyed a long history as a central construct in social psychology, investigated by both psychological and sociological social psychologists. Many theorists have explicitly or implicitly woven stigma into their explanations of stereotyping, prejudice, social justice, and social identity. Researchers have accumulated a wealth of information regarding the impact of stigmatized others (or "targets") on the affective and cognitive processes of perceivers, and a more modest but substantial amount of information regarding the impact of a stigma on the bearer. Researchers have also accumulated much knowledge on the social identity of stigmatized individuals, the consequences of membership in stigmatized groups, and coping with stigma (see Crocker, Major, & Steele, 1998, for a review).

Advances have also occurred in the definition and delineation of "stigma." Crocker et al. (1998) define stigma as the possession of (or the belief that one possesses) "some attribute, or characteristic, that conveys a social identity that is devalued in some particular social context" (p. 505). Stigmas may be visible (e.g., acne) or concealed (e.g., many cancers), concrete (e.g., a Star of David armband) or abstract (e.g., religion), inborn (e.g., skin color) or acquired (e.g., a prison uniform), simple (e.g., a birthmark) or complex (e.g., homosexuality), and so forth. Individuals may or may not be aware of *all* of their own stigmatizing characteristics (e.g., political liberalism or conservatism, gender), and even if they are aware, they may not continuously attend to them. Likewise, others (perceivers) may or may not be aware of the stigmatizing characteristics of those with whom they interact, and may not continuously attend to them even if they are aware.

The relative paucity of empirical data on stigma effects during actual social interaction constitutes a somewhat surprising gap in the stigma literature (Crocker et al., 1998). We know that nonstigmatized individuals negatively stereotype stigmatized others, avoid them, scapegoat them, and react to them in other derogatory ways. We also know that individuals sometimes categorize others in ways that stigmatize them so that others will devalue them (one only has to view political advertisements in the United States to realize this). Nonstigmatized individuals also experience negative affect in reaction to stigmatized people, including specific emotions such as disgust or fear. These facts point to the often antisocial nature of social interaction between nonstigmatized and stigmatized individuals, such as racial conflicts. In most cases, the "sociofugal" nature of such antisocial interaction precludes sustained or meaningful relationships: Physical or psychological distancing (flight) often occurs, though in some cases aggression (fight) ensues.

Why does stigma increase the likelihood of antisocial interaction? Cognitivistic explanations abound. In the context of social interaction, stigma may elicit negative stereotypes and schemas on the part of both stigmatized and nonstigmatized individuals, which work to poison the social context. The elicitation of negative stereotypes may even become automatic over time (Devine, 1989), increasing their insidious nature. Affectivistic explanations abound as well: Stigma elicits negative affect and emotions that individuals would rather avoid. We propose, however, that neither a purely cognitive nor a purely affective account provides the explanatory power necessary to understand the role of stigma in social interaction. Furthermore, we propose that understanding the role of stigma in social interaction requires more than a simple additive cognitive–affective framework.

We believe that we can best understand the role of stigma in social interaction within a motivational framework—one incorporating both cognitive and affective components, to be sure, but one that is more than simply the sum or even the interaction of these components. If we assume that "flight or fight" motivation contributes to the antisocial nature of social interactions involving stigma, then we can profitably venture into the area of motivation to understand more about it. What motivates psychological or physical flight in interactions involving stigmatized persons? What motivates aggression toward or by such persons? In a word, "threat" does. Threat, or the perception of possible physical or psychological harm, motivates individuals to protect themselves by flight (e.g., removal) or fight (e.g., retaliation and escalation).

We support the not particularly novel proposition (see also Crocker et al., 1998; Jones et al., 1984) that within the context of social interaction, stigmatized individuals typically but unwittingly threaten others. Threat can result primarily from cognitive processes, as when perception of a stigmatized other activates a threatening stereotype in the perceiver, automatically or otherwise. However, we propose that in many cases threat can also occur by virtue of the stigma itself—not because of the activation of threatening stereotypes, but because the stigma represents affective cues, including unlearned ones, that elicit threat directly.

We support the proposition that stigmatized individuals also experience threat in social interactions and that their experience of threat occurs via similar (i.e., cognitive and affective) processes. That stigmatized people experience threat more often than nonstigmatized people do hardly needs debate (Anderson, McNeilly, & Myers, 1993; Word, Zanna, & Cooper, 1974). That social interaction between stigmatized and nonstigmatized individuals often proves antisocial and sociofugal should not surprise us, given that such individuals mutually threaten one another.

THREAT (AND CHALLENGE) AS MOTIVATIONAL STATES

Our work (e.g., Blascovich & Mendes, 2000; Blascovich, Mendes, Hunter, Lickel, & Kowai-Bell, 2000; Blascovich & Tomaka, 1996; Tomaka, Blascovich, Kelsey, & Leitten, 1993) has focused on challenge and threat as motivational states resulting from individuals' evaluations[1] of situational demands and personal resources in what we have termed "motivated performance situations." Generally, when demands outweigh resources, threat results; when resources approximate or exceed demands, challenge results.

Motivated Performance Situations

Motivated performance situations are goal-relevant for performers and require instrumental cognitive-behavioral responses by them. The necessary goal relevance of motivated performance situations means that performers expect that the quality of their performance will provide meaningful input to their sense of self-worth. Hence, motivated performance situations necessarily involve self-evaluation at some level.

Motivated performance situations require active participation, in the sense that the performers must make appropriate cognitive-behavioral responses to maintain the structure and the integrity of the situation. For example, when taking an examination, students must answer questions. If they do not do so, the situation changes radically and no longer represents a motivated performance situation. When individuals stop answering questions, they disengage and no longer "take" the examination. The situation may still require coping, but no longer coping of an active or task-focused sort. We contrast motivated performance situations, with other kinds of situations, in which the individual's responses do not critically define and structure the integrity of the situation (such as watching a scary movie or a baseball game).

Motivated performance situations are ubiquitous in modern life. They may be primarily solitary and involve only the implicit presence of others (e.g., taking an examination alone, preparing a speech, solving a puzzle, or writing an article), or they may be primarily interactive (e.g., arguing with a significant other, negotiating with one's boss or subordinate, making a sales pitch, playing games, and engaging in sports). Motivated performance situations may be metabolically demanding (e.g., may require large muscle movements) or nonmetabolically demanding. We have focused on nonmetabolically demanding performance situations.

Evaluations

As mentioned above, threat and challenge result from the confluence of demand and resource evaluations. Demand evaluations involve the perceptions or assessments of (i.e., the experience of) *danger, uncertainty,* and *required effort* inherent in the particular motivated performance situation. At present, we choose not to specify an exact calculus for demand evaluations using these dimensions. They may be additive, interactive, or synergistic. Or evaluations of high demand on any one of these dimensions may trigger high overall demand evaluations. Perceptual cues associated with danger, uncertainty, and required effort undoubtedly contribute to demand evaluations.

Resource evaluations involve the perceptions or assessments of (i.e., the experience of) *knowledge and abilities* relevant to situational performance, *dispositional characteristics,* and *external support.* Again, we choose not to specify an exact calculus for resource evaluations. Again, they may be additive, interactive, or synergistic, or may be such that high resource evaluations on one dimension trigger high overall resource evaluations. Perceptual cues associated with knowledge and abilities, dispositional characteristics, and external support undoubtedly contribute to resource evaluations.

Individuals may make demand and resource evaluations consciously and/or unconsciously. Hence, individuals may make demand or resource evaluations or both without awareness. Conscious and unconscious appraisals may occur in parallel and may inform each other. Unconscious evaluations may be reflexive or learned.

Importantly, evaluations may involve affective (i.e., feeling) processes, semantic (i.e., cognitive) processes, or both. Zajonc (1999) demonstrates clearly that affective processes can occur independently of cognitive ones. LeDoux (1996) confirms and extends Zajonc's notions, suggesting that affective and cognitive systems, though independent, may actually influence one another. Figure 11.1 illustrates the incorporation of conscious and unconscious, affective and cognitive processing into the evaluation process described above.

We also note the iterative nature of the evaluation process. Prior to, during, and following task performance, an individual continuously reevaluates the situation, because neither the individual nor the situation remains static during motivated performance situation episodes. Each may affect the other, and external events may intervene. What begins as a demanding situation for an individual may become less demanding, or vice versa. For example, a doctoral student may be more threatened by some questions during a dissertation defense than by others. Similarly, what begins as a motivated performance situation for which an individual perceives few resources may become one in which he or she perceives

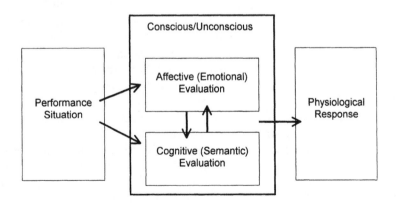

FIGURE 11.1. Evaluation model.

many. For instance, a speaker may feel more resourceful as the result of positive audience feedback.

Threat occurs when, as a result of the individual's evaluations, resources do not meet situational demands. For example, playing chess against a player who is clearly better than oneself results in a state of threat. *Challenge* occurs when, as a result of the individual's evaluations, resources meet situational demands. For example, playing chess against an opponent who is perceived as worse or slightly better than oneself results in a state of challenge. Cases of gross imbalance, such as extremely high levels of demands compared to resources (e.g., playing chess against Bobby Fischer) or extremely high levels of resources compared to demands (e.g., playing chess against an inexperienced young child) typically do not provide information meaningful to one's sense of self-worth, thus making the situation nonevaluative or non-goal-relevant, and hence nonmotivated. In such situations, threat and challenge states do not occur.

PHYSIOLOGICAL MARKERS OF CHALLENGE AND THREAT

Among physiological response systems, the cardiovascular system appears particularly attuned to challenge and threat. Although we would not argue against the proposition that the sensitivity of cardiovascular responses derives from an adaptive advantage inherent in the evolution of the "visceral" brain (i.e., the midbrain and the medial cortex) and its role in "fight or flight" responses, such a proposition, though consistent with the rationale here, remains logically unnecessary to it.

We have delineated two key cardiovascular response patterns evoked during goal-relevant, motivated performance situations. Based upon the psychophysiological theory and research of Paul Obrist (1981) as well as that of Richard Dienstbier (1989), we have developed physiological indexes of challenge and threat on the basis of patterns of neurally and hormonally controlled cardiovascular responses.

Increases in sympathetic–adrenomedullary (SAM) activity mark challenge. Neural stimulation of the myocardium enhances cardiac performance by means of sympathetically enhanced ventricular contractility (evidenced by faster preejection period, or PEP) and increased stroke volume, which (together with unchanged or increased heart rate) increases cardiac output (CO). Coterminously, adrenal medullary release of epinephrine dilates arteries in the large skeletal muscle beds and bronchi, thereby decreasing systemic vascular resistance (expressed as total peripheral resistance, or TPR). These responses result in relatively unchanged blood pressure. This challenge pattern mimics cardiovascular performance during metabolically demanding aerobic exercise tasks and represents the efficient mobilization of energy for coping.

Increased SAM activity combined with increased pituitary adrenal cortical (PAC) activity marks threat. PAC activity inhibits SAM release of epinephrine. Though faster PEP and increases in stroke volume, heart rate, and CO occur, they do so without accompanying decreases in TPR (i.e., vasodilation). Rather, no changes or even slight increases in TPR occur, resulting typically in relatively large increases in blood pressure. Figure 11.2 illustrates both the challenge and threat patterns of cardiovascular responses.

Self-Report Responses

We believe that physiological (i.e., cardiovascular) responses provide continuous, covert, online, unambiguous evidence of challenge and threat states for individuals within the context of relatively nonmetabolically demanding motivated performance situations. Whether individuals can self-report these states or their component evaluations veridically before, during, or after a performance situation depends on the degree to which affective and semantic appraisal processing occurs consciously, as well as the extent to which individuals concern themselves with self-presentation. We believe that much more measurement error can occur when investigators attempt to index appraisals via self-report rather than physiologically, though such reports can and do provide important information.

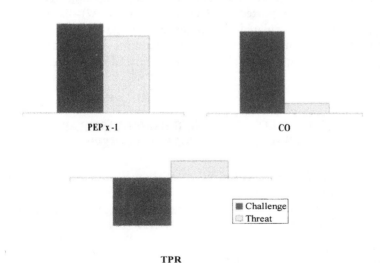

FIGURE 11.2. Cardiovascular patterns of challenge and threat. PEP, preejection period; CO, cardiac output; TPR, total peripheral resistance.

Cardiovascular Markers of Challenge and Threat: Validating Evidence

We have validated the specified cardiovascular response patterns as indexes of challenge and threat by conducting three types of studies: correlational, experimental, and manipulated physiology. Briefly (see Blascovich & Tomaka, 1996, for a more detailed description), all three types of studies point to the validity of the cardiovascular markers. The correlational studies (see Tomaka et al., 1993) demonstrated that participants who self-reported more resources than demands after receiving task instructions, but prior to performing a mental arithmetic task in a motivated performance situation, evidenced the predicted (see Figure 11.2) challenge pattern of responses (i.e., increased cardiac performance [faster PEP and increased CO] coupled with reduced TPR), and that participants who self-reported more demands than resources evidenced the predicted (see Figure 11.2) threat pattern of responses (i.e., increased cardiac performance coupled with slightly increased TPR). Our experimental study (reported in Tomaka, Blascovich, Kibler, & Ernst, 1997)—in which we induced threat and challenge via instructional set and nonverbal cues (i.e., vocal tone), using the same performance situation and task as in the correlational studies—also confirmed the validity of our cardiovascular markers. Those in the manipulated threat and challenge conditions produced the expected self-reported pretask evaluation patterns, and also evidenced the predicted cardiovascular threat and challenge patterns (see Figure 11.2). Finally, in a set of manipulated physiology studies (also reported in Tomaka et al., 1997)—in which we independently manipulated the cardiovascular patterns to determine whether evaluations followed from the patterns—we found that the physiological manipulations did not affect demand and resource evaluations.

STIGMA RESEARCH USING CARDIOVASCULAR CHALLENGE AND THREAT MARKERS

We have begun to examine the effects of stigmas during motivated performance situations involving interactions between nonstigmatized and stigmatized individuals. This work suggests that stigmas affect challenge and threat motivation from both perspectives.

Nonstigmatized Individuals' Perspective

In one study (Blascovich et al., 2000, Study 1), we recorded appropriate cardiovascular measures of nonstigmatized individuals interacting with stigmatized individuals. In this study, female dyads interacted in a motivated performance situation involving a speech. Ostensibly each dyad consisted of two naive undergraduate participants, though in reality and unknown to the real participant, we employed one of the undergraduates as a confederate. We manipulated whether or not the nonstigmatized female interacted with a stigmatized or a nonstigmatized female (the confederate). In the former condition, confederates bore a large, visible port-wine facial birthmark. In the latter condition, confederates bore no birthmark. We kept confederates unaware of experimental conditions by applying facial makeup to them in both conditions (either translucent powder for the nonstigmatized condition, or appropriate colored powder for the stigmatized condition) and removing all reflective surfaces from their environment.

We introduced each confederate and participant after they arrived at our laboratory. Subsequently, they briefly exchanged information about themselves (including age, major, hometown, etc.), according to a specifically designed protocol. We then took the participant and confederate to separate experimental/physiological recording rooms. There we applied appropriate physiological sensors (impedance cardiographic, electrocardiographic, and blood pressure) to the real participant. Following a baseline recording period, the participant received instructions that she would soon work together on a cooperative task with the other participant, but first would have to deliver a speech on the topic of "Working Together" for the other participant's review. We allowed the participant 1 minute to prepare the speech and 3 minutes to deliver the speech.

Significant differences in cardiovascular patterns emerged during the speech between participants interacting with stigmatized confederates and those interacting with nonstigmatized confederates. As Figure 11.3 illustrates, participants interacting with facially stigmatized confederates exhibited the cardiovascular markers of threat—specifically, increases in cardiac activity (especially PEP) and increases in vascular tone (i.e., TPR). Participants interacting with nonstigmatized confederates exhibited our cardiovascular markers of challenge—specifically, increases in cardiac activity coupled with decreases in vascular tone.

Stigmatized Individuals' Perspective

In a second study (Mendes, Blascovich, Kowai-Bell, & Seery, 1999), we recorded appropriate cardiovascular measures of stigmatized individuals interacting with nonstigmatized individuals. In this study, female dyads interacted in a motivated performance situation including a speech similar to the one described in the first study. Ostensibly each dyad again consisted of two naive undergraduate participants, though in reality and unknown to the real participant, we employed one of the undergradu-

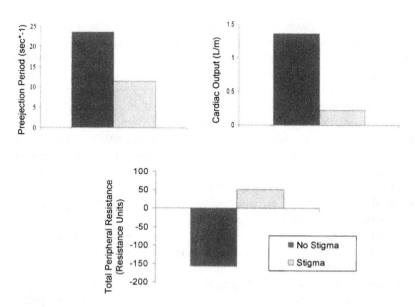

FIGURE 11.3. Cardiovascular reactivity during the first minute of the speech delivery task.

ates as a confederate. In this study, however, we used facial birthmarks to manipulate whether or not the real participants (not the confederates) were stigmatized or nonstigmatized. In the former condition, we led real participants to believe that they bore a large, visible port-wine facial birthmark. In the latter condition, we led them to believe that they bore no birthmark.

We implemented this manipulation and kept confederates unaware of the manipulation in the following way. We explained to female participants that we were studying the effects of stigma during interactions. We further elaborated that in the experimental condition we would apply makeup that would resemble a port-wine facial birthmark, and that in the control condition we would apply translucent powder. In fact, we always applied translucent powder. After completing several preexperiment questionnaires, we showed each participant a digital photo of herself (with or without a computer-generated birthmark, according to the condition to which she had been randomly assigned) and a photo of the other "participant" (the confederate). The participant and confederate then met each other and exchanged background information. Because the real participants did not actually bear the facial stigma, we kept the confederates unaware of experimental conditions. Following each interaction, we separated the participant and confederate and returned them to separate experimental/physiological recording rooms, where we applied sensors to the real participant. In this study, the participant and the confederate communicated via a 27" television monitor and intercom. As in the earlier study, the participant delivered a speech on the topic of "Working Together." Unlike the perceiver study, however, the "live" connection allowed for a "face-to-face" speech delivery.

The cardiovascular responses collected during the speech task revealed a main effect for stigma condition. Participants who believed that they bore a facial birthmark exhibited physiological threat (i.e., increases in cardiac activity and an increase in vascular tone), whereas nonstigmatized participants exhibited a challenge response (increases in cardiac activity and a decline in vascular tone).

STIGMAS AS EVALUATION CUES

The results of these studies confirm that stigma can engender threat in motivated performance situations involving interactions between stigmatized and nonstigmatized individuals. Although we have not tested any mediators of threat, we believe that these mediators involve demand and resource evaluations as suggested by our biopsychosocial model. Furthermore, we believe that many stigma-relevant factors can directly and indirectly influence such evaluations. Here we provide a nonexhaustive discussion of these factors.

We want to note that we use the term "evaluation cues" to mean information derived from the situation that may elicit cognitive or affective responses or meaning. Evaluation cues may take the form of any type of direct sensory input (e.g., visual, auditory, olfactory) or semantic information or knowledge. As we have discussed above, these cues may be primarily affective or cognitive. Furthermore, the relevance of these cues for demand and resource evaluations may be learned or unlearned. Finally, individuals may process these cues consciously or unconsciously.

Typically, sensory inputs provide cues relating to visible or unconcealed stigmas, such as race, physical deformity, ethnicity, gender, obesity, and so forth. Explicit data or information provide cues to concealed stigmas, such as homosexuality, religion, hidden diseases, or the like. Sometimes, physical markers such as emblems (e.g., a lavender triangle, a Star of David, a scarlet "A") provide sensory inputs for concealed stigmas. We maintain that individuals use these sensory and informational cues in making evaluations leading either to challenge or threat motivation during motivated performance tasks involving stigmatized individuals. That these cues affect nonstigmatized individuals in interactions involving stigmatized others appears obvious. That these cues elicit reactions, especially nonverbal ones, from nonstigmatized others that affect stigmatized others also appears fairly obvious. However, that these cues can affect stigmatized individuals themselves, even though self-generated, appears less obvious but no less significant.

Here we organize our discussion of stigmas as evaluation cues into two main categories (the first reflecting nonstigmatized participants' perspective, and the second reflecting stigmatized participants' perspective) and two subcategories within each of these (one reflecting demand evaluations, and a second reflecting resource evaluations). We have chosen this organizational scheme for didactic and heuristic purposes, rather than to impose a neatly defined structure on an admittedly somewhat fuzzy set of concepts and constructs. Note that we focus the discussion here on situations involving live interactions between stigmatized and nonstigmatized individuals.

Stigmas as Evaluation Cues to Nonstigmatized Interactants during Motivated Performance Situations

As described above, challenge and threat motivations result from the confluence of demand and resource evaluations. We first explicate our notions of how stigmas affect demand and resource evaluations of nonstigmatized individuals, limiting our discussion, as noted above, to interactions with stigmatized others in motivated performance situations.

Demand Evaluations

We maintain that three components—danger, uncertainty, and required effort—contribute to overall demand evaluations. As we have suggested above and elsewhere (Blascovich & Mendes, 2000), no exact calculus exists for how individuals factor component demand evaluations into an overall evaluation; they may factor additively, interactively, or synergistically, or any one component evaluation may exceed some threshold triggering threat.

Danger. The often-made argument (see Crocker et al., 1998; Goffman, 1963; Jones et al., 1984; Stephan & Stephan, 1985) that stigmatized individuals threaten others bolsters our contention that sensory input and other explicit information derived from stigmas increase the perception of danger on the part of nonstigmatized interactants. Several theories suggest ways in which stigmas may lead to perceptions of danger.

Evolutionary psychologists maintain that humans have evolved innate mechanisms or modules to assist in their adaptation to their environments (Barkow, Cosmides, & Tooby, 1992). The detection of disease via visible markers of physical abnormalities may arguably have evolved to protect individuals from potentially dangerous others. Because many visible stigmas (e.g., leprosy lesions) represent such markers or are similar (e.g., facial birthmarks) to such markers, evolutionary psychological theory would predict that individuals' sense of danger will be raised during interactions with individuals bearing them. Terror management theorists maintain that stigmas, whether apparent via the senses or via knowledge, increase the perceived dissimilarity of others, thereby threatening the cultural world view of nonstigmatized individuals and creating mortality salience to a greater or lesser extent (Becker, 1973; Greenberg, Pyszczynski, & Solomon, 1986). Social dominance theorists (Sidanius & Pratto, 1993) maintain that to the extent that stigmas indicate that individuals are members of culturally inferior groups, they represent a danger to the dominant or powerful groups in a culture. Still other theories suggest that interacting with devalued others, including stigmatized others, creates intergroup anxiety or tension (Devine, in press; Stephan & Stephan, 1985; Wilder, 1993). To the extent that such anxiety represents aversive psychological states themselves, interactions with stigmatized others can be regarded as dangerous.

Uncertainty. Nonstigmatized individuals remain relatively unfamiliar with interactions involving stigmatized individuals because of the relative infrequency of outgroup compared to ingroup interactions (Hamilton & Bishop, 1976). Interactions within motivated performance contexts, where individuals may have to cooperate or compete on some task, may well amplify this sense of novelty and unfamiliarity on the part of nonstigmatized individuals. Hence, the novelty of stigmatized individuals as interaction partners increases the uncertainty of the situation over and above what the actual performance task brings to bear on the situation. Jones et al. (1984, p. 46) note that this property of stigma (cf. disruptiveness) is less well defined than the others, but state that "any condition that makes appropriate interpersonal interaction patterns uncertain or unpredictable . . . has the capacity to be disruptive." Interaction with stigmatized others can make nonstigmatized individuals uncertain or ambivalent as to the course of appropriate behaviors.

Required Effort. Not surprisingly, the amount or degree of effort required in any motivated performance situation relates to overall demand evaluations, including ones involving social interaction. From the perspective of a nonstigmatized individual, interaction with a stigma-

tized other in a motivated performance situation may increase perceptions of required effort for a number of reasons.

First, the increased uncertainty and lack of familiarity that interaction with a stigmatized other brings to a socially interactive motivated
performance situation (see immediately above) requires more effort than
one not involving a stigmatized other. Nonstigmatized interactants must
devote increased attention to the motivated performance situation—including partners' and their own behaviors, especially the subtle nonverbal cues that govern two-way communication—simply because of lack
of familiarity or lack of communicative schemas (Gundykunst, 1984)
with such interaction partners. Increased effort in this regard may also
be necessary, as many visible stigmas (such as those associated with disease and deformity) are aversive in nature, and in many cases nonstigmatized individuals may want to suppress and or disguise their own nonverbal reactions connoting negative affect such as disgust or dislike
(Devine, Evett, & Vasquez-Suson, 1996). Frable, Blackstone, and Scherbaum (1990) have demonstrated that nonstigmatized individuals manifest considerably more effort, in the form of initiating conversation, talking and smiling more, and encouraging reciprocity, during interactions
with visibly stigmatized others.

Second, interactions with stigmatized others may involve additional
or hidden agendas on the part of nonstigmatized individuals—that is, ones
over and above the overt agenda inherent to successful performance within the motivated performance situation. At one extreme, nonstigmatized
individuals may strive to present themselves or to appear unaffected by
interaction partners' stigmas, so as not to appear prejudiced against the
stigmatized group (Archer, 1985; Devine et al., 1996; Stephan & Stephan,
1985). This requires more effort in terms of self-monitoring on the part of
nonstigmatized interactants. At the other extreme, nonstigmatized interactants, as members of higher-status groups than their partners, may seek
to justify or preserve this imbalance (see Jost & Banaji, 1996; Sidanius, in
press). Such an agenda would require nonstigmatized interactants to strive
to perform in a clearly superior fashion to their stigmatized partners. Katz
(1981) has suggested that at least some nonstigmatized individuals may
experience ambivalence alternating between self-presentational and socially dominating agendas, and such ambivalence would require even
more mental effort in the situation.

Third, because stigmas may evoke relevant negative stereotypes
even in nonprejudiced individuals, interactions with members of stigmatized may require stereotype suppression and replacement on the part of
nonstigmatized individuals (Devine, 1989). Although this activity serves
an adaptive purpose, it also constitutes an additional task not present
during interactions with nonstigmatized individuals.

Resource Evaluations

We maintain that three components—knowledge and abilities, dispositions, and external support—contribute to overall resource evaluations.

Knowledge and Abilities. Self-perceptions of pertinent knowledge
and abilities provide the most apparently relevant component of resource
evaluations on the part of actors in motivated performance situations. If
one must take a math exam, then mathematical ability becomes relevant. If
one must give a topical speech or a lecture, then substantive knowledge of
the topic becomes relevant, as do speaking skills or abilities. Yet the
knowledge and abilities required in socially interactive motivated performance situations extend beyond task knowledge and technical abilities.
One must consider not only task-relevant knowledge and abilities, but social interaction knowledge and abilities, in motivated performance situations involving nonstigmatized and stigmatized individuals.

1. *Task-relevant knowledge and abilities.* One might assume that
task-relevant knowledge and abilities remain unaffected by the stigmatized status of an interaction partner. However, several factors undermine such an assumption. First, the cognitive resources that might otherwise be applied solely to the motivated performance task may be co-opted
by non-task-related demands (e.g., stereotype and emotional suppression) in interactions between nonstigmatized and stigmatized individuals
(see above), thereby diminishing the cognitive resources that the nonstigmatized interactants can apply to the task. Second, nonstigmatized
interactants may question their own typically unquestioned knowledge
and abilities because of social comparison pressures to perform noticeably better than members of socially devalued (i.e., stigmatized) groups.
Even in a cooperative motivated performance situation, one in which
joint performance determines overall outcomes (i.e., success and failure),
such influences may operate. In a competitive motivated performance
situation, the pressures on nonstigmatized interactants may reach even
greater proportions. Third, the nature of a motivated performance situation can affect knowledge and ability evaluations. In both cooperative
and competitive motivated performance situation, one must consider not
only one's own knowledge and abilities but also those of one's partner.
Hence, a nonstigmatized interactant must judge his or her stigmatized
partner's knowledge and abilities. Negative performance stereotypes
about the stigmatized partner could easily drive the nonstigmatized partner's evaluation of joint knowledge and abilities down in a cooperative
situation, but the evaluation of his or her own knowledge and abilities
up in a competitive situation.

2. *Social interaction knowledge and abilities.* As we have noted, research reviews (e.g., Jones et al., 1984) have identified a dimension of
"disruptiveness to communication" that accompanies interactions involving nonstigmatized and stigmatized individuals. A nonstigmatized
individual may perceive that he or she does not know the most appropriate way to communicate with stigmatized individuals. In this sense, one
may consider interactions between stigmatized and nonstigmatized persons "intercultural interactions" (Wiseman, 1995). For example, members of different ethnic groups may possess (or believe they possess) different conversational and interaction styles. Insofar as nonstigmatized
individuals perceive that members of stigmatized groups possess conversational and interpersonal norms differing from their own group's, they
may perceive low knowledge and abilities in terms of interaction skills
within motivated performance contexts involving stigmatized others.
Again, Frable et al. (1990) demonstrated more compensatory behavior
by nonstigmatized individuals during interactions, but, importantly, the
stigmatized interactants paid a price for their partners' behavioral compensation: The stigmatized persons received lower attractiveness ratings
(i.e., less likable and lower in intelligence) from the nonstigmatized persons.

Dispositions. The consideration of dispositions as a component
within overall resource evaluations remains somewhat speculative at this
point. Nevertheless, it seems likely that dispositions may influence resource evaluations on the part of nonstigmatized individuals within motivated performance situations involving stigmatized others. Relevant
dispositions may include both general dispositions and ones more relevant to stigmatized others.

Certain dispositions contribute to resource evaluations in general.
Some theorists group a limited number of dispositions together as defining a sort of trait-like resilience or generalized self-confidence (e.g.,
Shrauger, 1975). In our challenge–threat model, high self-esteem, dispositional justice beliefs, and a generalized sense of control collectively
create a dispositional tendency for individuals to believe they possess the
resources to succeed in motivated performance situations in general. To
the extent that nonstigmatized individuals are likely to be more resilient
or self-confident in motivated performance situations involving stigmatized others, then they may be relatively predisposed toward high overall
resource evaluations. However, evidence on such dispositional differences between nonstigmatized and stigmatized individuals appears
mixed at best (Crocker & Major, 1989).

More specific dispositional tendencies on the part of nonstigmatized interactants may also contribute to overall resource appraisals. To the extent that highly racist or prejudiced individuals more strongly endorse or have more accessible negative performance stereotypes and schemas, they are more likely to make differential knowledge and ability evaluations when interacting with stigmatized others. Hence, negative performance stereotypes about a stigmatized partner could more easily drive a highly racist individual's evaluation of joint knowledge and abilities down in a cooperative situation, but his or her evaluation of relevant personal abilities up in a competitive situation, compared to the evaluations of a nonstigmatized individual low in racism. One could make the opposite predictions for highly empathic individuals. Authoritarianism, belief in a just world, and the like are other candidate dispositions that may influence the resource appraisals of nonstigmatized individuals.

External Support. The availability of direct external support to interactants within the context of motivated performance situations varies as a function of structural opportunities for such support. External support may take the form of socially supportive others, or it may take the form of some other types of resources, such as task practice opportunities or specific skills training.

Some situations may be purely dyadic and permit little if any direct social support. Other situations may involve multiple interactants (e.g., a spelling bee). To the extent that nonstigmatized individuals predominate in such a situation, they should feel more comfortable and supported by the implicit audience (i.e., other nonstigmatized competitors) than stigmatized competitors should. To the extent that motivated performance situations permit supportive (or nonsupportive) audiences, external support may be relatively high or low, depending on the nature and makeup of the audience. Presumably, a predominance of nonstigmatized others should increase the sense of external support on the part of nonstigmatized performers. Even without explicit audiences, interactive motivated performance situations may be structured so that nonstigmatized others occupy nonperformance roles (such as those of evaluators, judges, experimenters, teachers, etc.), increasing the sense of well-being of the nonstigmatized interactants.

To the extent that nonstigmatized individuals belong to more socially valued and dominant groups, they are more likely to enjoy the benefits of external resources in terms of training and practice relevant to the cultural values of the dominant group. Hence, if the motivated performance task itself is one valued by or culturally biased in favor of the dominant group, nonstigmatized individuals should be advantaged.

Summary

Clearly, stigmas serve as cues that generally increase demand evaluations on the part of nonstigmatized individuals, including increases in evaluations of danger, uncertainty, and required effort. Regarding danger, many theories converge to suggest that stigmas elicit perceptions of danger on the part of nonstigmatized individuals. Regarding uncertainty, interactive motivated performance situations increase perceptions of uncertainty as a function of novelty, unpredictability, and ambivalence for nonstigmatized interactants. Regarding required effort, stigmas cue increased perceptions of effort as a function of mindfulness, hidden agendas, and activated stereotypes.

Stigmas may also serve as cues that influence resource evaluations on the part of nonstigmatized individuals. However, unlike the hypothesized increase in demand evaluations by these individuals, stigma cues may increase or decrease resource evaluations on their part. Regarding knowledge and abilities, we argue that stigma cues generally decrease nonstigmatized persons' knowledge and ability evaluations, primarily because of the taxing of their cognitive resources in terms of attentional demands engendered by stigmatized others, as well as deficiencies in their communicative schemas. Regarding dispositional resources, some (e.g., high self-esteem, strong justice beliefs, high sense of control) provide nonstigmatized others with a sense of resilience across motivated performance situations, whereas others (e.g., racism and authoritarianism) have mixed effects, depending on the cooperative or competitive nature of a motivated performance task. Regarding external support, all other things being equal, one might expect that nonstigmatized individuals should benefit from greater resources by virtue of their membership in relatively socially valued groups.

Overall, because evaluations of demand should increase, and because evaluations of resources may not offset such demands (and in many cases may actually be lower), motivated performance situations involving stigmatized others should prove threatening to nonstigmatized performers.

Stigmas as Evaluation Cues to Stigmatized Interactants during Motivated Performance Situations

As suggested above, stigmas may also affect demand and resource evaluations on the part of stigmatized individuals in motivated performance situations involving nonstigmatized individuals. In this regard, a stigma may serve as a distal or indirect cue, evoking a response from a nonstigmatized interactant that serves as a proximal cue to a stigmatized individual; for example, an obese (distal stigma cue) person may notice a look of disgust (proximal cue) from his or her nonstigmatized interactant. A stigma may also serve as a proximal cue to a stigmatized individual; for example, an obese person may be disgusted directly by his or her own perceived physical image within the interaction.

Demand Evaluations

Crocker, Major, and Steele (1998) delineate a number of what they call "predicaments of the stigmatized." We recast these and others unmentioned by these authors under our rubric of danger, uncertainty, and required effort.

Danger. The evaluation of danger on the part of stigmatized interactants increases as a function of experience with prejudice and discrimination, negative aspects of social identity, and stereotype threat. Stigmatized individuals learn through experience that the potential for prejudice and discrimination exists in all social interactions involving nonstigmatized others, including motivated performance situations (Goffman, 1963; Jones et al., 1984). Hence, the potential for danger in social interactions involving both types of individuals is typically greater for stigmatized than for nonstigmatized individuals. Frable et al.'s (1990) data demonstrating that stigmatized individuals are more vigilant in social interactions involving nonstigmatized others suggest a heightened sense of danger on the part of stigmatized individuals. Furthermore, awareness of a devalued social identity places a person's sense of self-worth and collective self-esteem at risk (Crocker et al., 1998); hence, the social identity of stigmatized individuals relative to nonstigmatized individuals is endangered in motivated performance situations. Finally, stereotype threat (Steele & Aronson, 1995) places stigmatized individuals within motivated performance situations at risk of confirming negative stereotypes of their group. In this regard, their performance puts not only themselves as individuals in peril, but also their stigmatized group.

Uncertainty. Although stigmatized individuals may find interactions with nonstigmatized individuals more familiar than the reverse (Frable, Platt, & Hoey, 1998), certain aspects of interactive motivated performance situations may still increase situational uncertainty for them. In the first place, unless their stigma is one with a distinct physical marker that the nonstigmatized others are unambiguously able to perceive, stigmatized individuals may be uncertain as to whether nonstigmatized others are aware of their stigma. Frable and colleagues'

(1990) data indicating that individuals with either concealed or unconcealed stigmas are more vigilant in social interactions involving nonstigmatized individuals support this notion.

Moreover, stigmatized individuals often face the uncertainty of whether or not they are interacting with prejudiced or nonprejudiced others. Compounding this uncertainty, stigmatized individuals may have difficulty attributing causes for either the positive or negative responses of others to themselves or to their stigmatized status. Crocker and Major (1989) argue that such attributional ambiguity provides stigmatized individuals with an additional attributional explanation for outcomes, thereby increasing the uncertainty of the situation.

Required Effort. Although, as discussed above, required effort for nonstigmatized individuals probably increases in interactions involving stigmatized others, required effort may increase to an even greater extent for stigmatized others. Several lines of thought and research support this argument.

First, as nonstigmatized interactants must do with stigmatized others, stigmatized individuals must devote increased attention to nonstigmatized others during motivated performance situations. In the case of concealed stigmas, they must be sensitive to the responses of their nonstigmatized interactants, in order to determine whether or not the stigma is known. For presumably unknown stigmas, this continuous and effortful process involves a variety of strategies to keep the stigmas concealed (Kleck, 1968; Schneider & Conrad, 1980). In the case of visible or known stigmas, stigmatized interactants must monitor the responses of their interaction partners to determine the extent to which their stigmas influence the others—again, a continuous and effortful process. One might argue that this process is more taxing for stigmatized individuals than is the complementary process for nonstigmatized individuals (e.g., trying not to appear prejudiced), because stigmatized persons face potentially more difficult interaction partners (e.g., racists) than they are themselves; however, the comparative difficulty remains an empirical question.

Second, to achieve the implicit or explicit goals of an interaction (e.g., successful performance in a cooperative task), a stigmatized individual must often make extra efforts to facilitate the interaction by keeping it going. For example, visibly obese women have been shown to attempt to compensate for the negative attitudes of others by being particularly friendly and agreeable during social interactions (Miller, Rothblum, Felicio, & Brand, 1995).

Third, stigmatized individuals may need to expend extra effort to counteract the possibility of stereotype threat (Steele & Aronson, 1995; see discussion above). For example, because a performance mistake on the part of a stigmatized other is more likely to be attributed (and conform) to an existing negative group stereotype (i.e., the stigmatized group is unable to perform well on the task at hand) than to the individual him- or herself, stigmatized others must "try harder" not to make mistakes. Paradoxically, this extra effort may in the end reduce the quality of their overall performance. Stigmatized others may also try to distance themselves from their stigmatized group behaviorally through imitating the qualities of the nonstigmatized group (e.g., "passing") or through denial (Goffman, 1963), thereby adding self-presentational efforts to their task performance efforts.

Resource Evaluations

As they do for their nonstigmatized counterparts, knowledge and abilities, dispositions, and external support enter into the evaluation of resources for stigmatized individuals.

Knowledge and Abilities. Self-perceptions of pertinent knowledge and abilities provide the most apparently relevant component of resource evaluations for stigmatized individuals in motivated performance situations. As we have argued above, these pertinent knowledge and abilities include not only task-relevant ones, but also social interaction skills.

1. *Task-relevant knowledge and abilities.* One might assume that task-relevant knowledge and abilities are unaffected by stigmatized status. However, self-stereotyping challenges this assumption. To the extent that stigmatized individuals truly share a performance stereotype of their own group, these individuals will then evaluate their own task knowledge and abilities accordingly (Biernat, Vescio, & Green, 1996). In addition, to the extent that members of stigmatized groups have had weaker task-relevant substantive training or educational opportunities than their nonstigmatized interactants, they may accurately evaluate their level of task-relevant knowledge and abilities as low.

2. *Social interaction knowledge and abilities.* Stigmatized interactants may have underdeveloped interaction skills, especially with regard to interactions with nonstigmatized individuals, because of lack of experience in such social interactions. For example, Goldman and Lewis (1975) found that following telephone conversations, nonstigmatized interactants rated the verbal interaction skills of stigmatized (i.e., physically unattractive) college students less positively than those of nonstigmatized (i.e., attractive) college students, even though the raters were unaware of the stigmatized status. Miller, Rothblum, Barbour, Brand, and Felicio (1990) replicated this finding for obese and nonobese

women. Although it is not clear that stigmatized individuals always accurately perceive underdeveloped interaction skills on their own part, to the extent that they do, we would expect lower resource evaluations in terms of interaction skills in motivated performance situations involving others.

Dispositions. As it does for nonstigmatized individuals, the consideration of dispositions as a component within overall resource evaluations remains somewhat speculative with regard to stigmatized individuals. Nevertheless, it seems likely that dispositions may influence resource evaluations on the part of stigmatized individuals within motivated performance situations involving nonstigmatized others. Again, relevant dispositions may include both general dispositions and ones more relevant to stigma.

We would expect that stigmatized individuals with high resilience (high self-esteem, dispositional justice beliefs, and a generalized sense of control), like their nonstigmatized counterparts, may be relatively predisposed toward high overall resource evaluations. However, more specific dispositional tendencies on the part of stigmatized interactants may also contribute to overall resource appraisals. Anderson et al. (1993) suggest that certain stigmatized individuals evidence a dispositional style, "John Henryism," that affects their motives and behavior in motivated performance situations. "John Henryism" is a label for the dispositional belief that one needs only to work hard enough to overcome even overwhelming obstacles to succeed. We would expect that stigmatized individuals with this disposition would be likely to estimate their resources more highly than stigmatized individuals lacking such a dispositional tendency would do.

External Support. As it does for nonstigmatized individuals, the availability of direct external support to stigmatized interactants within the context of motivated performance situations varies as a function of structural opportunities for such support. Again, external support may take the form of socially supportive others, or it may take the form of some other types of resources—for example, task practice opportunities or specific skills training.

In situations permitting direct social support, stigmatized individuals should feel more comfortable and supported by the presence of stigmatized audience members. Indeed, Asch's (1962) classic work on conformity pressure suggests that the presence of even a single other stigmatized individual (i.e., another socially deviant individual) may prove supportive to a stigmatized performer in a motivated performance situation. Frable et al. (1998) found that the presence of similarly stigmatized others decreases anxiety and depression among stigmatized individuals. If similarly stigmatized others occupy nonperformance roles (such as those of evaluators, judges, experimenters, teachers, etc.), stigmatized others should feel more rather than less social support. Regarding nonsocial external resources, one would expect that stigmatized individuals as members of culturally devalued groups may have less training and practice on tasks relevant to the cultural values of the dominant group.

Summary

We have argued that stigmas serve as cues that generally increase demand evaluations on the part of stigmatized individuals, including increases in evaluations of danger, uncertainty, and required effort. Regarding danger, experience with prejudice and discrimination, a devalued social identity, and stereotype threat converge to suggest that stigmas elicit perceptions of danger on the part of stigmatized individuals. Lack of knowledge regarding their interaction partners' awareness of their stigma, and, even if the stigma is known, their interaction partners' level of prejudice toward their stigmatized group, increase perceptions of uncertainty for stigmatized interactants. The necessity of increased mindfulness in social interactions with nonstigmatized individuals, compensatory behaviors in such interactions, and stereotype threat increase the perceived level of required effort on the part of the stigmatized in motivated performance situations.

As they do for nonstigmatized individuals, stigmas can contribute positively or negatively to resource evaluations for stigmatized individuals. Regarding knowledge and skills, stigmatized individuals, as members of devalued social groups, may perceive themselves as having less substantive task-relevant knowledge and training and minimal interaction skills. Stigmatized individuals are as likely to benefit from positive dispositional influences (such as high self-esteem, justice beliefs, and sense of control) as nonstigmatized individuals, and may in some cases be predisposed to believe that they can prevail against overwhelming obstacles. Regarding external nonsocial support, stigmatized individuals as members of culturally devalued groups should have less training and practice in motivated performance tasks relevant to the cultural values of the dominant group. Hence, if the motivated performance task itself is one valued by or culturally biased in favor of the dominant group, stigmatized individuals should be disadvantaged.

Overall, because evaluations of demand should increase, and because evaluations of resources may not offset such demands (and in many cases may actually be lower), motivated performance situations involving interactions with nonstigmatized others should prove threatening to stigmatized performers.

FINAL THOUGHTS

Our empirical data based on covert cardiovascular indexes of threat suggest that both stigmatized and nonstigmatized individuals experience threat motivations when interacting with one another in motivated performance situations. Our theoretical analysis suggests many reasons why component demand and resource evaluations should lead to such threat motivations. One task that remains for us (and, we hope, for others) is to demonstrate the generality of the empirical threat effects to visible stigmas other than facial stigmas (such as skin color, ethnicity, gender, obesity, and physical unattractiveness) and to concealed stigmas (such as social status, sexual preference, and certain diseases). Another, more important task that remains is to test the demand and resource mediators we have suggested.

NOTE

1. We originally used the term "appraisals" to refer to individuals' calculations or determinations of demands and available resources. We now prefer "evaluations" for several reasons. First, we believe that the word "appraisals" implies purely cognitive and conscious assessments of demands and resources. In our most recent theoretical description of our biopsychosocial model (Blascovich & Mendes, 2000), we assert that both cognitive and affective, unconscious and conscious assessments of demands and resources occur. Second, readers often confuse our use of the term "appraisals" with that of Lazarus and Folkman (1984). Unlike ours, his presupposes demands and resources as part of a primary and secondary appraisal process. Although the theorizing of Lazarus and Folkman strongly influenced our formulation of the challenge and threat model, we believe that we extend the meaning of demands and resources from a purely cognitive perspective. In sum, we believe that "evaluations" is a more accurate and general term and covers both affective and cognitive, conscious and unconscious assessments of demands and resources.

REFERENCES

Anderson, N. B., McNeilly, M., & Myers, H. F. (1993). A biopsychosocial model of race differences in vascular reactivity. In J. J. Blascovich & E. S. Katkin (Eds.), *Cardiovascular reactivity to psychological stress and disease* (pp. 83–108). Washington, DC: American Psychological Association.

Archer, D. (1985). Social deviance. In G. Lindzey & E. Aronson (Eds.), *Handbook of social psychology: Vol. 2. Special fields and applications* (3rd ed., pp. 743–804). New York: Random House.

Asch, S. E. (1962). Issues in the study of social influences on judgment. In A. Berg

& B. M. Bass (Eds.), *Conformity and deviation* (pp. 143–158). New York: Harper.

Barkow, J. H., Cosmides, L., & Tooby, J. (1992). *The adapted mind*. New York: Oxford University Press.

Becker, E. (1973). *The denial of death*. New York: Free Press.

Biernat, M., Vescio, T. K., & Green, M. L. (1996). Selective self-stereotyping. *Journal of Personality and Social Psychology, 71*, 1194–1209.

Blascovich, J., & Mendes, W. B. (2000). Challenge and threat appraisals: The role of affective cues. In J. Forgas (Ed.), *Feeling and thinking: The role of affect in social cognition* (pp. 59–82). Cambridge, England: Cambridge University Press.

Blascovich, J., Mendes, W. B., Hunter, S. B., Lickel, B., & Kowai-Bell, N. (2000). *Perceiver threat in social interactions with stigmatized others*. Manuscript submitted for publication.

Blascovich, J., & Tomaka, J. (1996). The biopsychosocial model of arousal regulation. In M. P. Zanna (Ed.), *Advances in experimental social psychology* (Vol. 28, pp. 1–51). San Diego, CA: Academic Press.

Crocker, J., & Major, B. (1989). Social stigma and self-esteem: The self-protective properties of stigma. *Psychological Review, 96*, 608–630.

Crocker, J., Major, B., & Steele, C. (1998). Social stigma. In D. T. Gilbert, S. T. Fiske, & G. Lindzey (Eds.), *Handbook of social psychology* (4th ed., Vol. 2, pp. 504–553). Boston: McGraw-Hill.

Devine, P. G. (1989). Stereotypes and prejudice: Their automatic and controlled components. *Journal of Personality and Social Psychology, 56*, 5–18.

Devine, P. G. (in press). Processes of prejudice reduction: Obstacles and progress. In S. Oskamp & W. Crano (Eds.), *Reducing prejudice and discrimination*. Mahwah, NJ: Erlbaum.

Devine, P. G., Evett, S. R., & Vasquez-Suson, K. A. (1996). Exploring the interpersonal dynamics of intergroup contact. In R. M. Sorrentino & E. T. Higgins (Eds.), *Handbook of motivation and cognition: Vol. 3. The interpersonal context* (pp. 423–464). New York: Guilford Press.

Dienstbier, R. A. (1989). Arousal and physiological toughness: Implications for mental and physical health. *Psychological Review, 96*, 84–100.

Frable, D. E., Blackstone, T., & Scherbaum, C. (1990). Marginal and mindful: Deviants in social interactions. *Journal of Personality and Social Psychology, 59*, 140–149.

Frable, D. E., Platt, L., & Hoey, S. (1998). Concealable stigmas and positive perceptions: Feeling better around similar others. *Journal of Personality and Social Psychology, 74*, 909–922.

Goffman, E. (1963). *Stigma: Notes on the management of spoiled identity*. Englewood Cliffs, NJ: Prentice-Hall.

Goldman, W., & Lewis, P. (1975). Beautiful is good: Evidence that the physically attractive are more socially skillful. *Journal of Experimental Social Psychology, 13*, 125–130.

Greenberg, J., Pyszczynski, T., & Solomon, S. (1986). The causes and consequences of the need for self-esteem: A terror management theory. In R. F.

Baumeister (Ed.), *Public self and private self* (pp. 189–207). New York: Springer-Verlag.

Gundykunst, W. B. (1984). *Communicating with strangers: An approach to intercultural communications.* Reading, MA: Addison-Wesley.

Hamilton, D. L., & Bishop, G. D. (1976). Attitudinal and behavioral effects of initial integration of White suburban neighborhoods. *Journal of Social Issues, 32,* 47–67.

Jones, E. E., Farina, A., Hastorf, A. H., Markus, H., Miller, D. T., & Scott, R. A. (1984). *Social stigma: The psychology of marked relationships.* New York: Freeman.

Jost, J. T., & Banaji, M. R. (1994). The role of stereotyping in system-justification and the production of false consciousness. *British Journal of Social Psychology, 33,* 1–27.

Katz, I. (1981). *Stigma: A social psychological perspective.* Hillsdale, NJ: Erlbaum.

Kleck, R. (1968). Physical stigma and nonverbal cues emitted in face-to-face interaction. *Human Relations, 21,* 19–28.

Lazarus, R. S., & Folkman, S. (1984). *Stress, appraisal, and coping.* New York: Springer.

LeDoux, J. E. (1996). *The emotional brain: The mysterious underpinnings of emotional life.* New York: Simon & Schuster.

Mendes, W. B., Blascovich, J., Kowai-Bell, N., & Seery, M. (1999, June). *Cardiovascular reactivity as a function of perceptions of stigmatization.* Paper presented at the annual meeting of the American Psychological Society, Denver, CO.

Miller, C. T., Rothblum, E. D., Barbour, L., Brand, P., & Felicio, D. (1990). Social interactions of obese and nonobese women. *Journal of Personality, 58,* 365–380.

Miller, C. T., Rothblum, E. D., Felicio, D., & Brand, P. (1995). Compensating for stigma: Obese and nonobese women's reactions to being visible. *Personality and Social Psychology Bulletin, 21,* 1093–1106.

Obrist, P. A. (1981). *Cardiovascular psychophysiology: A perspective.* New York: Plenum Press.

Schneider, J. W., & Conrad, P. (1980). In the closet with illness: Epilepsy, stigma potential, and information control. *Social Problems, 28,* 32–44.

Shrauger, J. S. (1975). Responses to evaluation as a function of initial self-perceptions. *Psychological Bulletin, 82,* 581–596.

Sidanius, J. (in press). Social dominance: The interaction between gender and ethnic discrimination. In S. Oskamp & W. Crano (Eds.), *Reducing prejudice and discrimination.* Mahwah, NJ: Erlbaum.

Sidanius, J., & Pratto, J. (1993). The inevitability of oppression and the dynamics of social dominance. In P. Sniderman & P. E. Tetlock (Eds.), *Prejudice, politics, and race in America today* (pp. 173–211). Stanford, CA: Stanford University Press.

Steele, C. M., & Aronson, J. (1995). Stereotype threat and the intellectual test performance of African Americans. *Journal of Personality and Social Psychology, 69,* 797–811.

Stephan, W. G., & Stephan, C. W. (1985). Intergroup anxiety. *Journal of Social Issues, 41,* 157–175.

Tomaka, J., Blascovich, J., Kelsey, R. M., & Leitten, C. L. (1993). Subjective, physiological, and behavioral effects of threat and challenge appraisal. *Journal of Personality and Social Psychology, 18,* 616–624.

Tomaka, J., Blascovich, J., Kibler, J., & Ernst, J. M. (1997). Cognitive and physiological antecedents of threat and challenge appraisal. *Journal of Personality and Social Psychology, 73,* 63–72.

Wilder, D. A. (1993). The role of anxiety in facilitating stereotypic judgments of outgroup behavior. In D. M. Mackie & D. L. Hamilton (Eds.), *Affect, cognition, and stereotyping: Interactive processes in group perception* (pp. 87–109). San Diego, CA: Academic Press.

Wiseman, R. L. (1995). *Intercultural communication theory.* Thousand Oaks, CA: Sage.

Word, C. O., Zanna, M. P., & Cooper, J. (1974). The nonverbal mediation of self-fulfilling prophecies in interracial interaction. *Journal of Experimental Social Psychology, 10,* 109–120.

Zajonc, R. B. (2000). Nonconscious and noncognitive affect. In J. Forgas (Ed.), *Feeling and thinking: The role of affect in social cognition* (pp. 31–58). Cambridge, England: Cambridge University Press.

12

"Too Young, Too Old": Stigmatizing Adolescents and Elders

LESLIE A. ZEBROWITZ
JOANN M. MONTEPARE

> ... stigma involves not so much a set of concrete
> individuals who can be separated into two piles, the
> stigmatized and the normal, as a pervasive two-role social
> process in which every individual participates in both roles,
> at least in some connections and in some phases of life.
> —GOFFMAN (1963, pp. 137–138)

The truth of Goffman's insight is clearly evident when one considers age stigmas. We humans all pass through the adolescent stigma of being "too young," and, if we don't die a premature death, we also pass through the elderly stigma of being "too old." Attention to age as a universal stigmatizing condition can provide insights to social psychologists, who are interested in the nature of stigma, as well as to developmental psychologists, who are interested in the nature of adolescence and old age. In this chapter we examine the fit of age stigmas to the dimensions that have been used to characterize other stigmas. We also examine the stigmatizing experiences of those who are "too young" or "too old," the ways in which age-stigmatized people cope with those experiences, and the possible functions of age stigmas. Finally, we use the framework of age stigmas to suggest research topics of mutual interest to social and developmental psychologists. Because little social psychological or developmental research has directly tested the thesis that adolescence and old age can be understood as social stigmas, readers should be forewarned that our analysis is sometimes speculative.[1]

What does it mean to be "too young" or "too old"? It means that one's age identity is devalued—a state of affairs that has been viewed as an important defining feature of social stigma (Crocker, Major, & Steele, 1998). Devaluation of elderly people is shown in many ways. Our language disparages elderly persons with labels such as "old fogy," "hag," and "geezer" (Nuessel, 1982). Although the elderly segment of our population is the fastest-growing age group, we see relatively few images of older adults on television or in popular films and magazines. Even many psychology textbooks have given minimal attention to issues pertaining to aging adults (Whitbourne & Hulicka, 1990). Similarly, our cultural heroes and role models are rarely elderly adults, although there are exceptions, such as the astronaut John Glenn.[2] In addition, the competence of elderly adults is devalued in day-to-day domains ranging from driving an automobile to engaging in sexual relations to productivity in the workplace. They may also be declared incompetent to consent to medical procedures and to manage their finances. Like stereotyped perceptions of other stigmatized groups, these derogatory views of elderly people may not be applied to all members of the category. In particular, they may be more often applied to the general category than to known individuals, and they may be more often applied to the subcategory of "old-old" adults (those aged 75 and above) than to the subcategory of "young-old" adults (those aged 65 to 74). Nevertheless, even "young-old" people are devalued in comparison to young and middle-aged adults.

In contrast to the obvious devaluation of "too old" elders, the stigma suffered by "too young" adolescents is less recognized.[3] However, Lewin (1939) drew an analogy between adolescence and marginality in society, and adolescence, typically defined as the ages from 13 to 21, is in fact devalued in many social contexts. Simply on the basis of their age, adolescents are viewed as lacking the competence to see certain movies, vote, drive, drink alcohol, consent to medical procedures, earn a living, and have sexual relations. Moreover, because teenagers are branded as delinquent and trouble-prone, 146 of 200 major U.S. cities have utilized curfews that apply only to this age group (Berger, 1998). The marginality of adolescents is reflected in their complaints about the service they receive in restaurants and retail establishments. Although the following experience recalls complaints reported by Blacks in the United States, it was actually disclosed by an adolescent in response to the inquiry "Do stores discriminate against teenagers?"

I'm not allowed in the supermarket near our school anymore because whenever you go in, they make you take off your backpack. . . . I'm not going to leave my backpack at the front door where it could get stolen. So the security guard followed me around, and then the manager came out and yelled at me for wearing my backpack. It's not like I'm stealing. I've never stolen anything, and I've never been accused of it. I'm just buying my stuff. But the manager said, if you don't want to follow our rules, then you can leave. And I said, *Fine*. (Minton, 1998, p. 9)

It has been argued that a potentially stigmatizing attribute may cause people to be stigmatized in some contexts but not in others (Crocker et al., 1998). Similarly, certain social contexts may add to the devaluation and stigmatizing effects of being "too old" or "too young." For example, Luken (1987) has suggested that elderly people are especially likely to be stigmatized in contexts that involve physically or mentally demanding activities, such as performing strenuous exercises, using computers, and driving in heavy traffic. They will also be particularly stigmatized when chronological age is a pivotal discriminating marker, such as determining eligibility for participation in life or health insurance and retirement programs, or procuring reduced rates for public services. Adolescents are particularly apt to be stigmatized in contexts involving social or sexual activities that call attention to independent decision making and moral reasoning. They will also be particularly stigmatized when chronological age is a pivotal discriminating marker, such as determining eligibility for driving and marriage licenses, or gaining entrance to a bar or an R-rated movie.

Culture is a major social context that affects age stigmatization, and numerous comparative studies have shown that the stigma of being "too old" varies across cultures. In general, this research suggests that modernization and related social changes have contributed to the devaluation of the elderly. For instance, the respected role of elders as living storehouses of information has lost its status and value, with changes in technology that make their accumulated knowledge obsolete. Although the position of elderly individuals in traditional societies presents a favorable contrast to their position in more modernized societies, social scientists have been quick to point out that they may be less valued even within more traditional cultures (Fry, 1985; Keith, 1982). In particular, respect for elders may be displayed in conformity with custom and law rather than being genuine (Koyano, 1989). Consider, for instance, these complaints of elderly adults from agricultural villages of India:

Old people get respect on ritual occasions, but in everyday life those ideals are ignored. The truly aged retire into insignificance and fade away.

Many old people cannot sleep well because of worry and the unsympathetic attitude of their family around them. Old people may be spit upon, or even hit. (Harlan, 1968, pp. 474–475)

Ideas about the nature of adolescence have also been influenced by cultural developments. In particular, the widening gap between physical and social maturity in modern societies may exacerbate adolescent stigma by extending its duration. Because pubertal maturation occurs earlier in modernized societies than it did several generations ago, while the assumption of adult roles occurs later, there is a prolongation of the adolescent stigma of being denied the rights and responsibilities of adulthood despite physical maturity (Berger, 1998; Wyshak & Frisch, 1982). This stigmatization may be avoided in more traditional societies that have rites of passage to provide a clear transition from childhood to adulthood.

DIMENSIONS OF AGE STIGMAS

Jones and his colleagues (1984) have postulated several dimensions along which stigmatizing conditions can vary: "visibility," "aesthetic qualities," "disruptiveness," "peril," "controllability," "origin," and "course." The standing of a stigma on these dimensions influences its social consequences, with more adverse social interactions experienced by those with stigmas that are highly visible, aesthetically displeasing, disruptive of social interactions, perilous to others, and controllable. These dimensions can also be applied to age stigmas.

Age stigmas are highly visible. As is true for many other stigmas, those who are "too young" or "too old" possess objective features that mark their membership in the stigmatized category. These include not only chronological age, but also distinctive physical qualities (Chumlea, 1982; Sinclair, 1973). Elderly adults may be marked by slowed movements, stooped posture, white hair, wrinkled skin, and a trembling voice. As a result of the growth spurt signaling the onset of puberty, "adolescents grow a new body" (Petersen & Leffert, 1997, p. 6), and they may be temporarily marked by a big-footed, long-legged, and short-waisted appearance. Secondary sex characteristics also appear (e.g., coarser and darker body hair, deeper voice and facial hair in boys, breasts and increased body fat in girls). Many adolescents also experience the ravages of acne, which may become a mark of adolescence as revealed in *Zits,* a syndicated comic strip about this age period. Unlike the appearance qualities that mark elderly adults, those that mark adolescents are not always aesthetically displeasing. For example, the lean body builds and youthful faces of adolescent girls are highly valued in our society. Age stigmas may be more problematic for those adolescents and older adults who possess the most aesthetically displeasing age markers. However, regardless of their aesthetic qualities, the high visibility of age markers means that age stigmas can have an adverse effect on many social interactions.

As for other social stigmas, there are individual differences in the degree of visibility that may make some who are "too young" or "too old" more vulnerable than others to stigmatization on the basis of their age. Baby-faced adolescents or late-maturing adolescents will be more vulnerable than ones who look old for their age, and white-haired, deeply lined, and stooped elders will be more vulnerable than ones who look young for their age. Although the stigma of being an adolescent or an elderly person is visible, it also can be concealed to some extent. Dyes can alter hair color; makeup and plastic surgery can reduce facial wrinkles; various medications can hide or eliminate acne; and fake ID cards can allow adolescents to pass as mature adults.

Age stigmas can be disruptive to social interactions. Losses in hearing and declines in cognitive functioning and memory can disrupt social interaction with elders, as can the peril of death that older adults make salient. Although such disruptiveness may be more characteristic of interactions with those who are "too old," it can also be seen with regard to those who are "too young." For example, adolescents' egocentrism and self-consciousness, which may result in part from the maturation of certain cognitive abilities (Elkind, 1978), can make interaction with these youth difficult. It is also possible that the health and vitality of adolescents make the peril of death as salient to some middle-aged adults as does the deteriorating physical condition of elders. Age stigma may be most problematic for adolescents and elderly people whose appearance and psychological qualities are most disruptive of social interactions.

The progression of age is inexorable, but the physical markers of age and the stigmatizing conditions associated with maturation and aging can be seen as somewhat controllable. Adolescents can control their acne with antibiotics and creams, and, as we shall discuss later, they can compensate for their general stigmatized status in a variety of ways. The controllability of old-age stigma is also revealed in gerontologists' distinction between "primary" and "secondary" aging (Busse, 1987). Primary aging reflects basic, shared, inevitable sets of declines. For instance, the losses of hair pigment and of visual and auditory acuity correlate very strongly with chronological age and are probably the results of genetic or biological factors. Although these markers of age are not controllable in the sense of being preventable, they can be corrected by hair dyes, glasses, and hearing aids. Secondary aging, in contrast, is the product of controllable environmental influences and health habits, and is neither inevitable nor shared by all aging adults. Thus, for example, although the rates of heart disease, cancer, and osteoporosis are higher for elderly people, various risk factors (such as decades of smoking, drinking, and inactivity) contribute to their incidence (Berger, 1998). Adult men and women certainly share the belief that at least some of the consequences of aging are controllable, as evidenced by the time, money, and effort that many of them spend on cosmetics, dietary programs, nutritional supplements, and exercise equipment that claim to retard or reverse these consequences. While it may seem like good news that age-related stigmatizing conditions are sometimes controllable and perceived to be so by many individuals, the bad news is that people tend to respond more negatively to individuals with controllable stigmas (e.g., Crandall & Biernat, 1990; Weiner, Perry, & Magnusson, 1988).

Although certain aspects of age stigmas are not controllable, they do change and the course of these stigmas is highly predictable. Maturation eliminates the stigma of being "too young," and death eliminates the stigma of being "too old." The predictably changing course of age stigmas is unique. Other stigmas may change (e.g., a blind person may regain sight, a physically disabled person may regain mobility), but their course is never certain. One implication of this distinctive feature of age stigmas is that all individuals can anticipate the experience of being "too old" in their lifetimes. Such anticipation could foster the development of better coping mechanisms than are available to individuals who suffer from other stigmas. Moreover, the experience of being "too young" may provide a developmental testing ground for adaptive coping strategies. On the other hand, the mindless acceptance of elderly stereotypes from a young age may make adaptive coping even less likely for elders than for other stigmatized groups (Langer, 1989).

EXPERIENCES OF THOSE WHO ARE "TOO YOUNG" OR "TOO OLD"

Stereotypes, Prejudice, and Discrimination

Like those in other stigmatized groups, adolescents and elders experience prejudice and discrimination fueled by stereotypes of their traits and abilities. Stereotypes of elderly people can be traced to ancient times. For example, Aristotle (ca. 362 B.C./1927) made the following claims in his treatise "The Three Ages of Man": "Elderly men . . . are cowardly . . . are continually talking of the past . . . do not feel their passions much . . . are too fond of themselves . . . are querulous, and not disposed to jesting or laughter" (pp. 325–327).

Elderly stereotypes have been widely studied, and a common picture that has emerged from this work is one of physical, cognitive, and interpersonal deficiency (e.g., Pasupathi, Carstensen, & Tsai, 1995). Mirroring some of Aristotle's claims, elderly people are often perceived as feeble, slow-thinking, dependent, ill-tempered, depressed, self-centered, and demanding (Hummert, 1994a). Certain positive images of older adults have also been found. For instance, Brewer and Lui (1984) found that some older women may be viewed as nurturing "grandmothers," and some older men may be seen as distinguished "elder statesmen." Similarly, Hummert (1994a) found that while some older adults may be negatively characterized as the "despondent" type of elderly persons, others are positively characterized as the "Golden Ager" type. However, these positive images are more likely to be associated with younger-looking, -sounding, and -moving elderly adults, which is consistent with the premise that elderly adults whose age is most visible are the most vulnerable to being stigmatized (Hummert, 1994a, 1994b, 1999; Hummert, Garstka, & Shaner, 1997). More specifically, positive images are more likely to be associated with elderly adults who have minimal wrinkling and grey hair, whereas negative images are more likely to be associated with elderly adults who have wrinkles and grey hair. Similarly, certain negative age stereotypes are more pronounced for older men who are bald. They are perceived as less powerful and less aggressive than their hirsute peers (Muscarella & Cunningham, 1996). Just as elderly adults who look younger are viewed more positively than those who look older, those with more youthful-sounding voices are perceived more positively than those who sound older. Negative elderly stereotypes are also elicited by adults who walk slowly, drag their feet, and appear stiff-jointed. They are perceived as less powerful and less happy than their more youthful-walking peers (Montepare & Zebrowitz-McArthur, 1988).

Like stereotypes of the elderly, stereotypes about adolescents have existed since ancient times. Aristotle (ca. 362 B.C./1927) ascribed stereotypic qualities to youth, such as the following: "Young men have strong passions . . . show absence of self-control . . . are changeable and fickle . . . hot-tempered . . . trust others readily . . . are fonder of their friends, intimates, and companions than older men are . . . think they know everything . . . are fond of fun" (pp. 323–325).

Despite their long history, stereotypes of adolescents have been little studied, perhaps because they are so widely accepted. For example, an editorial cartoon in a recent issue of *The Boston Globe* mirrored some of Aristotle's claims, depicting adolescents as being self-absorbed and preoccupied with playing, partying, and possessions. Rather than evoking negative reactions from readers, as would be expected for stereotypic depictions of most social groups, a reader responded with the observation that this "is a sad but totally accurate portrayal of the typical American teenager's priorities" (Ferraguto, 1998, p. A12). Petersen (1988, p. 584) notes that such "powerful beliefs about adolescence have undermined systematic work. . . . Despite the paucity of research on this topic, most people believe they know what adolescence is like and are unreceptive to findings that challenge their beliefs." Beliefs about adolescents are well represented in folk psychology. Teenagers are viewed as belligerent, moody, irresponsible, and under the influence of raging hormones. Early writings in developmental psychology embodied such views of adolescence by characterizing this period as marked by storm and stress (Hall, 1904). Indeed, Anna Freud (1958) went so far as to view a calm adolescence as abnormal: "Adolescence is by its nature an interruption of peaceful growth, and . . . the upholding of a steady equilibrium during the adolescent process is in itself abnormal. . . . The adolescent manifestations come close to symptom formation of the neurotic, psychotic or dissocial order." This view persists in more recent descriptions of adolescents. For example, Ingersoll (1989) notes that parents who seek advice about their adolescent children often describe them as if they have some type of personality disorder, insofar as "at one moment their adolescent is friendly and cooperative, and the next he or she is hostile and belligerent" (p. 5).

Elderly people and adolescents cannot help being well aware of the widely shared stereotypes about their age groups, and evidence from several Western cultures indicates that both adolescents and elders actually endorse negative stereotypes about their own groups. Not only do people of all ages agree that social status is highest among middle-aged adults (Graham & Baker, 1989), but also adolescents, middle-aged adults, and elderly adults all agree that middle-aged adults are more socially at ease and pleasing to others than either adolescents or elders (Luszcz, 1983, 1985–1986; Luszcz & Fitzgerald, 1986). People of all ages also stereotype elderly adults as less personally satisfied and at peace with themselves than the other two age groups. However, the three age groups differed somewhat in their stereotypes about autonomy and instrumentality. All groups viewed middle-aged adults as highest in autonomy—that is, the group that is the most self-sufficient and contributes more than it receives from the social system. However, the group that was perceived as second in autonomy differed across age, showing ingroup favoritism. Elderly people viewed elders as more autonomous than adolescents, and adolescents viewed adolescents as more autonomous than elders. All groups also viewed elderly adults as the lowest in instrumentality—that is, the group that is the least adaptable and active in the pursuit of goals. However, ingroup favoritism again influenced the group that was perceived as second in instrumentality. Adolescents viewed adolescents as more instrumental than middle-aged adults, whereas elderly and middle-aged adults perceived little difference in the instrumentality of middle-aged adults and adolescents. To translate these findings into simple stereotype labels, it appears that elderly adults view their own age group as lower in status, less likable, more unhappy, more dependent, and less goal-oriented than nonstigmatized middle-aged adults, while adolescents view their own group as lower in status, less likable, and more dependent.

Stereotypes about elderly adults are manifested in patronizing behavior toward them. Rubin and Brown (1975) found that young adults not only evaluated fictitious elderly adults as less intellectually competent, but also used fewer words when explaining rules of a game to elderly targets. Montepare, Steinberg, and Rosenberg (1992) showed that young adults' voices became higher in pitch, more babyish-sounding, and more unpleasant when conversing with their grandparents than with their parents. Rodin and Langer (1980) examined the difficulty level of questions that middle-aged adults were willing to ask elderly targets, and found that they asked easier questions of elderly than of middle-aged targets, regardless of information provided about elderly targets' competence level.

Research has also documented discriminatory behavior toward aging adults in medical settings. Greene and colleagues (Greene, Adelman, Charon, & Hoffman, 1986; Greene, Adelman, Charon, & Friedmann, 1989) showed that physicians communicate with elderly patients in a less engaging, complex, and supportive manner than they do with younger adult patients. Similarly, Caporael and colleagues found that care providers in nursing homes talk in patronizing and condescending ways to elderly residents (Caporael, 1981; Caporael & Culbertson, 1986; Caporael, Lukaszewski, & Culbertson, 1983). Butler (1975) found that the elderly are provided with less rigorous clinical assessments when they report a complaint that is considered symptomatic of old age, even though many age-related diseases can be treated effectively (Grant, 1996). Similarly, elderly persons are less apt to be referred for psychiatric assessments than are younger persons, even when they report the same symptoms as younger persons (Hillerbrand & Shaw, 1990).

Discrimination against aging adults in the workplace has been well documented. Freedberg (1987) reported that nearly 27,000 age discrimination cases were filed with federal and state authorities in 1986, which was double the number of cases filed in 1980. Moreover, one-fourth of the cases filed by the Equal Employment Opportunity Commission in 1986 resulted from the Age Discrimination in Employment Act. Discrimination may also occur in more subtle ways, such as the invisibility of elderly people in the mass media. In general, television idealizes vigor, attractiveness, and competence, and portrays being "too old" as undesirable (Northcott, 1975). In line with the television ideal, considerable research attests to the underrepresentation of elders on television (Kubey, 1980; Robinson, 1989). For example, Northcott (1975) found that elderly people appeared in 1.5% of all portrayals on television, and mostly in minor roles. Moreover, Kubey (1980) notes that in comparison to any other age group, elders are more likely to be portrayed in comical roles that highlight stereotypes of their physical, cognitive, and sexual impotence. Although there have been some positive elderly characters in recent years (Bell, 1992), television's underrepresentation and largely negative representation of elderly people clearly convey a message of their marginalization to the viewing audience.

Discrimination against adolescents has not been the focus of systematic research, perhaps because this age group is rarely recognized as stigmatized, with stereotypes and differential treatment accepted as appropriate. Indeed, it has been noted that the belief that storm and stress are normative in adolescence may have thwarted treatment of adolescents experiencing psychological problems. Rutter, Graham, Chadwick, and Yule (1976) reported that "transient situational disorder" was the most common diagnostic category for adolescents seen at outpatient clinics and was very prevalent even among adolescent psychiatric inpatients. The fact is that the majority of adolescents do not experience significant psychological difficulties, and those who do often develop serious mental illness in adulthood (see Petersen, 1988, for a pertinent review). Thus, just as physicians may fail to provide aggressive treatment for cognitive difficulties in elderly people, viewing these as inevitable outcomes of aging, so may mental health professionals fail to provide appropriate treatment for psychological disturbances in adolescents, viewing these as "just a phase" (Arnett, 1999; Hartlage, Howard, & Ostrove, 1984, cited in Ingersoll, 1989).

Beliefs about adolescent storm and stress may have other negative consequences as well. In particular, some developmental theorists are concerned that such beliefs may lead parents to adopt authoritarian parenting strategies to offset expected difficulties in their teenagers' behavior (Arnett, 1999). Not only may developmental transitions be treated inappropriately, but the behavior of highly distressed or disturbed adolescents may be overgeneralized to the entire age category. Consider public responses to the recent outbreaks of violence in high schools. Some school systems have responded by proposing that all students carry mesh book bags that make their contents visible. Others have proposed dress codes that would require students to tuck in shirts, so that weapons cannot be hidden in waistbands (Sack, 1999). Although one can view these measures as efforts to protect high school students from harm, they also can be viewed as a discriminatory infringement on the civil rights of the vast majority of law-abiding youth. Surely no one would have proposed similar requirements for all mail carriers after the violent rampage of a U.S. postal worker several years ago, or similar requirements for all PhD candidates after one murdered his mentor. The reaction to adolescent killers reflects the view that adolescents are a psychologically unstable group of people—as opposed to the equally (if not more) plausible view that there are some highly disturbed adolescents, just as there are some highly disturbed mail carriers and PhD candidates.

Self-Concepts

There is some evidence that the self-concepts of those who are "too young" or "too old" incorporate age stereotypes. During an 8-year period following retirement, which often marks the onset of entry into the stigmatized elderly category, people showed a decreased likelihood of describing themselves as "ambitious," "assertive," "bossy," "competitive," and "shrewd." On the other hand, during an 8-year period following graduation from high school, when people were leaving the stigmatized adolescent category, they showed an increased likelihood of describing themselves in these terms (Thurnher, 1983).[4] Although, as noted earlier, ingroup favoritism does lead elders and adolescents to rate themselves and ingroup members higher than others rate them, adolescents nevertheless judge themselves to be lower in autonomy than middle-aged or elderly people judge themselves to be, and elderly people judge themselves to be lower in instrumentality than adolescents or middle-aged people judge themselves to be (Luzscz & Fitzgerald, 1986). Older adults also acknowledge impending developmental constraints by showing a decrease in optimism about the probability of successfully planning and accomplishing goals in life, in contrast to the sense of optimism and control about the future found in younger adults—what Taylor and Brown (1988) have referred to as positive illusions (Heckhausen, 1997).

Given that age stigmas may affect the degree to which adolescents and the elderly view themselves as possessing culturally valued attributes, one might also expect those who are "too young" or "too old" to suffer from low self-esteem and depression. However, as has been found for other stigmatizing attributes, adverse effects on self-esteem and well-being are elusive (see Crocker et al., 1998; and Crocker & Major, 1989, for pertinent reviews). The maintenance of self-esteem in those stigmatized by age or other qualities may result from various coping responses that are discussed below: disidentifying with the stigmatized age group, disengaging from the attributes that they are perceived to lack, or engaging in behaviors that overcome the devalued age identity.

There is little evidence for adverse effects of old-age stigma on self-esteem among elderly people. For instance, Thurnher (1983) found no changes in happiness when assessing self-ratings of "unhappy," "dissatisfied," "worried," and "jealous" during an 8-year period following retirement, when adults would be more fully experiencing the stigma of being "too old." Other researchers also have failed to find negative effects of retirement on the well-being of elderly persons (Ward, 1984a), although there is some evidence of an increase in suicide rates after age 70, as well as a higher rate of suicide among elders than among those who are young or middle-aged (McCall, 1991)—effects that have been attributed to serious illnesses and the loss of power in older men (Osgood, 1985). Similarly, research has failed to find convincing evidence for a general decline in self-esteem with age until the final phases of the life course, when serious health problems become an overriding concern (Brandstadter & Greve, 1994).

There is more evidence for adverse effects of age stigmas on self-esteem among adolescents than among the elderly, but the effects are small and inconsistent. Thurnher (1983) found no increases in happiness when assessing self-ratings of "unhappy," "dissatisfied," "worried," and "jealous" during an 8-year period following graduation from high school, when adolescents are leaving behind the stigma of being "too young." On the other hand, global measures of self-esteem show an increase between the ages of 13 and 23 (O'Malley & Bachman, 1983), suggesting that the greater the "too young" stigma, the lower the self-esteem. There also appears to be a slight rise in psychiatric disorders from childhood to adolescence; adolescents are slightly more likely to report depression than their mothers are; girls show increases in depression over the adolescent period; and the prevalence of suicide and suicide attempts also increases during this period (Diekstra, 1985; McGee, Feehan, Williams, & Anderson, 1992; Rutter et al., 1976). In addition to showing an increase during adolescence, suicide rates have been shown in some research to be higher among adolescent boys than among those who are young or middle-aged (McCall, 1991). It is noteworthy that the risk factors for psychological disturbance in childhood, such as educational difficulties and adverse family factors, do not predict psychological disturbance that shows up for the first time in adolescence (Rutter et al., 1976). This is consistent with the proposition that the stigma of adolescence may itself be a risk factor. There are, of course, many possible explanations for the reported relationships between age and psychological disturbance. However, it is possible that the stigma of being "too young" or "too old" contributes to the distress of certain vulnerable individuals.

As noted earlier, the stigma of being "too old" should be felt most acutely by those who look old for their age. Although there is little research bearing on this hypothesis, the lucrative hair replacement industry attests to the fact that this visible mark of old age is very troubling to men. In contrast to the greater stigmatization experienced by bald men, more babyfaced elderly adults, who look relatively young for their age, seem to suffer less from the stigma of being "too old." In particular, they report feeling fewer constraints in their lives than do their older-looking, maturefaced peers (Andreoletti, Zebrowitz, & Lachman, 1999).

Conversely, the adolescent stigma of being "too young" should be felt most acutely by those who look young for their age—babyfaced or late-maturing adolescents. Indeed, adults perceive physically immature adolescent boys as less attractive than their more mature peers (Johnson & Collins, 1988), and there is some evidence that late-maturing or babyfaced adolescent boys are more vulnerable to peer rejection, particularly in lower-socioeconomic-status (lower-SES) samples (Clausen, 1975; Zebrowitz & Lee, 1999). Late-maturing boys also have more negative body images (Cok, 1990; Crockett & Peterson, 1987; Blyth et al., 1981; Rodriguez-Tome et al., 1993; Simmons, Blyth, Van Cleave, & Bush, 1979; Tobin-Richards, Boxer, & Petersen, 1983). Adolescent boys' body dissatisfaction is strongly related to feeling too short (Duke-Duncan, Ritter, Dornbusch, Gross, & Carlsmith, 1985; Simmons & Blyth, 1987), which is not surprising, because height is one of the most salient indicators of age during the years from birth to maturity. Although late-maturing boys are unhappy with their appearance, no consistent effects of pubertal timing on overall self-esteem have been reported (see Alsaker, 1995, for a pertinent review; Brack, Orr, & Ingersoll, 1988; Brooks-Gunn & Ruble, 1983; Simmons & Blyth, 1987; Tschann et al., 1994; Zakin, Blyth, & Simmons, 1984).

Interestingly, whereas late maturation appears to exacerbate the stigma of being "too young" for adolescent boys, it is early maturation that is problematic for girls. In particular, early-maturing girls have more negative body images than their late-maturing peers (Crockett & Petersen, 1987). Although being too tall may be problematic for early-maturing girls, who tower over the boys, their body dissatisfaction has been found to be strongly related to feeling "too fat," although this effect may vary across cultures (Cok, 1990; Crockett & Petersen, 1987; Duke-Duncan et al., 1985; Rodriguez-Tome et al., 1993; Stattin & Magnusson, 1990). Not only do early-maturing girls experience an earlier loss of the prepubertal lean bodies that Western culture values so highly in women, but moreover the adult bodies of early maturers tend to be heavier than those of those who mature later (Brooks-Gunn, 1988; Jones & Mussen, 1958; Silbereisen & Kracke, 1993; Tanner, 1962). Although early-maturing girls are unhappy with their appearance, research has found inconsistent effects of early maturation on self-esteem and psychological distress (Alsaker, 1995; Ge, Conger, & Elder, 1996; Simmons, Blyth, & McKinney, 1983; Tschann et al., 1994). In sum, it appears that adolescent girls' self-concepts are more adversely affected by the stigma of being "too fat," which may be exacerbated by early maturation, than by the stigma of being "too young," which may be exacerbated by late maturation. This interesting interaction between sex and age stigmatization in adolescence may be reversed in old age.

Whereas the stigma of being "too young" may be worse for adolescent males, the stigma of being "too old" may be worse for elderly women. Sontag (1972) has proposed a "double standard of aging" and argued that society offers fewer rewards for aging women than for aging men because aging corrupts women's principal social asset—their physical beauty. Although early cross-sectional research suggested that aging takes a greater toll on women's than on men's attractiveness (Deutsch, Zalenski, & Clark, 1986; Kogan, 1979), research assessing the attractiveness of the same individuals across the lifespan has shown equivalent declines for men and women (Zebrowitz, Olson, & Hoffman, 1993). Nevertheless, equal declines in attractiveness may have more adverse social consequences for women than for men. Indeed, the aforementioned tendency for baby-faced elderly adults, who look relatively young for their age, to perceive fewer constraints in their lives was stronger for women than for men (Andreoletti et al., 1999). Thus older-looking women suffer more in comparison to their younger-looking peers than do older-looking men. Aging is also worse for women in other respects. The elderly stigma of being dependent is worse for old women than for old men, because old women are more likely to be poor: The estimated poverty rate for old women is 80% higher than that for old men (Cavanaugh, 1990). Women also live longer, which means that more women than men make it to the most stigmatized category of the "old-old": In the age group over 75, there are about 100 women for every 73 men (Cavanaugh, 1990). Living longer means that women are more likely to be deprived of a mate. This may contribute to the view of older women as "asexual," something that is less true for perceptions of older men. Although sexuality in older men may lead to derogatory labels such as "dirty old man," older men who take young wives also may be viewed as "studs." Tongues wag more disapprovingly when older women are involved with younger men. There may be awe, but no moral outrage, when 70- or even 80-year-old men marry younger women and father children. Quite the contrary is true for reactions to pregnancies in women between 50 and 60 who take advantage of recent advances in fertility technology.

BEHAVIORAL REACTIONS TO AGE STIGMAS

Stereotype Confirmation

A self-fulfilling prophecy effect occurs when the expectations created by age stigmas are realized. For example, stereotypes about adolescents or elders may lead to social interactions that elicit behavior confirming the expectancy that they will be low in autonomy or competence. Several models, grounded in communication accommodation theory, have been proposed to explain how this may occur in interactions with elderly people (e.g., Ryan, Giles, Bartolucci, & Henwood, 1986; Hummert, 1994a). These models emphasize that individuals may use overaccommodating, patronizing speech when interacting with elderly persons, in response to stereotypic expectations about their declining cognitive and communication skills. They also emphasize that expectations about elders will be guided in large part by distinctive physical cues or contextual cues that activate old-age stereotypes. For example, Hummert, Shaner, Garstka, and Clark (1998) found that individuals were more likely to construct patronizing social messages when they expected them to be received by an elderly adult fitting the negative "despondent" elderly stereotype as opposed to the positive "Golden Ager" stereotype. Moreover, patronizing messages were elicited more often when an elderly adult was envisioned in a hospital context as opposed to a community setting. Finally, these models suggest that such stereotype-driven communications with the elderly not only may affect their feelings of control and self-esteem, but also may impose constraints on their present and future behavior.

In one of the few studies that has attempted to test directly the full extent of these models, Harris, Moniz, Sowards, and Krane (1994) explored the self-fulfilling prophecy effects of age-adapted communication. Young adults engaged in a teaching task, modeled after the TV game show *$20,000 Pyramid,* with a partner who they believed was either a similar-age peer or an elderly woman. The young adult teachers' vocal behavior was recorded on videotape as they provided instructions and clues to their fictitious partner. Next, a naive group of young adults was yoked to the videotaped communications, and their performance and perceptions of their teachers were assessed. Consistent with the theoretical models described above, young adult teachers provided fewer clues and conceptual information, sounded more nervous, and were less friendly when communicating with the elderly target. Moreover, young adults exposed to the communications ostensibly delivered to an elderly woman performed less well on the task and felt more negatively about their teachers than those exposed to the communications delivered to a similar-age peer. Thus the expectancy that elderly people are incompetent and cantankerous may lead to social interactions that elicit confirmatory behavior.

Although self-fulfilling prophecy effects like those found by Harris et al. (1994) may sometimes occur in interactions with elderly people, there are factors in real-life social interactions that may work against consistent behavioral confirmation effects. In particular, behavioral confirmation is less likely when the expected behaviors are socially undesirable and when targets know that the perceiver has a negative expectation, both of which characterize expectancies based on old-age stigma. It is possible that elderly people's reactions to behaviors communicating these expectations will be quite different from the reactions shown by young adults who were treated as if they were elderly in the Harris et al. (1994) study. In particular, elderly people may have developed ways to compensate for the negative expectations that are revealed in others' behavior toward them. Such compensatory strategies have been shown by obese and unattractive individuals, who are also stigmatized, whereas behavioral confirmation effects are more consistently shown by those who are not unattractive but are treated as if they are (Miller & Myers, 1998; Miller, Rothblum, Felicio, & Brand, 1995; Miller & Rudiger, 1997; Snyder, Tanke, & Berscheid, 1977).

Although behavioral confirmation appears to be relatively rare, occurring only when perceivers have very strong expectations and when targets are uncertain about their own traits (e.g., Major, Cozzarelli, Testa, & McFarlin, 1988; Swann & Ely, 1984; see also Snyder, 1992), it is noteworthy that such target uncertainty may be relatively high for adolescents and elders because of the developmental changes they are experiencing. It has been found that children just entering school are more vulnerable to teacher expectancy effects regarding their academic abilities, presumably because they do not have well-formed concepts of their own abilities (Jussim, 1986). Similarly, those just entering physical maturity and late adulthood may be more vulnerable to self-fulfilling prophecy effects than are midlife adults. Indeed, adolescence is a developmental stage marked by significant uncertainty surrounding issues of identity vis-à-vis sexual, occupational, and social roles, with identity formation considered the most important developmental task of that period (Erikson, 1968). The changes in physical and social status experienced by elderly people may also make them uncertain about their identities and thus more vulnerable to expectancy effects. In fact, old age has been characterized as a life stage marked not only by a loss of formal roles, but also by the absence of general socialization for an old-age role (Ward, 1984a). Because identity may be in flux for adolescents and elders, self-fulfilling prophecy effects may be more common for these age groups than for others.

Stereotype Disconfirmation

Another possible outcome of age stigmas is a self-defeating prophecy effect. Such an effect occurs when stereotypes lead to social interactions that elicit behaviors that are the opposite of those expected. There are two ways this can happen. One is that a person holding such expectancies engages in social interactions that themselves defeat the prophecy. For example, a physician may explain a medication regimen very carefully to an elderly individual, who is expected to suffer from cognitive deficits, with the consequence that the elderly person becomes more capable of executing the regimen than a middle-aged adult would be. A second mechanism is that the target of the expectancies defeats them because the social interactions produced by the expectancies are negative. For example, an adolescent boy who is expected to be low in autonomy may reject this low-status identity and compensate by becoming highly self-sufficient. Such outcomes are discussed below in connection with coping mechanisms.

Stereotype Threat

Another path to behavioral effects of stereotypes is "stereotype threat" (Steele & Aronson, 1995). In Goffman's (1963) words, "minor failings or incidental impropriety may . . . be interpreted as a direct expression of his stigmatized differentness" (p. 15). More specifically, awareness of age stereotypes may cause adolescents and elderly persons to be concerned that their behavior will confirm others' stereotyped views. Several possible consequences may follow from these concerns. One is that stereotypes will be confirmed due to the adverse effects of stereotype threat on performance. For example, even when Scholastic Aptitude Test scores are controlled for, Black students perform less well than White students on tests that are described as assessing intellectual ability—a performance dimension that evokes stereotype threat in Blacks, due to the stereotypical view that they are intellectually inferior. On the other hand, when stereotype threat is not activated because the same tests are described as nondiagnostic of ability, then the performance of Black students is equivalent to that of Whites (Steele & Aronson, 1995). Similarly, elderly people who are well aware of stereotypes about age-related declines in cognitive capacities may perform more poorly on tests of memory and other cognitive functions when they perceive that their abilities are under scrutiny than when stereotype threat is absent.

Research has found strong effects of implicit self-stereotyping on memory performance in elderly people. More specifically, Levy (1996) found that when either negative or positive images of aging were evoked in elderly adults with a priming task, these images had a significant impact on these adults' memory performance. When positive stereotypes were activated, elderly adults' memory performance improved on four types of memory tasks. On the other hand, when negative stereotypes were activated, memory performance worsened. Interestingly, these effects were obtained when stereotypes were manipulated implicitly by a prime, but not when they were manipulated by explicit false-positive or false-negative feedback. One possible explanation for these divergent findings is that explicit positive feedback was discounted by older adults due to strongly enculturated negative images of aging and memory, whereas implicit positive feedback was able to bypass these cultural stereotypes. Another possible explanation is that older adults engaged in behaviors to compensate for explicit negative feedback, such as higher effort, whereas implicit negative feedback did not engage such compensatory mechanisms. The fact that neither explicit nor implicit feedback had effects on younger adults in this study is consistent with the argument that stereotype threat causes impaired performance. Young adults would not be concerned that their behavior would confirm others' stereotyped views of their poor memories.

COPING WITH AGE STIGMAS

Researchers have identified a variety of coping strategies utilized by those who are stigmatized. These fall into the categories of "secondary compensation" (i.e., changing the way one feels about outcomes that the stigma affects) and "primary compensation" (i.e., engaging in behaviors that facilitate achieving desired outcomes despite the stigma) (Miller & Myers, 1998). Both types of strategies are shown by people who are stigmatized on account of their age.

Secondary Compensation

One way that people can cope with a social stigma is to change the way they feel about their outcomes. Such secondary compensation mechanisms include "psychological disengagement," whereby stigmatized individuals disengage their self-esteem from their outcomes in the domains in which they are expected to perform poorly, and "disidentification," whereby stigmatized individuals cease to value these domains (Crocker & Major, 1989; Crocker et al., 1998; Major, Spencer, Schmader, Wolfe, & Crocker, 1998; Miller & Myers, 1998).

Evidence pertinent to psychological disengagement in the elderly can be found in research showing that the link between people's self-esteem and how old they think they are perceived to be differs for adolescents and elderly adults. Adolescents' self-esteem is highly tied to how old they believe they are regarded by others: The older they think they are perceived to be, the higher their self-esteem. In contrast, older adults' self-esteem is more strongly linked to how physically and psychologically old they feel (Montepare, 1996). Thus older adults disengage their self-esteem from others' perceptions of their chronological age, tying it more to their competencies.

Evidence of psychological disidentification with domains in which poor performance is expected can be found in both adolescents and elders. In particular, elderly adults and adolescents place less value on the goal of "giving love and security to others" than do middle-aged adults, which is consistent with the stereotype that elders and adolescents are not even self-sufficient, much less capable of giving to others (Luzcsz & Fitzgerald, 1986). In comparison to middle-aged adults, elderly adults also designate fewer goals related to work and finances; this is consistent with their diminished opportunities in our society for success in these domains (Heckhausen, 1997). Similarly, adolescents place less value on job satisfaction than do middle-aged adults, which is consistent with the fact that such a goal is probably not attainable for them (Luzcsz & Fitzgerald, 1986). In addition, Pliner, Chaiken, and Flett (1990) found that with increases in age, women considered their physical appearance to be a less important personal attribute—a belief that would compensate for age-related declines in attractiveness (e.g., Zebrowitz, Olson, & Hoffman, 1992).[5]

Not only may stigmatized individuals disengage from the values and goals that they are prevented from attaining, but they may also develop a strong substitute identification with values and activities unique to their own groups. Indeed, responses on a social distance scale revealed that each age group prefers members of the ingroup over all others (Luszca & Fitzgerald, 1986). This preference is particularly marked among adolescents, who make a point of setting themselves apart from young adults through various appearance qualities, including clothing, hairstyles, and (nowadays) tatoos and body piercings. The adolescent subculture also embraces music and literature that are shunned by adults. Although the particular qualities that distinguish adolescents may vary from generation to generation, the differences between adolescents and adults persist. However, research suggests that this generation gap does not extend to significant values. Parents and their adolescent children have more similar values and attitudes than do adolescents and their peers (Kandel & Lesser, 1972; Lerner, Karson, Meisels, & Knapp, 1975; Rutter et al., 1976).

Favorable social comparisons is another secondary compensation mechanism that can protect the self-esteem of those who are stigmatized by being "too young" or "too old." For example, negative reactions to the low autonomy experienced by adolescents and elders can be ameliorated by within-age comparisons. Similarly, negative reactions to the declines in functioning experienced by elderly people can be ameliorated by "social downgrading"—comparing oneself positively to a negatively biased view of one's reference group. Indeed, Heckhausen and Brim (1997) found that although younger, middle-aged, and older adults all believed that their peers' problems were more serious than their own, social downgrading was particularly pronounced in older adults, especially when they evaluated the seriousness of personal problems involving work, leisure, marriage, and stress. Relatedly, O'Gorman (1980) demonstrated that older adults who had personally experienced problems in particular life domains were more likely to ascribe more serious problems in these domains to age peers. Moreover, Brandstadter and Greve (1994) found not only that many elderly adults typically made such self-protecting comparisons when threatened by perceived developmental losses, but also that more favorable comparisons were linked to fewer depressive tendencies. Adolescents and the elderly may actively promote such comparisons by selectively choosing with whom they interact. In fact, Steinberg (1984) reports that American adolescents spend more time talking with peers on a daily basis than engaging in any other activity. And when adolescents work in part-time jobs, they are more likely to work with others their age. Elderly people may also actively promote within-age comparisons by opting to live in age-homogeneous settings, such as retirement communities and age-segregated apartments, and to participate in age-segregated social activities (Ward, 1984b).

Another secondary compensation mechanism is the use of self-protective causal attributions. When elderly people or adolescents are treated with disrespect, they may attribute these outcomes to prejudice and discrimination against their age groups, rather than taking it to reflect their personal lack of merit. Some empirical support for such attributions is found in interviews with unemployed older workers about their unemployment experiences (Rife & First, 1989). When asked why they were unable to find another job, a majority stated reasons other than a lack of available jobs or personal inadequacies such as low skills or poor health. Rather, many asserted that their unemployment was a result of their age and a devaluation of the skills of older workers. Although there may be truth to their claims, many respondents could not report specific instances of discrimination; this is consistent with the possibility that these claims reflected secondary compensation. It should be noted that, as is true for attributions to other stigmatizing qualities, causal attributions to one's age group can be double-edged swords.

When elderly people or adolescents receive positive outcomes, they may suffer attributional ambiguity. For example, adolescents and elderly people who suffer from stereotype threat concerning their competence may wonder whether praise of their performance is honest or patronizing.

An extreme form of secondary compensation is to disidentify with the stigmatized group altogether and to "pass" as a member of the nonstigmatized group. In Goffman's (1963) words, "Because of the great rewards of being considered normal, almost all persons who are in a position to pass will do so on some occasion by intent" (p. 74). Such disidentification is unusual in this age of "political correctness." It has become relatively rare for Blacks to try to pass as White, gays as straight, or Jews as Christian, or for women to take pride in being told that they "think like a man." But adolescents remain quite happy to pass for 21, and many 70-year-olds prefer passing for 60 to being labeled "old-timers." Consistent with the double standard of aging, old women are more reluctant to tell their age than old men are. The tendency for adolescents and elders to deny their age is not merely a self-presentation strategy; it seems to be internalized. Indeed, when asked how old they feel, adolescents report feeling older than their chronological ages and elderly adults report feeling younger (Heckhausen, 1997; Montepare & Lachman, 1989). Moreover, many adolescents prefer to label themselves "young adults," and many elderly adults prefer to call themselves "senior citizens," "retired persons," or "mature adults" (Montepare & Lachman, 1983; Ward, 1984a). Heckhausen (1997) has also found that aging adults perceive their own developmental goals to be more consistent with the goals of adults younger than themselves, presumably because comparisons to a nonelderly, nonstigmatized reference group serves to elevate aging adults' self-image. Just as the elderly may attempt to deny their age, adolescents may endeavor to deny their youth by aspiring to developmental goals and responsibilities typically associated with older, more mature persons who hold a higher, more desirable social status (Heckhausen, 1997; Montepare & Clements, 1995). Such effects are properly viewed as secondary compensation only when they reflect internalized changes in group identification. When they reflect changes in behavior designed to achieve desirable outcomes that are typically reserved for nonstigmatized individuals, then they should be viewed as primary compensation effects.

Primary Compensation

> The stigmatized individual can also attempt to correct his condition indirectly by devoting much private effort to the mastery of areas of activity ordinarily felt to be closed on

incidental and physical grounds to one with his
shortcoming. This is illustrated by the lame person who
learns or re-learns to swim, ride, play tennis, or fly an
airplane, or the blind person who becomes expert at skiing
and mountain climbing.

—GOFFMAN (1963, p. 10)

In addition to the possibility of coping with their stigmas by changing
how they feel about various negative outcomes, stigmatized individuals
may engage in behaviors that enable them to achieve desired outcomes
in spite of their stigmas. This strategy has been called "primary compensation" (Miller & Myers, 1998). As adolescents attempt to negotiate the
transition from childhood to adulthood, their primary interest is the development of autonomy (e.g., Adams, Montemayor, & Gullotta, 1996).
Thus adolescents may lie about their age to achieve independence from
adult control, be it control over their access to movies, alcohol, or particular jobs. They may also engage in delinquent behavior in an effort to
attain adult privileges. Moffitt (1993) has argued that the gap between
biological and social maturity that adolescents experience may lead them
to act out in the attempt to gain adult privileges such as sex, parenthood,
drinking, and ownership of material goods. Because these privileges are
not readily attainable, many adolescents resort to delinquent behavior to
attain them. In addition to serving a primary compensation function, delinquent behavior may provide secondary compensation by bolstering
self-esteem. Indeed, people who experienced a publicly degrading situation (perhaps simulating the experience of a stigma) were more likely to
go along with a subsequent suggestion to steal something (Van Duuren
& Di Giacomo, 1996), and those engaging in mild delinquent behavior
may also have high self-esteem (Silbereisen & Noack, 1988). These findings are consistent with evidence that stigmatized individuals may offset
deficiencies in one area by bolstering other aspects of the self (Steele,
1988).

As noted earlier, the adolescent stigma of being "too young" may
be particularly keen for babyfaced adolescents, because babyfaced people of all ages are perceived as more socially and intellectually weak than
their more maturefaced peers (see Montepare & Zebrowitz, 1998, and
Zebrowitz, 1997, for pertinent reviews). As a result, babyfaced adolescents may be particularly motivated to behave in ways that will bridge
the maturity gap and achieve adult privileges. Consistent with this suggestion, Zebrowitz, Andreoletti, Collins, Lee, and Blumenthal (1998,
Study 3) found that lower-SES babyfaced adolescent boys were more
likely than their maturefaced peers to be delinquent, particularly when
the boys were also short. Moreover, within the group of delinquents,
those who were more babyfaced committed more crimes. Being baby-

faced has also been found to increase the likelihood of behavior that can compensate for the lack of adult privileges among nondelinquent adolescents. Zebrowitz, Collins, and Dutta (1998) found that middle-SES babyfaced adolescent boys were more assertive and hostile than their maturefaced peers, according to assessments made by judges who had never met the boys but who had access to data gathered from the boys, their families, and school records. Items such as "values independence," "rebellious," "pushes limits," and "skeptical" contributed to the assertiveness measure, while items such as "negativistic," "self-indulgent," "deceitful," "condescending," "distrustful," and "irritable" loaded on the hostility measure. Such behavior seems aimed at compensating for the particularly low autonomy and low status that babyfaced adolescents experience.

The compensatory assertive and contentious behavior of babyfaced adolescents can yield prosocial as well as antisocial effects. Babyfaced soldiers who served in the military during World War II and the Korean War were more likely to win a military award (Collins & Zebrowitz, 1995). This outcome suggests courageous and heroic behavior that could bridge the maturity gap.[6] Babyfaced adolescent boys from middle-SES samples had higher educational attainment than their maturefaced peers, thus bridging the maturity gap by showing their intellectual competence (Zebrowitz, Andreoletti, et al., 1998, Study 1). Babyfaced adolescent boys from lower-SES and delinquent samples also showed higher academic achievement than their maturefaced peers, but this was true only for boys who were above average for those samples in SES or IQ (Zebrowitz, Andreoletti, et al., 1998, Study 2). It thus appears that babyfaced boys show positive compensation effects that can bridge the maturity gap by achieving more competence only when they are able to do so by virtue either of their intelligence or a minimally favorable socioeconomic environment. Babyfaced adolescents who lack the social background or intelligence to compensate for the expectation that they will be intellectually weak fulfill those expectations with lower academic performance than their maturefaced peers.

Like babyfaced boys, late-maturing boys may be particularly likely to respond to the stigma of adolescence with primary compensation behaviors. Although research has revealed somewhat inconsistent effects of pubertal timing, there is some evidence that late-maturing boys are more rebellious toward their parents, lower in submissiveness, at higher risk for drinking problems, and higher in intellectual curiosity (for pertinent reviews, see Alsaker, 1995, 1996; Connolly, Paikoff, & Buchanan, 1996; and Northcraft & Hastorf, 1986). Like the behavior of babyfaced adolescents, such behavior may compensate for the particularly low autonomy and low status that late-maturing adolescents experience. Some of these behaviors may also serve to maintain the general self-esteem of these boys, which, as noted earlier, appears to be comparable to that of early-maturing boys. Interestingly, positive compensation effects in the domain of academic performance are absent for late-maturing boys from lower-SES backgrounds, just as they are for babyfaced boys from such backgrounds. Late-maturing boys from lower-SES backgrounds show lower academic ability and are less likely to want to complete college; these findings, coupled with lower expectations from their parents, suggest a self-fulfilling prophecy effect (Dornbusch, Gross, Duncan, & Ritter, 1987).

Neither being babyfaced nor maturing late appears to increase compensatory behavior among adolescent girls. Indeed, early-maturing girls have been found to show more problem behaviors (e.g., Caspi, Lynam, Moffitt, & Silva, 1993; Silbereisen, Petersen, Albrecht, & Kracke, 1989; Stattin & Magnusson, 1990). Although there are many possible explanations for this finding, it could reflect in part compensation for the stigma of being "too fat," which appears to be more problematic for early-maturing girls than is the stigma of being "too young" for late maturers.[7] Babyfaced adolescent girls and late-maturing girls may show no stronger reactions to the maturity gap than their maturefaced peers, because the way babyfaced and late-maturing adolescents are treated is more congruent with a feminine gender identity than with a masculine one. Not only are perceptions of babyfaced people and children paralleled by perceptions of women (see Friedman & Zebrowitz, 1992); it has also been argued that women's self-concepts incorporate elements consistent with the babyface stereotype, such as likability and connection to others, in contrast to men's self-concepts, which emphasize power and self-sufficiency (see Cross & Madson, 1997, for a pertinent review). Just as adolescent girls are less likely than boys to compensate for being babyfaced or maturing late, they may be less likely than boys to compensate for the general adolescent stigma of being "too young." Consistent with this suggestion, girls do not show the same pattern of delinquent behavior at adolescence as boys do. More specifically, although there is a steady increase in the number of delinquent acts among boys and girls across the adolescent years, boys are consistently more likely than girls to admit to having committed nontrivial offenses, and the seriousness of boys' delinquent acts increases with age (Gold & Petronio, 1980).

Like adolescents, elderly people may show primary compensation effects. Such effects have been described by Baltes and Baltes (1990) as a process of selective optimization with compensation, whereby aging adults devise alternative behavioral strategies to compensate for age-related declines in ability. More specifically, in order to cope with the undeniable physical and cognitive losses of later adulthood, and the reactions that these losses may evoke from others, elderly adults may set about rethinking their goals, reassessing their abilities, and making behavioral adjustments necessary to accomplish what they want despite the limitations and declines brought on by old age. Thus, for example, an elderly man who aims to continue driving may decide to avoid driving during rush hours, to take certain routes to avoid busy intersections, and to record specific directions to avoid getting lost (Johnson & Bear, 1993).

Heckhausen (1997) has proposed that elderly people will show "primary control" effects (analogous to primary compensation effects), whereby they selectively focus on goals that allow the greatest control and possibility of success. Consistent with this premise, Heckhausen found that older adults were not only less likely than young and middle-aged adults to aspire to work- and finance-related goals, as noted above, but also more likely to aspire to more attainable goals related to health and leisure. Moreover, within various domains older adults were more likely to strive to avoid losses rather than to achieve gains, again showing primary compensation by selecting more attainable goals (Heckhausen, 1997).[8]

Whether compensation effects among elderly persons also occur with respect to social skills and abilities is an interesting question. For example, might negative expectations regarding elderly people's communication skills lead them to engage in certain compensation strategies? Research has shown that, compared to younger adults, older adults report a greater tendency to lose track of the topic during conversations and more difficulty recalling factual information. As well, they are more likely to feel that other people speak too fast and too softly, making it difficult to sustain interaction. Older adults may attempt to compensate for these difficulties by taking charge of the conversation and steering it toward more familiar and personal topics, repeating what they say, and talking at a slower pace. Such compensation effects are certainly consistent with stereotypes of older adults' expressive and receptive language skills, if not with actual differences in their conversational practices (Ryan, See, Meneer, & Trovato, 1992).

Although elderly adults do show primary compensation, some theorists have suggested that the frequency of such coping strategies may be age-dependent (Brandtstadter & Greve, 1994; Brandtstadter, Wentura, & Greve, 1993; Heckhausen & Schulz, 1993). With advancing age, it may become increasingly difficult for some elderly adults to make use of primary compensation strategies, and the costs of maintaining desired levels of performance may eventually outweigh the expected benefits for these individuals. Thus they may be more likely to rely on secondary compensation strategies, which involve the psychological adjustment of goals and self-evaluative standards. In contrast to older adults, some adolescents may be more likely to use primary compensation strategies (such as delinquent behavior), because the constraints imposed by the adolescent stigma are more external than internal.

Like babyfaced adolescents, elderly people who are marked by physical signs of age, such as white hair and lined faces, may suffer most acutely from the stigma of their age. Although their greater stigmatization may make these individuals feel more constraints on their behavior, they may also compensate for those constraints and achieve more control over various outcomes than their younger-looking peers. Whether older-looking elderly people, like babyfaced adolescents, are more prone to show primary compensation effects is an interesting question. As is true for adolescents, the answer is likely to depend upon other factors, such as their ability to compensate for the view of elderly people as low in power and competence. Among elderly people who are high in IQ or in good health, those who look particularly old may make a greater effort to compensate, showing less intellectual decline than those who are younger-looking. On the other hand, the reverse may be true among elderly people who are low in IQ or in poor health, with those who look particularly old being more vulnerable to self-fulfilling prophecy effects. Although a study of the relationship between being babyfaced and perceiving control did not provide evidence for greater compensation effects by older-looking elderly people, additional research is needed to examine the moderating effects of IQ or health (Andreoletti et al., 1999).

FUNCTIONS OF AGE STIGMAS

Why are adolescents and elderly people devalued? Some of the functions that have been invoked to explain devaluation elicited by other stigmas fit these age stigmas as well (see Crocker et al., 1998; Goffman, 1963; Jones et al., 1984). One is the function of self-enhancement. By derogating the power and competence of those who are "too young" or "too old," individuals in young and middle adulthood can enhance their own feelings of power and competence. Adolescents and elderly people are logical targets for self-enhancing derogation by young and middle-aged adults because they may in fact be relatively low in power and/or competence. Many adolescents have not yet achieved their full physical power, and many elderly people are losing theirs. Many adolescents have not yet achieved their full intellectual competence, and many elders are losing theirs. This analysis suggests that derogation of those who are "too young" or "too old" should be more pronounced among young and middle-aged adults whose self-esteem is threatened, as has been shown for derogation of other stigmatized groups (see Wills, 1981; Wylie, 1971).

System justification may also be served by derogating adolescents and elders. People in these age groups suffer a relatively low status in society: They may be denied employment opportunities, denied opportunities for sexual satisfaction, denied the privilege of managing their own finances or legal affairs, and/or denied the privilege of living on their own. A function of derogatory stereotypes about these age groups may be to explain and to justify their disadvantaged position in society. The strength of this function of age stereotypes is underscored by the fact that the lower status of adolescents, if not elderly people, is viewed as appropriate. Age stereotypes, like other group stereotypes, qualify as hierarchy-legitimating myths (Pratto, Sidanius, Stallworth, & Malle, 1994). Empirical support for this function can be gleaned from research by Ahammer and Baltes (1972), who found that middle-aged adults were more likely to hold stereotypic views of adolescents and older adults than persons in these two age groups were to hold such views of middle-aged adults. These authors interpreted middle-aged adults' stereotypic perceptions as being motivated by their desire to set themselves apart from older and younger generations, in order to justify their position in the distribution of power in society. Consistent with this explanation, Neugarten (1968) interviewed over 2,000 adults and found that middle-aged men and women regarded themselves as the norm bearers and decision makers in a society controlled by their age peers. Moreover, middle-aged adults perceived their age stage as qualitatively different from younger and older age periods, and as marked by a heightened sensitivity to their position and role in the social structure.

Terror management is another function of stigmatization that fits age stigma. People may be stigmatized because they exacerbate the existential anxiety that is caused by the fear of death and a meaningless existence (Solomon, Greenberg, & Pyszczynski, 1991). Elderly people may be devalued because they remind people of their mortality and the inescapable possibility of death. Indeed, Collette-Pratt (1976) has found that negative attitudes toward death were a significant predictor of devaluation of old age, especially among young and middle-aged adults. Elders may also be devalued because they challenge the meaning that is imposed on existence in Western culture, where people are viewed as being in control of their own destiny and as deriving purpose in life through their work. Adolescents may be devalued both because their youthful vitality reminds middle-aged people of their own aging and mortality, and also because they challenge their world view—in this case, by deviating from accepted cultural norms. Of course, there is a chicken–egg question here: Are adolescents devalued because they deviate from accepted norms, or do they deviate from accepted norms because they are devalued? Both causal links may be true.

CONCLUSIONS

Although separated in time by at least five decades, adolescence and old age share a number of common features in our society. Not yet having fully achieved adulthood, adolescents are devalued for being "too young." And, having moved beyond the prime of adulthood, elderly people are devalued for being "too old." Each of these stigmatized conditions is highly visible, often aesthetically unappealing, somewhat disruptive of social interactions, partially uncontrollable, and threatening to the values of young or middle-aged adults. Those who suffer from these age stigmas experience stereotypes, prejudice, and discrimination. They respond in part by internalizing society's negative views, and they may show behavioral confirmation effects. But those who are "too young" or "too old" also show positive coping mechanisms. They may psychologically disengage from arenas in which they are expected to fall short, and they may identify with activities unique to their own groups. They may compare themselves with similar-age others, so as not to suffer unduly from upward social comparison. They resist the labels "too young" or "too old" by thinking of themselves as closer to what is viewed as the prime of life and, when possible, by "passing" for more valued ages. Adolescents and the elderly also engage in behaviors other than "passing" in order to achieve desired outcomes in spite of the stigma, thereby compensating directly for real or perceived inadequacies.

The social–developmental framework of this chapter emphasizes that no individual who achieves his or her full life expectancy can avoid being a member of a stigmatized group. As such, some aspects of stigmatization are part of the social-psychological processes of normal development, as opposed to unique phenomena experienced by particular individuals. This has important implications for social psychologists' understanding of stigma, as well as for developmental psychologists' understanding of adolescence and old age. The effort to understand what social and psychological forces can produce stigmatization of social categories that are so dissimilar and so familiar as adolescence and old age will contribute much to our overall comprehension of stigma. So will greater attention to the short- and long-term implications of moving into and out of stigmatized groups, which is characteristic of age stigmas. For example, making salient to people the inevitability of their own stigmatization may increase tolerance for other stigmatized groups (Galanis & Jones, 1986).

Developmental psychologists' understanding of cognitive, emotional, and behavioral changes in adolescents and older adults may be enriched by greater attention to the possible contributions of their stigmatizing experiences. Although researchers have acknowledged the potential role of age-graded expectancies in the development of adolescents and older adults, they have rarely focused on links between specific components of stigmatization and aspects of coping or well-being (e.g., Nurmi, 1993). For example, discrimination against adolescents may give rise to delinquent behavior as a primary compensation strategy (Moffitt, 1993). Considering commonalities between adolescence and old age may enrich developmental theories in other ways. For example, psychologists concerned with adult development have been very interested in the question of how positive views of the self are achieved in the elderly years (see, e.g., Baltes & Baltes, 1990; Brandstadter & Greve, 1994; Heckhausen, 1997; Carstensen & Freund, 1994). Although many appreciate that such views are intimately tied to individuals' personal experiences over time, the search for connections between experiences during the early and later years of development has been limited. The present chapter suggests at least one way in which these experiences may be functionally related. The stigma of adolescence may provide a developmental testing ground for coping strategies that will become essential determinants of well-being much later in life.

The social–developmental framework in which stigma has been considered not only underscores the general value of social psychologists' considering developmental issues and developmental psychologists' considering social issues, but also highlights specific research questions concerning the dimensions, consequences, functions, and moderators of age stigmas. For example, the fact that a target's sex appears to moderate an age stigma raises the interesting question of what other target attributes may serve as moderators of these and other stigmas—be they those that Goffman (1963) categorized as "abominations of the body," "blemishes of individual character," or the "tribal identities" of race, nation, and religion (see also Eagly & Kite, 1987). With respect to the dimensions of age stigmas, it would be interesting to examine the extent to which people view the processes of maturation and aging as controllable, and the impact of these perceptions on stigmatization of those who are "too young" or "too old." It is also of interest to examine the extent to which stigmatizing experiences can indeed be controlled by the various aids and ploys people use to conceal their age. With respect to the consequences of age stigmas, a great deal has yet to be learned about the range and limits of self-fulfilling and self-defeating prophecy effects guided by age stereotypes and moderated by self-perceptions and competencies. Questions regarding coping with age stigmas are also plentiful. For example, an understanding of individual differences in the outcomes of stigmatizing experiences would benefit from identifying the factors that lead to the use of primary versus secondary compensation mechanisms. With respect to the functions of age stigmas, a closer examination of the role played by self-enhancement may provide interesting insights into why those who are "too young" and "too old" are derogated, as well as how age stigmas may be attenuated for all of us who too must face their challenges.

NOTES

1. Several theorists in social gerontology have conceptualized the aging process as a response to social stigma (see Ward, 1984a). However, the present discussion differs from previous approaches by taking a more lifespan developmental approach and a more intrapsychic, individual level of analysis of process and outcome.

2. It is interesting to note, however, that John Glenn is admired precisely because his behavior does not conform to expectations about elderly adults.

3. An exception is Westman (1991), who has discussed prejudice and discrimination against children ("juvenile ageism"), some of which is also pertinent to adolescents.

4. One might suggest that the changes in self-descriptions shown by retired adults and high school graduates reflects a movement out of or into paid employment, rather than the acceptance of elderly stereotypes and the rejection of adolescent stereotypes, respectively. But traits like "competitive," "assertive," and "shrewd" can be manifested in many arenas besides the workplace. Thus changes in employment status per se seem inadequate to account for the changes in self-views on these traits.

5. One might suggest that elderly individuals and adolescents simply have different values from those of other age groups, and that these values are not connected to their inability to attain certain goals. Although this hypothesis cannot be rejected, it may reflect stereotyped views of elderly people and adolescents.

6. An alternative explanation is that this finding reflects a contrast effect, whereby whatever courageous actions babyfaced men took received more recognition because the contrast with the perception of babyfaced individuals as warm, dependent, and submissive made these actions more salient.

7. Interestingly, Caspi et al. (1993) found that the tendency for early-maturing girls to show higher levels of delinquent behavior was limited to girls in mixed-sex schools. Although this could well reflect an adverse influence of older boys on early-maturing girls in the mixed-sex setting, it might also reflect a greater need to compensate for the stigma of being "too fat" in a mixed-sex setting.

8. To some readers, compensation effects may be reminiscent of social gerontologists' "disengagement" theory (Cummings & Henry, 1961). This theory

maintained that in order to cope successfully with losses in social roles and contacts, elderly people are compelled to disengage or withdraw from their past social worlds and develop more passive lifestyles. However, we agree with critics of disengagement theory, who view compensation effects as active restructuring and optimization of available resources rather than as passive withdrawal.

REFERENCES

Ahammer, I. M., & Baltes, P. B. (1972). Objective versus perceived age differences in personality: How do adolescents, adults, and old people view themselves and each other? *Journal of Gerontology, 27,* 46–51.

Adams, G. R., Montemayor, R., & Gullotta, T. P. (Eds.). (1996). *Psychosocial development during adolescence.* Thousand Oaks, CA: Sage.

Alsaker, F. D. (1995). Timing of puberty and reactions to pubertal changes. In M. Rutter (Ed.), *Psychosocial disturbances in young people: Challenges for prevention* (pp. 37–82). Cambridge, England: Cambridge University Press.

Alsaker, F. D. (1996). Annotation: The impact of puberty. *Journal of Child Psychology and Psychiatry, 37,* 249–258.

Andreoletti, C., Zebrowitz, L.A., & Lachman, M.E. (1999, June). *Physical appearance and perceived control in young, middle-aged, and older adults.* Poster session presented at the annual meeting of the American Psychological Society, Denver, CO.

Aristotle. (1927). The three ages of man, from the *Rhetoric.* In W.D. Ross (Ed.), *Aristotle: Selections* (pp. 323–327). New York: Scribner's. (Original work composed ca. 362 B.C.)

Arnett, J. J. (1999). Adolescent storm and stress, reconsidered. *American Psychologist, 54,* 317 - 326.

Baltes, P. B., & Baltes, M. M. (1990). Psychological perspective on successful aging: The model of selective optimization with compensation. In P. B. Baltes & M. M. Baltes (Eds.), *Successful aging: Perspective from the behavioral sciences* (pp. 1–34). Cambridge, England: University Press.

Bell, J. (1992). In search of a discourse on aging: The elderly on television. *The Gerontologist, 32,* 305–311.

Berger, K. S. (1998). *The developing person through the life span.* New York: Worth.

Blyth, D. A., Simmons, R. G., Bulcroft, R., Felt, D., Van Cleave, E. F., & Bush, D. M., (1981). The effects of physical development on self-image and satisfaction with body-image for early adolescent males. In R.G. Simmons (Ed.), *Research in community and mental health* (Vol. 2, pp. 43–73). Greenwich, CT: JAI Press.

Brack, C. J., Orr, D. P., & Ingersoll, G. (1988). Pubertal maturation and adolescent self-esteem. *Journal of Adolescent Health Care, 9,* 280–285.

Brandstadter, J., & Greve, W. (1994). The aging self: Stabilizing and protective processes. *Developmental Review, 14,* 52–80.

Brandstadter, J., Wentura, D., & Greve, W. (1993). Adaptive resources of the aging self: Outlines of an emergent perspective. *International Journal of Behavioral Development, 16,* 323–349.

Brewer, M. B., & Lui, L. N. (1984). The primacy of age and sex in the structure of person categories. *Social Cognition, 7,* 262–274.

Brooks-Gunn, J. (1988). Antecedents and consequences of variations in girls' maturational timing. *Journal of Adolescent Health Care, 9,* 365–373.

Brooks-Gunn, J., & Ruble, D. N. (1983). The experience of menarche from a developmental perspective. In J. Brooks-Gunn & A. C. Petersen (Eds.), *Girls at puberty: Biological and psychosocial perspectives* (pp. 155–177). New York: Plenum Press.

Busse, E. W. (1987). Primary and secondary aging. In G. L. Maddox (Ed.), *The encyclopedia of aging* (p. 534). New York: Springer.

Butler, R. N. (1975). *Why survive?: Being old in America.* New York: Harper & Row.

Caporael, L. R. (1981). The paralanguage of caregiving: Babytalk to the institutionalized aged. *Journal of Personality and Social Psychology, 40,* 876–884.

Caporael, L. R., & Culbertson, C. (1986). Verbal response modes of babytalk and other speech at institutions for the aged. *Language and Communication, 6,* 99–112.

Caporael, L. R., Lukaszewski, M., & Culbertson, G. (1983). Secondary babytalk: Judgments by institutionalized elderly and their caregivers. *Journal of Personality and Social Psychology, 44,* 746–754.

Carstensen, L. L., & Freund, A. M. (1994). Commentary: The resilience of the aging self. *Developmental Review, 14,* 81–92.

Caspi, A., Lynam, D., Moffitt, T. E., & Silva, P. A. (1993). Unraveling girls' delinquency: Biological, dispositional, and contextual contributions to adolescent misbehavior. *Developmental Psychology, 29,* 19–30.

Cavanaugh, J. C. (1990). *Adult development and aging.* Belmont, CA: Wadsworth.

Chumlea, C. W. (1982). Physical growth during adolescence. In B. B. Wolman (Ed.), *Handbook of developmental psychology* (pp. 471–485). Englewood Cliffs, NJ: Prentice-Hall.

Clausen, J. A. (1975). The social meaning of differential physical and sexual maturation. In S. E. Dragastin & G. H. Elder (Eds.), *Adolescence in the life cycle: Psychological change and social context* (pp. 25–47). Washington, DC: Hemisphere.

Cok, F. (1990). Body image satisfaction in Turkish adolescents. *Adolescence, 25,* 409–413.

Collette-Pratt, C. (1976). Attitudinal predictors of devaluation of old age in a multigenerational sample. *Journal of Gerontology, 31,* 193–197.

Collins, M. A., & Zebrowitz, L. A. (1995). The contributions of appearance to occupations outcomes in civilian and military settings. *Journal of Applied Social Psychology, 25,* 129–163.

Connolly, S. D., Paikoff, R. L., & Buchanan, C. M. (1996). Puberty: The interplay of biological and psychosocial processes in adolescence. In G. R. Adams, R. Montemayor, & T. P. Gullotta (Eds.), *Psychosocial development during adolescence* (pp. 259–299). Thousand Oaks, CA: Sage.

Crandall, C., & Biernat, M. (1990). The ideology of anti-fat attitudes. *Journal of Applied Social Psychology, 20,* 227–243.

Crocker, J., & Major, B. (1989). Social stigma and self-esteem: The self-protective properties of stigma. *Psychological Review, 96,* 608–630.

Crocker, J., Major, B., & Steele, C. (1998). Social stigma. In D. T. Gilbert, S. T. Fiske, & G. Lindzey (Eds.), *Handbook of social psychology* (4th ed., Vol. 2, pp. 504–553) Boston: McGraw-Hill.

Crockett, L. J., & Petersen, A. C. (1987). Pubertal status and psychosocial development: Findings from the Early Adolescence Study. In R. M. Lerner & T. T. Foch (Eds.), *Biological–psychosocial interactions in early adolescence: A lifespan perspective* (pp. 173–188). Hillsdale, NJ: Erlbaum.

Cross, S. E., & Madson, L. (1997). Models of self: Self construals and gender. *Psychological Bulletin, 122,* 5–37.

Cummings, E., & Henry, W. (1961). *Growing old: The process of disengagement.* New York: Basic Books.

Deutsch, F. M., Zalenski, C. M., & Clark, M. E. (1986). Is there a double standard of aging? *Journal of Applied Social Psychology, 16,* 771–785.

Diekstra, R. F. W. (1995). Depression and suicidal behaviors in adolescence: Sociocultural and time trends. In M. Rutter (Ed.), *Psychosocial disturbances in young people: Challenges for prevention* (pp. 212–246). Cambridge, England: Cambridge University Press.

Dornbusch, S. M., Gross, R. T., Duncan, P. D., & Ritter, P. L. (1987). Stanford studies of adolescence using the National Health Examination Survey. In R. M. Lerner & T. T. Foch (Eds.), *Biological–psychosocial interactions in early adolescence* (pp. 189–206). Hillsdale, NJ: Erlbaum.

Duke-Duncan, P. D., Ritter, P. L., Dornbusch, S. M., Gross, R. T., & Carlsmith, J. M. (1985). The effects of pubertal timing on body image, school behavior, and deviance. *Journal of Youth and Adolescence, 14,* 227–235.

Eagly, A., H., & Kite, M.E. (1987). Are stereotypes of nationalities applied to both women and men? *Journal of Personality and Social Psychology, 53,* 451–462.

Erikson, E. H. (1968). *Identity: Youth and crisis.* New York: Norton.

Elkind, D. (1978). Understanding the young adolescent. *Adolescence, 13,* 127–134.

Ferraguto, M. (1998, March 17). Cartoon depicting teen brain is accurate. *Boston Globe,* p. A12.

Freedberg, S. P. (1987, October 13). Forced exits?: Complaints confront way of age-discrimination suits. *The Wall Street Journal,* p. 37.

Freud, A. (1958). Adolescence. *Psychoanalytic Study of the Child, 13,* 255–278.

Friedman, H., & Zebrowitz, L. (1992). The contribution of typical sex differences in facial maturity to sex role stereotypes. *Personality and Social Psychology Bulletin, 18,* 430–438.

Fry, C. (1985). Culture, behavior, and aging in the comparative perspective. In R. Birren & W. Schaie (Eds.), *Handbook of the psychology of aging* (pp. 216–244). New York: Van Nostrand Reinhold.

Galanis, C. M. B., & Jones, E. E. (1986). When stigma confronts stigma: Some conditions enhancing a victim' tolerance of other victim. *Personality and Social Psychology Bulletin, 12*, 169–177.

Ge, X., Conger, R. D., & Elder, G. H., Jr. (1996). Coming of age too early: Pubertal influences on girls' vulnerability to psychological distress. *Child Development, 67*, 3386–3400.

Goffman, E. (1963). *Stigma: Notes on the management of spoiled identity.* Englewood Cliffs, NJ: Prentice-Hall.

Gold, M., & Petronio, R. J. (1980). Delinquent behavior in adolescence. In A. Adelson (Ed.), *Handbook of adolescent psychology* (pp. 495–535). New York: Wiley.

Graham, I. D., & Baker, P. M. (1989). Status, age and gender: Perceptions of old and young people. *Canadian Journal on Aging, 8*, 255–265.

Grant, L. (1996). Effects of ageism on individual and health care providers' responses to healthy aging. *Health and Social Work, 21*, 9–15.

Greene, M., Adelman, R., Charon, R., & Friedmann, E. (1989). Concordance between physicians and their older and younger patients in the primary care medical encounter. *The Gerontologist, 29*, 808–813.

Greene, M., Adelman, R., Charon, R., & Hoffman, S. (1986). Ageism in the medical encounter: An exploratory study of doctor–elderly patient relationship. *Language and Communication, 6*, 113–124.

Hall, G. S. (1904). *Adolescence: Its psychology and its relations to physiology, anthropology, sociology, sex, crime, religion, and education* (2 vols.). New York: Appleton.

Harlan, W. H. (1968). Social status of the aged in three Indian villages. In B. L. Neugarten (Ed.), *Middle age and aging* (pp. 469–478). Chicago: University of Chicago Press.

Harris, M. J., Moniz, A. J., Sowards, B. A., & Krane, K. (1994). Mediation of interpersonal expectancy effects: Expectancies about the elderly. *Social Psychology Quarterly, 57*, 36–48.

Heckhausen, J. (1997). Developmental regulation across adulthood: Primary and secondary control of age-related changes. *Developmental Psychology, 33*, 176–187.

Heckhausen, J., & Brim, O. G. (1997). Perceived problems for self and others: Self-protection by social downgrading throughout adulthood. *Psychology and Aging, 12*, 610–619.

Heckhausen, J., & Schulz, R. (1993). Optimization by selection and compensation: Balancing primary and secondary control in life-span development. *International Journal of Behavioral Development, 16*, 287–304.

Hillerbrand, E., & Shaw, D. (1990). Age bias in a general hospital: Is there ageism in psychiatric consultation? *Clinical Gerontologist, 2*, 3–13.

Hummert, M. L. (1994a). Stereotypes of the elderly and patronizing speech. In M. L. Hummert, J. M. Wiemann, & J. F. Nussbaum (Eds.), *Interpersonal communication in older adulthood* (pp. 162–184). Newbury Park, CA: Sage.

Hummert, M. L. (1994b). Physiognomic cues and activation of stereotypes of the elderly in interaction. *International Journal of Aging and Human Development, 39*, 5–20.

Hummert, M. L. (1999). Vocal characteristics of older adults and stereotyping. *Journal of Nonverbal Behavior, 23,* 111–132.

Hummert, M. L., Garstka, T. A., & Shaner, J. L. (1997). Stereotyping of older adults: The role of target facial cues and perceiver characteristics. *Psychology and Aging, 12,* 107–114.

Hummert, M. L., Shaner, J. L., Garstka, T. A., & Clark, H. (1998). Communication with older adults: The influence of age stereotypes, context, and communicator age. *Human Communication Research, 25,* 124–151.

Ingersoll, G. M. (1989). *Adolescents.* Englewood Cliffs, NJ: Prentice-Hall.

Johnson, B. M., & Collins, W. A. (1988). Perceived maturity as a function of appearance cues in early adolescence: Ratings by unacquainted adults, parents, and teachers. *Journal of Early Adolescence, 8,* 357–372.

Johnson, C. I., & Baer, B. M. (1993). Coping and a sense of control among the oldest old. *Journal of Aging Studies, 7,* 67–80.

Jones, E. E., Farina, A., Hastorf, A. H., Markus, H., Miller, D. T., & Scott, R. A. (1984). *Social stigma: The psychology of marked relationships.* New York: Freeman.

Jones, M., & Mussen, P. (1958). Self-conceptions, motivations, and interpersonal attitudes of early- and late-maturing girls. *Child Development, 29,* 491–501.

Jussim, L. (1986). Self-fulfilling prophecies: A theoretical and integrative review. *Psychological Review, 93,* 429–445.

Kandel, D. B., & Lesser, G. S. (1972). *Youth in two worlds.* San Francisco: Jossey-Bass.

Keith, J. (1982). *Old people as people.* Boston: Little, Brown.

Kogan, N. (1979). A study of age categorization. *Journal of Gerontology, 34,* 358–367.

Koyano, W. W. (1989). Japanese attitudes toward the elderly: A review of research findings. *Journal of Cross-Cultural Gerontology, 4,* 335–345.

Kubey, R. (1980). Television and aging: Past, present, and future. *The Gerontologist, 20,* 16–35.

Langer, E. (1989). *Mindfulness.* Reading, MA: Addison-Wesley.

Lerner, R. M., Karson, M., Meisels, M., & Knapp, J. R. (1975). Actual and perceived attitudes of late adolescents: The phenomenon of the generation gap. *Journal of Genetic Psychology, 126,* 197–207.

Levy, B. (1996). Improving memory in old age through implicit self-stereotyping. *Journal of Personality and Social Psychology, 71,* 1092–1107.

Lewin, K. (1939). Field theory and experiment in social psychology: Concepts and methods. *American Journal of Sociology, 44,* 868–897.

Luken, P. C. (1987). Social identity in later life: A situational approach to understanding old age stigma. *International Journal of Aging and Human Development, 25,* 177–193.

Luszcz, M. A. (1983). An attitudinal assessment of perceived intergenerational affinities linking adolescence and old age. *International Journal of Behavioral Development, 6,* 221–231.

Luszcz, M. A. (1985–1986). Characterizing adolescents, middle-aged, and elderly adults: Putting the elderly into perspective. *International Journal of Aging and Human Development, 22,* 105–121.

Luszcz, M. A., & Fitzgerald, K. M. (1986). Understanding cohort differences in cross-generational, self, and peer perceptions. *Journal of Gerontology, 41,* 234–240.

Major, B., Cozzarelli, C., Testa, M., & McFarlin, D. B. (1988). Self-verification versus expectancy confirmation in social interaction: The impact of self-focus. *Personality and Social Psychology Bulletin, 14,* 346–359.

Major, B., Spencer, S., Schmader, T., Wolfe, C., & Crocker, J. (1998). Coping with negative stereotypes about intellectual performance: The role of psychological disengagement. *Personality and Social Psychology Bulletin, 24,* 34–50.

McCall, P. L. (1991). Adolescent and elderly white male suicide trend: Evidence of changing well-being? *Journal of Gerontology: Social Sciences, 1,* 543–551.

McGee, R., Feehan, M., Williams, S., & Anderson, J. (1992). DSM-III disorders from age 11 to age 15 years. *Journal of the American Academy of Child and Adolescent Psychiatry, 31,* 50–59.

Miller, C. T., & Myers, A. M. (1998). Compensating for prejudice: How heavyweight people (and others) control outcomes despite prejudice. In J. K. Swim & C. Stangor (Eds.), *Prejudice: The target's perspective* (pp. 191–218). San Diego, CA: Academic Press.

Miller, C. T., Rothblum, E. D., Felicio, D., & Brand, P. (1995). Compensating for stigma: Obese and nonobese women's reactions to being visible. *Personality and Social Psychology Bulletin, 21,* 1093–1106.

Miller, C. T., & Rudiger, L. (1997, October). *Compensation for prejudice: How the stigmatized obtain desired outcomes despite prejudice.* Paper presented at the annual meeting of the Society of Experimental Social Psychology, Toronto.

Minton, L. (1998, February 22). Fresh voices. *Parade Magazine,* p. 9.

Moffitt, T. (1993). Adolescence-limited and life-course-persistent antisocial behavior: A developmental taxonomy. *Psychological Review, 100,* 674–701.

Montepare, J. M. (1996). An assessment of adults' perceptions of their psychological, physical, and social ages. *Journal of Clinical Geropsychology, 2,* 117–128.

Montepare, J. M., & Clements, A. (1995, April). *"The denial of youth": Implications for age identification in young adult men and women.* Paper presented at the meeting of the Eastern Psychological Association, Boston.

Montepare, J. M., & Lachman, M. E. (1983, April). *Subjective age identification from adolescence to old age.* Paper presented at the meeting of the Society for Research in Child Development, Detroit, MI.

Montepare, J. M., & Lachman, M. E. (1989). "You're only as old as you feel": Self-perceptions of age, fears of aging, and life satisfaction from adolescence to old age. *Psychology and Aging, 4,* 73–89.

Montepare, J. M., Steinberg, J., & Rosenberg, B. (1992). Characteristics of vocal communication between young adults and their parents and grandparents. *Communication Research, 19,* 479–492.

Montepare, J. M., & Zebrowitz, L. A. (1998). Person perception comes of age: The salience and significance of age in social judgment. In M. P. Zanna (Ed.), *Advances in experimental social psychology* (Vol. 30, pp. 93–161). San Diego, CA: Academic Press.

Montepare, J. M., & Zebrowitz-McArthur, L. A. (1988). Impressions of people created by age related qualities of their gait. *Journal of Personality and Social Psychology, 55,* 547–556.

Muscarella, F., & Cunningham, M. R. (1996). The evolutionary significance and social perception of male patterned baldness and facial hair. *Ethology and Sociobiology, 17,* 99–117.

Neugarten, B. L. (1968). The awareness of middle age. In B. L. Neugarten (Ed.), *Middle age and aging* (pp. 93–99). Chicago: University of Chicago Press.

Northcott, H. (1975). "Too young, too old": Age in the world of television. *The Gerontologist, 15,* 184–186.

Northcraft, G., & Hastorf, A. (1986). Maturation and social behavior: A framework for the analysis of deviance. In C. P. Herman, M. P. Zanna, & E. T. Higgins (Eds.), *The Ontario Symposium: Vol. 3. Physical appearance, stigma, and social behavior* (pp. 221–244). Hillsdale, NJ: Erlbaum.

Nuessel, F. H. (1982). The language of ageism. *The Gerontologist, 22,* 273–276.

Nurmi, J. (1993). Adolescent development in an age-graded context: The role of personal beliefs, goals, and strategies in the tackling of developmental tasks and standards. *International Journal of Behavioral Development, 16,* 169–198.

O'Gorman, H. J. (1980). False consciousness of kind: Pluralistic ignorance among the aged. *Research on Aging, 2,* 105–128.

O'Malley, P. M., & Bachman, J. G. (1983). Self esteem: Change and stability between age 13 and 23. *Developmental Psychology, 19,* 257–268.

Osgood, N. J. (1985). *Suicide in the elderly.* Rockville, MD: Aspen.

Pasupathi, M., Carstensen, L. L., & Tsai, J. L. (1995). Ageism in interpersonal settings. In B. Lott & D. Maluso (Eds.), *The social psychology of interpersonal discrimination* (pp. 160–182). New York: Guilford Press.

Petersen, A. C. (1988). Adolescent development. *Annual Review of Psychology, 39,* 583–607.

Petersen, A.C., & Leffert, N. (1995). What is special about adolescence? In M. Rutter (Ed.), *Psychosocial disturbances in young people: Challenges for prevention* (pp. 3–36). Cambridge, England: Cambridge University Press.

Pliner, P., Chaiken, S., & Flett, G. (1990). Gender differences in concern with body weight and physical appearance across the life span. *Personality and Social Psychology Bulletin, 16,* 263–273.

Pratto, F., Sidanius, J., Stallworth, L. M., & Malle, B. F. (1994). Social dominance orientation. A personality variable predicting social and political attitudes. *Journal of Personality and Social Psychology, 67,* 741–763.

Rife, J. C., & First, R. J. (1989). Discourage older workers: An exploratory study. *International Journal of Aging and Human Development, 29,* 195–203.

Robinson, J. D. (1989). Mass media and the elderly: A uses and dependency interpretation. In J. F. Nussbaum (Ed.), *Life-span communication: Normative processes* (pp. 319–338). Hillsdale, NJ: Erlbaum.

Rodin, J., & Langer, E. (1980). Aging labels: The decline of control and the fall of self-esteem. *Journal of Social Issues, 36,* 12–29.

Rodriguez-Tome, H., Bariaud, F., Cohen Zardi, M. F., Delmas, C., Jeanvoine, B., & Szylagyi, P. (1993). The effects of pubertal changes on body image and relations with peers of the opposite sex in adolescence. *Journal of Adolescence, 16,* 421–438.

Rubin, K. H., & Brown, I. D. (1975). A life-span look at person perception and its relationship to communicative interaction. *Journal of Gerontology, 30,* 461–468.

Rutter, M., Graham, P., Chadwick, O. F. D., & Yule, W. (1976). Adolescent turmoil: Fact or fiction? *Journal of Child Psychology and Psychiatry, 17,* 35–56.

Ryan, E. B., Giles, H., Bartolucci, G., & Henwood, K. (1986). Psycholinguistic and social psychological components of communication by and with the elderly. *Language and Communication, 6,* 1–24.

Ryan, E. B., See, K. S., Meneer, W. B., & Trovato, D. (1992). Age perceptions of language performance among younger and older adults. *Communication Research, 19,* 423–443.

Sack, K. (1999, May 24). Schools add security and tighten dress, speech, and civility rules. *The New York Times,* pp. 1, 23.

Silbereisen, R. K., & Kracke, B. (1993). Variation in maturational timing and adjustment in adolescence. In S. Jackson & H. Rodriguez-Tome (Eds.), *Adolescence and its social worlds* (pp. 67–94). Hillsdale, NJ: Erlbaum.

Silbereisen, R. K., & Noack, P. (1988). On the constructive role of problem behavior in adolescence. In N. Bolger, A. Caspi, G. Downey, & M. Moorehouse (Eds.), *Person in conflict: Developmental processes* (pp. 152–180). Cambridge, England: Cambridge University Press.

Silbereisen, R. K., Petersen, A. C., Albrecht, H. T., & Kracke, B. (1989). Maturational timing and the development of problem behavior: Longitudinal studies in adolescence. *Journal of Early Adolescence, 9,* 247–268.

Simmons, R. G., & Blyth, D. A. (1987). *Moving into adolescence: The impact of pubertal change and school context.* New York: Aldine de Gruyter.

Simmons, R. G., Blyth, D. A., & McKinney, K. (1983). The social and psychological effects of puberty on white females. In J. Brooks-Gunn & A. C. Petersen (Eds.), *Girls at puberty: Biological and psychosocial perspectives* (pp. 229–272). New York: Plenum Press.

Simmons, R. G., Blyth, D. A., Van Cleave, E., & Bush, D. (1979). Entry into early adolescence: The impact of school structure, puberty, and early dating on self-esteem. *American Sociological Review, 44,* 948–967.

Sinclair, D. (1973). *Human growth after birth.* New York: Oxford University Press.

Snyder, M. (1992). Motivational foundations of behavioral confirmation. In M. P. Zanna (Ed.), *Advances in experimental social psychology* (Vol. 25, pp. 67–114). San Diego, CA: Academic Press.

Snyder, M., Tanke, E., & Berscheid, E. (1977). Social perception and interpersonal behavior: On the self-fulfilling nature of social stereotypes. *Journal of Personality and Social Psychology, 35,* 656–666.

Solomon, S., Greenberg, J., & Pyszczynski, T. (1991). Terror management theory of self-esteem. In C. R. Snyde & D. Forsyth (Eds.), *Handbook of social and clinical psychology: The health perspective* (pp. 21–40). New York: Pergamon Press.

Sontag, S. (1972). The double standard of aging. In A. R. Laurence & D. T. Jaffer

(Eds.), *Readings in adult psychology: Contemporary perspectives* (pp. 285–294). New York: Harper & Row.

Stattin, H., & Magnusson, D. (1990). *Pubertal maturation in female development.* Hillsdale, NJ: Erlbaum.

Steele, C. M. (1988). The psychology of self-affirmation: Sustaining the integrity of the self. In L. Berkowitz (Ed.), *Advances in experimental social psychology* (Vol. 21, pp. 261–302). San Diego, CA: Academic Press.

Steele, C. M., & Aronson, J. (1995). Stereotype threat and the intellectual test performance of African Americans. *Journal of Personality and Social Psychology, 53,* 797–811.

Steinberg, L. D. (1984). The varieties and effects of work during adolescence. In M. Lamb, A. Brown, & B. Rogoff (Eds.), *Advances in developmental psychology* (Vol. 3, pp. 1–37). Hillsdale, NJ: Erlbaum.

Swann, W. B., Jr., & Ely, R. (1984). A battle of wills: Self-verification versus behavioral confirmations. *Journal of Personality and Social Psychology, 53,* 1287–1302.

Tanner, J. M. (1962). *Growth at adolescence* (2nd ed.). Oxford: Blackwell.

Taylor, S. E., & Brown, J. D. (1988). Illusion and well-being: A social psychological perspective on mental health. *Psychological Bulletin, 103,* 193–210.

Thurnher, M. (1983). Turning points and developmental change: Subjective and "objective" assessments. *American Journal of Orthopsychiatry, 53,* 52–60.

Tobin-Richards, M. H., Boxer, A. M., & Petersen, A. C. (1983). The psychological significance of pubertal change. Sex differences in perceptions of self during early adolescence. In J. Brooks-Gunn & A. C. Petersen (Eds.), *Girls at puberty: Biological and psychological perspectives* (pp. 127–154). New York: Plenum Press.

Tschann, J. M., Adler, N. E., Erwin, C. E., Jr., Millstein, S. G., Turner, R. A., & Kegeles, S. M. (1994). Initiation of substance use in early adolescence: The roles of pubertal timing and emotional distress. *Health Psychology, 13,* 326–333.

Van Duuren, F., & Di Giacomo, J. P. (1996). Degrading situations and antisocial behavior: An experimental approach to delinquency. *European Journal of Social Psychology, 26,* 763–776.

Ward, R. A. (1984a). *The aging experience.* New York: Harper & Row.

Ward, R. A. (1984b). The marginality and salience of being old: When is age relevant? *The Gerontologist, 24,* 227–232.

Weiner, B., Perry, R. P., & Magnusson, J. (1988). An attributional analysis of reactions to stigma. *Journal of Personality and Social Psychology, 24,* 14–21.

Westman, J. C. (1991). Juvenile ageism: Unrecognized prejudice and discrimination against the young. *Child Psychiatry and Human Development, 21,* 237–256.

Whitbourne, S. K., & Hulicka, I. M. (1990). Ageism in undergraduate psychology texts. *American Psychologist, 45,* 1127–1136.

Willis, P. (1977). *Learning to labor.* New York: Columbia University Press.

Wills, T. A. (1981). Downward comparison principles in social psychology. *Psychological Bulletin, 90,* 245–271.

Wylie, R. (1971). *The self-concept: A critical survey of pertinent research literature.* Lincoln, NE: University of Nebraska Press.

Wyshak, G. L., & Frisch, R. E. (1982). Evidence for a secular change in age of menarche. *New England Journal of Medicine, 306,* 1033–1035.

Zakin, D. F., Blyth, D. A., & Simmons, R. G. (1984). Physical attractiveness as a mediator of the impact of early pubertal changes for girls. *Journal of Youth and Adolescence, 13,* 439–450.

Zebrowitz, L. A. (1997). *Reading faces: Window to the soul?* Boulder, CO: Westview Press.

Zebrowitz, L. A., Andreoletti, C., Collins, M. A., Lee, S. Y., & Blumenthal, J. (1998). Bright, bad, babyfaced boys: Appearance stereotypes do not always yield self-fulfilling prophecy effects. *Journal of Personality and Social Psychology, 75,* 1300–1320.

Zebrowitz, L. A., Collins, M. A., & Dutta, R. (1998). The relationship between appearance and personality across the life span. *Personality and Social Psychology Bulletin, 24,* 736–749.

Zebrowitz, L. A., & Lee, S. Y. (1999). Appearance, stereotype incongruent behavior, and social relationships. *Personality and Social Psychology Bulletin, 25,* 569–584.

Zebrowitz, L. A., Olson, K., & Hoffman, K. (1993). Stability of babyfaceness and attractiveness across the life span. *Journal of Personality and Social Psychology, 64,* 453–466.

13

Stigma and Self-Fulfilling Prophecies

LEE JUSSIM
POLLY PALUMBO
CELINA CHATMAN
STEPHANIE MADON
ALISON SMITH

This chapter reviews the role of stigmas in creating self-fulfilling prophecies that serve to justify and maintain those stigmas. To date, there has been no comprehensive review of research on stigma and self-fulfilling prophecies; in fact, there has been very little empirical research specifically framed as examining the self-fulfilling potential of many stigmas. Therefore, we draw on and integrate ideas from three main literatures for this review: (1) the stigma literature, even when it has not addressed self-fulfilling prophecies; (2) the self-fulfilling prophecy literature, even though it has rarely explicitly addressed stigmas; and (3) the stereotype and prejudice literatures, because prejudice and negative stereotypes are two potential manifestations of stigmas that can trigger self-fulfilling prophecies.

After a brief introductory section in which we define our key terms, we review and critically evaluate the empirical research suggesting that self-fulfilling prophecies contribute to the maintenance of social stigmas and the inferior status of stigmatized individuals. To do so, we first present a brief overview of the early research on self-fulfilling prophecies. Second, we review and critically evaluate research on the role of self-fulfilling prophecies in maintaining beliefs about stigmatized individuals in dyadic interactions. Dyadic interactions involve two individuals at a time (teacher–student, employer–employee, etc.). The overwhelming majority of empirical studies of self-fulfilling prophecies has focused on dyadic interactions. This section focuses largely on stereotypes and prejudice because they so often go hand in glove with stigmas (e.g., Crocker, Major, & Steele, 1998; Goffman, 1963; Steele, 1992). In the context of both the strengths and weaknesses of the empirical research, we evaluate the extent to which stigmas are likely to be self-fulfilling in dyadic interactions. In addition, we discuss some of the factors that may moderate (increase or reduce) stigma-triggered dyadic self-fulfilling prophecies. After this review, we draw broad conclusions about the state of, and limitations of, social science knowledge regarding the contribution of dyadic self-fulfilling prophecies to the maintenance of social stigmas.

Some of the most powerful self-fulfilling prophecies, however, may not occur at the level of interactions between individuals. Instead, as argued in Merton's (1948) original article describing the self-fulfilling prophecy, broad sociological forces may be far more important than are dyadic interactions. Ironically, however, sociological-level self-fulfilling prophecies have received almost no direct empirical attention. Furthermore, many of the specific examples of self-fulfilling prophecies cited in Merton's (1948) analysis are no longer relevant today (we discuss this in more detail later). Therefore, the last major section of this chapter draws upon research in education, social psychology, sociology, and anthropology in an attempt to update Merton's (1948) analysis, and to show how his fundamental ideas regarding self-fulfilling prophecies at a broader sociological level of analysis are still relevant as we enter the 21st century.

STIGMAS, STEREOTYPES, PREJUDICE, DISCRIMINATION, AND SELF-FULLFILLING PROPHECIES

A "stigma" is an attribute or condition that is devalued or derogated by many individuals in a culture (Crocker et al., 1998; Goffman, 1963). Typically, a stigma involves a web of affects, beliefs, and behaviors. For example, many people may feel revolted by an extremely obese person (affect); many people may assume that obese persons are lazy or lack discipline (belief); and many may avoid them (behavior). However, this chapter does not address how and why people stigmatize others. Instead, our focus is on one process involving stigmatization—self-fulfilling prophecies.

A "self-fulfilling prophecy" occurs when an initially erroneous social belief leads to its own fulfillment (Merton, 1948). Self-fulfilling prophecies, therefore, may at least sometimes help sustain a social stigma and appear to provide justification for continuing to derogate some group. This is because when a self-fulfilling prophecy occurs, people actually behave in a manner that confirms the initially erroneous belief. Self-fulfilling prophecies may be particularly pernicious sources of stigma maintenance, because stigmatizers can point to the actual behavior of those in the stigmatized group as "evidence" for the appropriateness of derogating them. Stigmas overlap to a great extent with stereotypes, prejudice, and discrimination. People often discriminate against, derogate, and despise those who are stigmatized. Thus we often draw on theory and research on self-fulfilling prophecies in those areas to provide insights into stigmas.

There are, however, some important differences between stigmas on the one hand and stereotypes, prejudice, and discrimination on the other. First, a stigma by definition is negative, whereas discrimination, stereotypes, and prejudice may all be positive (people may treat, like, or view members of some groups very positively—see, e.g., Allport, 1958; Jussim, McCauley, & Lee, 1995). Even if people do not despise or derogate other groups, they may like and favor their own groups. Similarly, people may stereotype librarians as introverted, but this does not necessarily mean that they stigmatize them.

Second, although stigmas based on race or religion clearly do involve intergroup relations, some types of stigmas may not involve intergroup relations. For example, people may despise criminals, be revolted by major physical deformities, and avoid persons with serious mental illness—but these reactions do not seem to stem from group-based interests and identities to the same extent as do, for example, reactions to foreigners or people of another race. Thus, in this chapter, we also address the extent to which stigmas other than those involving intergroup relations are likely to be self-fulfilling.

In order to understand the potential role of self-fulfilling prophecies in stigma, it is first necessary to understand self-fulfilling prophecies. Therefore, we first briefly review some of the early research on self-fulfilling prophecies.

SELF-FULFILLING PROPHECIES: HISTORICAL OVERVIEW

The concept of the self-fulfilling prophecy was first proposed by sociologist Robert Merton (1948), who applied the idea to phenomena as diverse as test anxiety and bank failures. The self-fulfilling prophecy, however, did not receive much empirical attention until Rosenthal's pio-

neering work on experimenter effects. This work showed that researchers may (intentionally or not) act in such a way as to evoke from their
research subjects (animal and human) behavior that confirms their expectations. For example, one study focused on psychology students who
were training rats to run a maze (Rosenthal & Lawson, 1964). Half the
students were led to believe that their rats were especially smart; the
other half were led to believe that their rats were especially dumb. In
fact, there were no differences between the rats in the different groups
(students were randomly assigned to rats). Nonetheless, the "smarter"
rats learned the maze more quickly than the "dumber" rats. Students'
beliefs about their rats' intelligence were self-fulfilling.

Despite the importance of the experimenter effects studies, it was
Rosenthal and Jacobson's (1968a) seminal and controversial "Pygmalion study" that launched self-fulfilling prophecies as a major social
and scientific phenomenon. Rosenthal and Jacobson led teachers to believe that some students in their classes were "late bloomers"—students
destined to show sudden and dramatic increases in IQ over the course of
the school year. In fact, these students had been selected at random. Results showed that, especially in the earlier grade levels, the "late bloomers" gained more in IQ than the other students. Although Rosenthal and
Jacobson (1968a) induced teachers to develop positive expectations, the
implications for social problems seemed obvious. The summary of this
study that appeared in *Scientific American* (Rosenthal & Jacobson,
1968b) was titled "Teacher Expectations for the Disadvantaged," presumably because of (1) its apparent relevance to understanding why students from low-socioeconomic-status (low-SES) backgrounds often had
difficulties at school, and (2) its potential relevance for alleviating those
social problems. Rosenthal and Jacobson (1968b) suggested that induc-
ing teachers to develop high expectations was at least as effective as programs requiring far more money and effort, such as Head Start.

This study was heavily criticized at the time (e.g., Elashoff & Snow,
1971) and remains controversial today (e.g., Wineburg, 1987; Rowe,
1995). Many critics questioned the very existence of the self-fulfilling
prophecy phenomenon (for reviews, see Harris, 1989; Jussim, Smith,
Madon, & Palumbo, 1998; and Rosenthal, 1974). Consequently, it
sparked numerous attempts at replication and was the prototype for
hundreds of follow-up experiments. However, the controversy ended
with Rosenthal and Rubin's (1978) meta-analysis of the first 345 studies, which conclusively documented the existence of self-fulfilling prophecies.

With the basic phenomenon firmly established, many researchers
began studying the social and psychological processes underlying self-
fulfilling prophecies. Virtually all major reviews (e.g., Brophy & Good,

1974; Darley & Fazio, 1980; Jussim, 1986) agree that three main steps are necessary for a self-fulfilling prophecy to occur: (1) Perceivers develop erroneous expectations; (2) perceivers' expectations influence how they treat targets; and (3) targets react to this treatment with behavior that confirms the expectation.

The role of self-fulfilling prophecies in contributing to the long-term maintenance of inaccurate social beliefs may now be obvious: Through self-fulfilling prophecies, initially false beliefs become objectively true. Thus Rosenthal and Lawson's (1963) students' "smart" rats really did run mazes more quickly; and Rosenthal and Jacobson's (1968a, 1968b) "late bloomers" really did obtain higher IQ test scores. Thus, even if the basis for a stigma is initially inaccurate, if the stigma is self-fulfilling, people can then point to the "evidence" as "support" for their stigmatizing beliefs. Theoretically, therefore, initially inaccurate beliefs may be maintained indefinitely. Consequently, we next review research documenting how various stigmas may lead to self-fulfilling prophecies that sustain the stigmas.

Following Rosenthal's early work, most of the subsequent research on self-fulfilling prophecies focused on dyadic interactions. In the last 30 years, there has been a great deal of research addressing self-fulfilling prophecies in dyadic interactions. Next, therefore, we review that research with a particular focus on understanding how stigmas may become self-fulfilling.

DYADIC PROCESS: HOW AND WHY MIGHT STIGMAS BE SELF-FULFILLING?

Following the tradition in the self-fulfilling prophecy literature (e.g., Darley & Fazio, 1980; Jones, 1986; Jussim, 1991), we designate one person the "perceiver" and the other the "target." The perceiver may hold an expectation about, or stigmatize, the target. This distinction is artificial, because in any given situation, each person is both perceiver and target. Furthermore, each person may stigmatize the other. For example, in an interracial interaction, a White perceiver may stigmatize an African American target as intellectually inferior; the African American may stigmatize the White as racist. Nonetheless, the perceiver–target distinction is useful, because when we discuss the role of stigmas in creating self-fulfilling prophecies, it makes clearer just whose expectations may be influencing whom.

Another value of this distinction between perceivers and targets is that it highlights the possibility of at least two broad classes of self-fulfilling prophecies produced by stigmas: those triggered by erroneous beliefs held by the perceiver, and those triggered by erroneous beliefs held by the target. The next sections address each of these types of stigma-induced self-fulfilling prophecies.

Perceiver-Initiated Self-Fulfilling Prophecies

Although there has been little empirical research on the self-fulfilling potential of various stigmas, there has been considerable research in the related area of the self-fulfilling potential of various social stereotypes. Negative stereotyping (holding unfavorable beliefs about a group) is one manifestation of many stigmas. Therefore, we review the research on stereotypes and self-fulfilling prophecies in order to understand the extent to which stigmas may be self-fulfilling.

In this chapter, we define "stereotypes" as perceivers' beliefs about social groups and their individual members (see also Ashmore & Del Boca, 1981). Therefore, we distinguish stereotypes (beliefs) from "prejudice," which we define as liking or disliking of social groups and their individual members. This distinction is important, because one may hold an accurate belief about a group and still dislike that group; conversely, one can hold an inaccurate belief about a group and still like the group. It is clear that there is often little overlap between stereotypes and prejudice when they are defined in this manner (Eagly & Mladinic, 1989).

There has been far less research on the potentially self-fulfilling nature of prejudice, perhaps because prejudice does not fit a self-fulfilling prophecy analysis quite as well as do stereotypes. That is, the self-fulfilling prophecy starts with a false belief (Merton, 1948; Jussim, 1991; Rosenthal & Jacobson, 1968a), and accuracy is not relevant to likes and dislikes. Nonetheless, it is possible that a perceiver's prejudice triggers an interaction sequence that undermines the objective performance, competencies, and qualities of the target of prejudice. And because many stigmas have an affective quality (many stigmatized persons are regarded not only as inferior, but as repulsive), an analysis of the role of prejudice in leading to self-fulfilling prophecies may also contribute to understanding stigma. Thus, after addressing the potential for stereotypes to trigger self-fulfilling prophecies, we also address the role of prejudice in triggering self-fulfilling prophecies.

Stereotypes

There are at least three major classes of social stigmas (Goffman, 1963). "Tribal identities" refer to stigmas involving nationality, ethnicity, and religion. "Abominations of the body" include physical deformities (e.g., facial scars) and diseases. "Blemishes of individual character" include mental illnesses, criminality, homosexuality, and addictions. Typically, derogatory stereotypes accompany each stigma. Therefore, we next review the role of stereotypes in creating stigma-maintaining self-fulfilling prophecies.

Ethnicity. Negative ethnic stereotypes are perhaps the prime example of Goffman's (1963) tribal stigmas. Such stereotypes are often used to justify oppression or exploitation of one group by another (Jost & Banaji, 1994). Are ethnic stereotypes self-fulfilling? The answer may seem "obvious." In the United States, the dominant ethnic group (Whites) holds negative stereotypes about many ethnic minority groups; Whites treat members of ethnic minority groups less favorably than they treat other Whites; and thus members of minority groups receive lower-quality education and lower-paying jobs (if any).

Undoubtedly, this sequence may sometimes occur. And the desire to understand social sources of inequality may underlie much research on self-fulfilling prophecies. However, we are aware of only two studies implicating self-fulfilling prophecies in ethnic inequalities (Chen & Bargh, 1997, which we discuss later; and Word, Zanna, & Cooper, 1974). In the first of Word et al.'s (1974) classic experiments, White perceivers interviewed targets for a job. In fact, however, targets were confederates who had been carefully trained to engage in the same set of behaviors with each subject. For half of the subject/perceivers, the confederate targets were Black; for the other half of the subject/perceivers, the confederate targets were White. The main dependent variables were interviewers' nonverbal behaviors.

Consistent with a self-fulfilling prophecy, perceivers were colder to Black targets than to White targets. Interviewers sat further away from Black targets, had more speech dysfluencies when talking to them, and conducted shorter interviews. This, however, only showed that White perceivers treated Black interviewees differently than they treated White interviewees; it did not show that this treatment actually undermined the performance of the Black interviewees.

Therefore, Word et al. (1974) conducted a second experiment in which confederates were trained to interview subject/applicants in either of two ways: (1) the cold style received by the Black interviewees in Study 1, or (2) the warm style received by the White interviewees in Study 1. All subject/applicants in this study were White. Results showed that the applicants treated coldly, as were the Black applicants in Study 1, actually performed more poorly in the interview (as rated by independent judges) than did the applicants treated warmly. The type of treatment accorded Black applicants in Study 1 undermined the actual interview performance of White applicants in Study 2. Thus Whites' stereotypes were fulfilled.

The implications of the research on ethnicity and self-fulfilling prophecies are extremely limited in several ways. First, the Word et al. (1974) article remains one of only two research reports examining influences of ethnic stereotypes on target behavior (the other is discussed when we address prejudice). The study needs replication: Would the pattern hold today, at colleges and universities other than Princeton University (where it was conducted), and among nonstudent samples? Our view is that this is an extremely narrow base from which to reach any firm conclusions.

Second, the existence of social and economic inequalities is a phenomenon to be explained. Although it may be consistent with a self-fulfilling prophecy explanation, it does not provide prima facie evidence that all, or even most, ethnic differences result from self-fulfilling prophecies. In fact, one of the few studies to assess empirically the validity of Whites' racial stereotypes found that Whites actually tend to underestimate differences between Blacks and other Americans (McCauley & Stitt, 1978). This result suggests that self-fulfilling prophecies would often operate to *reduce* ethnic inequalities.

Third, throughout U.S. history, many ethnic groups (e.g., Asians, Irish, Jews) have been the target of intensely negative stereotypes (and prejudice and discrimination), but have nonetheless attained educational and occupational success comparable to or beyond that of most Whites (Marger, 1991). Thus, although dyadic self-fulfilling prophecies may contribute to ethnic differences, the magnitude of that contribution is probably modest, and they are certainly only one among many contributors.

Gender. Gender may operate, at least sometimes, as a stigmatizing attribute. Girls' and women's worth may be devalued in some domains; men's and boys' worth may be devalued in other domains. Therefore, it may be valuable to understand the role of gender-based self-fulfilling prophecies in creating, exacerbating, or maintaining sex differences and traditional sex roles. Both experimental and naturalistic studies have documented the potentially self-fulfilling nature of gender stereotypes. First we discuss the experiments, and then we review the naturalistic studies.

Zanna and Pack (1975) led female students to believe that they would be interacting with either a desirable or an undesirable man, who held either traditional or nontraditional gender role stereotypes. These female students expressed more traditional gender role attitudes and scored more poorly on an anagrams test when they believed they would interact with a desirable man holding traditional gender role attitudes (in comparison to when they believed they would interact with either of the undesirable men or with a desirable man holding nontraditional gender role attitudes). In a follow-up study (von Baeyer, Sherk, & Zanna, 1981), women actually met with a male job interviewer who (they were informed) held either sexist or nonsexist attitudes. When anticipating a sexist interviewer, the women arrived wearing more makeup and accessories, and were less likely to make eye contact. They were also more likely to respond to questions concerning marriage and children in traditionally feminine ways.

These studies show that when women want something from sexist men, they may alter their behavior to confirm traditional stereotypes about women. These studies did not provide evidence that men act on their gender stereotypes in such a way as to evoke stereotype-confirming behavior from women. Providing such evidence, however, was exactly the purpose of the next experiment.

Skrypnek and Snyder (1982) examined the role of men's gender stereotypes in influencing the behavior of women. Because interactants were in different rooms, they could not see one another. Therefore, Skrypnek and Snyder (1982) were able to manipulate the target's supposed gender. Male perceivers received a questionnaire allegedly completed by their partner; this questionnaire indicated that the partner (target) was either male or female. In fact, however, all targets were female.

By using an electronic signaling system, male perceivers negotiated a division of 24 pairs of tasks with their partners (these tasks were rated by independent judges for the degree to which they were masculine or feminine). Both individuals simultaneously indicated their first choice. If they both chose the same task, they then engaged in a series of negotiations to decide upon the final division.

Results provided clear evidence of self-fulfilling prophecies. Perceivers initially chose more masculine tasks for themselves when they believed the target was female than when they believed the target was male. In addition, they were more likely to accept the less preferred task when they believed they were negotiating with a man. These actions clearly influenced the female targets. Those targets labeled "male" ultimately accepted marginally significantly more masculine tasks, and the targets labeled "female" ultimately accepted working on significantly more feminine tasks. Thus the (female) targets came to behave in a manner consistent with males' beliefs about their gender.

Although there are only three experimental studies (Skrypnek & Snyder, 1982; von Baeyer et al., 1981; and Zanna & Pack, 1975) of gender and self-fulfilling prophecies, all show that beliefs about gender and gender-related behaviors can be self-fulfilling. Of course, experimental studies only show that gender-related beliefs and stereotypes *can* be self-fulfilling; they do not show that such beliefs typically *are* self-fulfilling under naturalistic conditions. Fortunately, however, numerous naturalistic studies have addressed exactly this issue.

An early study examined whether teachers' beliefs about sex differences in ability to learn how to read might be self-fulfilling. Palardy (1969) started with a pool of 42 first-grade teachers and identified two groups: (1) One group believed that boys and girls learn to read equally well ("Group A"); and (2) a second group believed that girls learn to read more quickly than boys ("Group B"). Even though student IQ was statistically controlled for, girls had higher reading achievement test scores than boys, but only in the classes in which teachers believed girls learned to read more quickly.

Another early study (Doyle, Hancock, & Kifer, 1972) focused on three primary predictions: (1) that first-grade teachers would have higher expectations for girls than for boys; (2) that these different expectations would be erroneous; and (3) that erroneous expectations would be self-fulfilling. All three predictions were supported. Although there were no differences in boys' and girls' mean IQ scores (103.0 and 102.8, respectively), teachers estimated that boys had mean IQ scores of 99.9 and girls had mean scores of 104.5 (a difference that was statistically significant). Teachers *underestimated* the IQs of nearly 59% of the boys, and they *overestimated* the IQs of nearly 57% of the girls.

Doyle et al. (1972) then divided students into two groups: those whose IQ scores teachers overestimated or underestimated. The main outcome variable, reading achievement scores, was then submitted to a discrepancy (over- vs. underestimated IQ) × sex analysis of covariance using actual IQ scores as a covariate (this controlled for differences between students that existed prior to the assessment of teacher expectations). Results were consistent with a self-fulfilling prophecy: Despite slightly lower IQ scores, girls had higher reading achievement scores, and the effect for discrepancy was highly significant. Students with a mean IQ of 98 (those in the overestimated group, who were disproportionately girls) actually outperformed those with a mean IQ of 107 (those in the underestimated group, who were disproportionately boys).

Another naturalistic study focused on the self-fulfilling effects of over 1,000 mothers' gender stereotypes on their children's self-perceptions of ability in math, sports, and social activities (Jacobs & Eccles, 1992). The investigators found that the children's sex interacted with their mothers' gender stereotypes: The children felt they had more ability when their sex corresponded to the sex that their mothers believed was generally superior. For example, boys evaluated their math ability more highly than girls evaluated their own math ability when their mothers believed that boys were better at math (this pattern was reversed among the minority of mothers who felt that girls were better at math). However, their results also showed that the children were not completely (or even mostly) at the mercy of their mothers' stereotypes. Children's actual skills in these areas were consistently stronger predictors of self-perceptions than were mothers' stereotypes.

Taken together, the laboratory and naturalistic studies provide clear and strong evidence that gender stereotypes may be self-fulfilling. The experimental studies showed that whether perceivers' beliefs about targets' gender or targets' beliefs about perceivers' gender stereotypes were manipulated, self-fulfilling prophecies occurred. These studies provided strong evidence of a possible causal influence of gender stereotypes on targets. However, they suffered from the problems with ecological validity typical of most experiments (they were artificial laboratory studies, experimenters deceived subjects, etc.). These limitations, however, were themselves overcome by the naturalistic studies, which showed self-fulfilling effects of gender stereotypes both in classrooms and in the home.

Gender stereotypes are at least partially self-fulfilling, which serves to maintain those stereotypes. Many of the self-fulfilling prophecies found in the research described above either advantaged males over females (e.g., Jacobs & Eccles, 1992; Skrypnek & Snyder, 1982) or operated to sustain beliefs supporting lower status for women (von Baeyer et al., 1981; Zanna & Pack, 1975). Thus self-fulfilling prophecies may contribute to the continuing inequalities in power, status, and resource distribution between men and women.

However, the self-fulfilling prophecies found in these studies did not always favor males over females. The teacher expectation studies (Doyle et al., 1972; Palardy, 1969) consistently showed self-fulfilling prophecies advantaging girls over boys. These results are consistent with research on stereotypes showing that, even in sixth-grade math classes, teachers see girls as performing more highly than boys (Jussim, Eccles, & Madon, 1996; Madon, Jussim, & Eccles, 1997). Although boys generally do better in math and science starting in junior high school, girls do better overall than boys (receive higher grades; are less likely to receive a diagnostic label, such as "learning-disabled" or "emotionally disturbed"; etc.) throughout elementary, secondary, and postsecondary education (Jussim et al., 1998; Kimball, 1989). Although societal advantages may ultimately favor males over females and more than compensate for the disadvantages males face in school, it is at least possible that many boys do face something like a low-grade stigma throughout their school years.

Socioeconomic Status. Abundant evidence shows that people hold higher expectations for individuals from middle-SES backgrounds than for individuals from lower-SES backgrounds (Dusek & Joseph, 1983; Jussim, Coleman, & Lerch, 1987). Nonetheless, we are aware of only two studies that have examined whether these expectations are self-fulfilling. Perhaps the most dramatic and best-known of such studies was performed by Rist (1970). Rist observed that by the eighth day of class, a kindergarten teacher had divided her class into three groups— supposedly "smart," "average," and "dumb" groups. Each group sat at its own table (Tables 1, 2, and 3, respectively). Furthermore, the main difference between the students was not intelligence; there were no mean differences in IQ scores among the three tables on a test administered at the end of the school year. Instead, the main difference was SES. In comparison to the other students, the students at Table 1 came from homes that had higher incomes, were less likely to be supported by welfare, and were more likely to have both parents present; the children themselves were cleaner and more likely to dress appropriately. There were comparable differences between the students at Tables 2 and 3. Table 1 was positioned closest to the teacher, and she proceeded to direct nearly all of her time and attention to those students. In addition, she was generally friendlier and warmer to the "smart" students. Consequently, Rist (1970) interpreted his study as documenting strong self-fulfilling prophecies.

The differences Rist (1970) observed in teacher treatment of middle-SES versus lower-SES students would be inappropriate and Unjustified even if there were real differences in the intelligence of the children at the different tables. Nonetheless, despite Rist's (1970) conclusions, the study provided no evidence of self-fulfilling prophecy. Although Rist provided a wealth of observations concerning teacher treatment, he provided few regarding student performance. The only objective performance data that he provided were the IQ test scores, which showed that by the end of the school year there were *no* significant differences among the students at the three tables. Thus, although the teacher may have held very different expectations for middle- versus lower-SES students, and even though the teacher may have treated students from different backgrounds very differently, this had no effect on students' IQ scores (see Jussim & Eccles, 1995, for a more detailed critique of this study).

A naturalistic study that included over 10,000 students (Williams, 1976) provided a much more rigorous analysis of the role of SES in educational self-fulfilling prophecies. Williams (1976) used path-analytic techniques to assess relations among teacher expectations, students' previous and future achievement, and SES. Consistent with most studies examining SES, Williams (1976) found that teachers held higher expectations for students from upper-SES backgrounds. However, SES differences in teacher expectations evaporated after students' previous levels of performance were controlled for. This means that, rather than student SES backgrounds' biasing teacher expectations, teachers accurately perceived genuine differences in achievement among students from differing SES backgrounds. Of course, accurate expectations do not create self-fulfilling prophecies.

A colleague once described the Rist (1970) study as "a real tearjerker," and we cannot help agreeing. Nonetheless, the less well-known Williams (1976) study is much stronger than Rist's (1970) study on almost all important scientific grounds. Rist relied primarily on his own subjective and potentially biased observations, whereas Williams relied on school records and questionnaires; Rist focused on 30 students, whereas Williams focused on over 10,000 students; Rist claimed to provide strong evidence of self-fulfilling prophecy but actually provided none, whereas Williams (1976) rigorously tested for bias and self-fulfilling prophecy and failed to find any. We do not doubt that SES may sometimes lead to self-fulfilling prophecies. However, with respect to drawing conclusions about the current state of our knowledge about SES, the Williams (1976) study deserves dramatically more weight than that of Rist (1970).

Physical Attractiveness. Except perhaps in the extreme, physical unattractiveness probably would not qualify as one of Goffman's (1963) "abominations of the body." Nonetheless, the types of injuries, diseases, and birth defects that can be categorized as abominations of the body also dramatically damage one's physical attractiveness. This is important, because although we know of no research directly examining the self-fulfilling nature of abominations of the body, there has been considerable research on the self-fulfilling nature of physical attractiveness. This research is reviewed next.

Many people hold considerably less favorable perceptions of physically unattractive individuals and treat them more negatively than they treat more attractive individuals (see reviews and meta-analyses by Eagly, Ashmore, Makhijani, & Longo, 1991, and Feingold, 1992). For example, people like unattractive individuals less and believe that they have less socially desirable traits than their attractive counterparts. Because of expectations that unattractive people are, for example, less warm or less socially skilled than their attractive peers, unattractiveness is in some manner also a characterological stigma that is manifested in defective behavior and personality.

Despite the numerous studies on expectations related to attractiveness, we are aware of only three studies that have empirically examined whether such beliefs may be self-fulfilling. In a classic study (Snyder, Tanke, & Berscheid, 1977), male perceivers received a photograph of a female with whom they would soon be interacting. The photograph showed a woman who was either physically attractive or unattractive (this was determined through a pilot test, in which judges rated the women's photographs). In fact, male–female interaction partners were randomly assigned to attractiveness condition. They then had a telephone conversation (they were in different rooms). The main findings were that male perceivers were warmer and friendlier to female targets who they (erroneously) believed were more attractive, and these females reciprocated with similarly high levels of warmth and friendliness.

A study by Andersen and Bern (1981) obtained results that conflicted with Snyder et al.'s (1977) findings. In addition to using a nearly identical methodology (interactants in different rooms had a phone conversation, perceivers were provided with false photographs of their partners in order to manipulate physical attractiveness, etc.), they extended Snyder et al.'s (1977) paradigm in two ways: (1) They included both male and female perceivers and targets, and (2) perceivers' gender identity was assessed. This study found no significant differences between the behavior of the supposedly attractive and unattractive female targets who interacted with male perceivers. Male beliefs about the attractiveness of their female partners did not lead to a self-fulfilling prophecy.

Partial evidence of a self-fulfilling prophecy emerged in the behavior of male targets who interacted with sex-typed female perceivers. These male targets did behaviorally confirm the expectations associated with physical attractiveness: The supposedly attractive males were rated as friendlier and more socially skilled. Males who had androgynous female partners, however, showed the reverse pattern: supposedly unattractive males were rated as more socially attractive, responsive, and confident than their attractive counterparts.

Another study (Frieze, Olson, & Russell, 1991) focused on the relation between physical attractiveness and income among about 700 people who had recently earned MBA degrees (and who are hereafter referred to as "MBAs"). This study is included here because the authors framed their predictions almost entirely in self-fulfilling prophecy terms. On the basis of research such as Snyder et al.'s (1977) study, Frieze et al. (1991) predicted that attractive MBAs would receive higher starting salaries than unattractive MBAs, and that these differences would increase over time.

Their results partially supported this prediction. Attractive men received significantly higher starting salaries than unattractive men, but attractiveness was not significantly related to the starting salaries of women. More attractive and less overweight men received significantly higher starting salaries, but again there were no effects of attractiveness or weight for women. Physical attractiveness significantly predicted subsequent salaries for both men and women, and the salary differential between attractive and unattractive MBAs increased over time.

Several aspects of the Frieze et al. (1991) study, however, undermine the self-fulfilling prophecy interpretation of their results. First there was no assessment of employers' expectations for individual employees. Therefore, whether the relation between physical attractiveness and income was mediated by employers' physical attractiveness stereotypes is unknowable from their data. Second, their results seemed to provide considerable evidence of accuracy. Work experience consistently predicted income to a greater extent than did attractiveness or weight.

Third, their analyses probably suffered from at least one important omitted variable. Research consistently shows that physically attractive adults are more socially skilled than less attractive adults (e.g., Goldman & Lewis, 1977; see the meta-analysis by Feingold, 1992). It seems likely that more socially skilled MBAs would deserve and actually receive higher salaries than less socially skilled MBAs. Thus attractiveness may predict MBAs income because it is a proxy for social skill, rather than because of self-fulfilling prophecies.

Although the development of individual differences in social skill is beyond the scope of the present chapter, we may wonder where these differences come from. Isn't it possible that self-fulfilling prophecies create a difference where none previously existed? Although it is possible, the mere existence of social skill differences provides neither empirical evidence nor logical justification for supporting a self-fulfilling prophecy explanation (or any other explanation). There are many plausible alternative explanations for why social skill differences between the attractive and unattractive exist. Furthermore, current evidence indicates that the expectancy explanation is one of the *weakest* accounts for those differences (see Feingold's [1992] meta-analysis).

Obesity. Similar to unattractive individuals, obese people are also stigmatized on the basis of bodily flaws. Clearly, they are subjected to disdain and discrimination in their daily lives—perhaps moreso than unattractive individuals, who may have (or be perceived to have) less control over their physical appearance.

People who are obese encounter discrimination in education (e.g., Canning & Mayer, 1966), employment (e.g., Rothblum, Brand, Miller, & Oetjen, 1990), and social life (e.g., Miller, Rothblum, Barbour, Brand, & Felicio, 1990). Compared to their normal-weight peers, they are less likely to attend elite colleges (Canning & Mayer, 1966; Crandall, 1991), less likely to get hired (Larkin & Pines, 1979), and more likely to have a hard time finding dates (Millman, 1980). Obesity is associated with a variety of negative outcomes, including lower SES (e.g., Sobal & Stunkard, 1989) and low self-esteem (e.g., Wadden, Foster, Brownell, & Finley, 1984). Negative attitudes toward obese people exist in the United States among members of many ethnic and socioeconomic groups; among health professionals, including doctors, nurses, and psychologists; among children as young as age 6; and even among obese people themselves (e.g., Allon, 1982; Crandall & Biernat, 1990; Goodman, Richardson, Dornbusch, & Hastorf, 1963; Staffieri, 1967; Wadden & Stunkard, 1985).

Although we know of no research that has directly examined whether obese individuals become targets of self-fulfilling prophecies, indirect evidence strongly suggest they do. For example, obese students have been underrepresented at elite colleges and universities (e.g., Canning & Mayer, 1966). This may occur because parents are less likely to provide financial support for college to their heavy daughters than to their thin daughters, regardless of their ability to provide such support (Crandall, 1991, 1995). Perhaps parents believe that their obese daughters are not capable of high levels of success or do not deserve to attend such a school, and thus are less willing to support them. As a consequence, their daughters may be less able to attend these schools, so that ultimately they do not reap the professional and economic benefits of attending these institutions. In this way, parental beliefs associated with obesity may become a self-fulfilling prophecy.

Crandall (1991, 1995) provided some evidence that parental beliefs may be responsible for this phenomenon: Politically conservative parents provide less financial assistance to their heavy daughters than to their thinner daughters. Because earlier research has found a significant relationship between political conservatism and negative attitudes toward obesity (Crandall & Biernat, 1990), Crandall (1995) employed political attitudes as a measure of anti-fat attitudes and concluded that anti-fat attitudes predicted parental financial support. However, parental expectations were not directly measured. Instead, the daughters provided the reports of parental political attitudes. In addition, there were no measures of the daughters' actual life outcomes (college attendance, occupational success, etc.). Although it is quite possible that parents' expectations became self-fulfilling for their obese daughters, empirical evidence for this phenomenon is weak.

Attention-Deficit/Hyperactivity Disorder. Attention-deficit/hyperactivity disorder (ADHD) probably qualifies as a characterological stigma in Goffman's (1963) typology. The ADHD label represents a devalued social identity based on flaws in a person's behavior (and, to a lesser extent, personality). ADHD is characterized by difficulty with impulse control, difficulties focusing one's attention on anyone task, and excessive and inappropriate restlessness (American Psychiatric Association, 1994), Because perceivers tend to overemphasize the role of an actor's disposition in determining behavior (Ross, 1977), we consider the label of ADHD a primarily characterological stigma.

Social scientists commonly emphasize the pernicious effects of applying diagnostic labels (e.g., " ADHD," "handicapped," "learning-disabled," "emotionally disturbed," "schizophrenic") to people (e.g., Jones et al., 1984; Rist & Harrell, 1982; Rosenhan, 1973). Diagnostic labels are essentially social stereotypes—categories of psychological and physical infirmities, within which there is considerable variation among individuals. Many complaints about labels focus on their inaccuracy or their tendency to bias evaluations and judgments. Although these issues are beyond the scope of this chapter (see Jussim, Madon, & Chatman, 1994, for a review), researchers often suggest or imply that inaccurate labels create self-fulfilling prophecies.

Nonetheless, we are aware of only two highly similar studies that have addressed this issue empirically with the label of ADHD. Both examined the self-fulfilling effects of the ADHD label on peer interactions among elementary school boys (Harris, Milich, Corbitt, Hoover, & Brady, 1992; Harris, Milich, Johnston, & Hoover, 1990). Results from the two studies showed broad effects of the expectancy on both the perceivers and targets. Perceivers "observed" more ADHD-like symptoms, were less friendly, and talked less to targets labeled as having ADHD. They also gave ADHD-labeled targets less credit for strong test performance. ADHD-labeled targets enjoyed the interaction less, felt they did less well on the task, accepted less credit for good performance and felt that their partners were "meaner."

The research by Harris et al. (1992), however, also helps put these findings in some context. They used a "balanced-placebo" design: Perceivers' expectations were manipulated orthogonally to targets' actual diagnostic status. That is, targets either were or were not diagnosed as having ADHD. Regardless of their actual ADHD status, however, half the targets were labeled as having ADHD and half were not. Thus Harris et al. (1992) were able to sort out expectancy effects from genuine differences between targets with ADHD and "normal" targets. In general, for both perceivers and targets, the effects of actually being diagnosed with ADHD were substantially larger than the differences between *being labeled* as having ADHD or not. Thus this study shows that although the label may contribute to a cycle of negative peer interactions for children with ADHD, most differences between children with ADHD and their "normal" peers are genuine and do not exist primarily in the mind of perceivers.

Mental Illness. Mental illness is one of Goffman's (1963) classic characterological stigmas. Individuals who have a mental illness are perceived to have personality and behavioral defects. People dislike, derogate, hold negative stereotypes about, and discriminate against others who have or are perceived to have a mental illness (Farina, 1982).

However, research showing that people dislike, derogate, and otherwise treat those with mental problems unfavorably (e.g., Rosenhan, 1973) does not provide evidence of a self-fulfilling prophecy, which requires the stigma to change targets' behavior. We are aware of only one study that has directly examined the role of the stigma of mental illness in creating a self-fulfilling prophecy. Sibicky and Dovidio (1986) had pairs of undergraduate subjects participate in a getting-acquainted conversation. In half of the pairs, perceivers were led to believe that their partners were psychotherapy clients; in the other half of the pairs, perceivers were told that their partners were introductory psychology students. Before the conversation, perceivers who would interact with psychotherapy clients rated their partners more negatively than those paired with psychology students did. Independent judges found that perceivers with counseling partners also behaved more negatively during the conversation. Last, independent judges rated the "psychotherapy clients" more negatively than the "psychology students."

Some mental illnesses are so extreme, such as schizophrenia and severe forms of bipolar disorders, that self-fulfilling prophecies probably contribute little to such conditions. Nonetheless, the negative treatment that often accompanies stigma may indeed either exacerbate some of the milder forms of mental illness, or at least render improvement more difficult.

Stereotypes, Stigmas, and Self-Fulfilling Prophecies: Conclusions. It is abundantly clear that at least sometimes, negative stereotypes can be self-fulfilling. Research has demonstrated this for race, sex, physical attractiveness, and labels associated with mental illness; the results regarding obesity also raise the specter of stigma-maintaining self-fulfilling prophecies. Nonetheless, except for sex, there have been relatively few studies (rarely more than one or two) that have assessed whether stereotypes are self-fulfilling. And at least sometimes (as in the case of physical attractiveness), those results have been inconsistent. Other times, even though the research shows stereotypes leading to self-fulfilling prophecies, those self-fulfilling prophecies do not always favor only one group (as in the case of sex). Furthermore, it is also clear that self-fulfilling prophecies can rarely account for large differences between social groups, and that many differences between groups derive from sources other than self-fulfilling prophecies (e.g., Jussim, 1991; Jussim et al., 1996). Thus, although some stigmas may create self-fulfilling prophecies that help maintain and reinforce those stigmas, other factors (such as cultural values and world views, institutional practices, segregation, etc.) probably play more significant roles in the maintenance of most stigmas than do self-fulfilling prophecies in dyadic interactions.

Prejudice

At least sometimes, prejudice may be a more important self-fulfilling prophecy trigger than stereotypes. As noted earlier, we define "prejudice" as how much one likes or dislikes social groups and their individual members. Disliking (disgust, revulsion, disdain, etc.) is one of the classic aspects of stigma (e.g., Crocker et al., 1998; Goffman, 1963). That liking of groups (prejudice) differs from beliefs about groups (stereotypes) is easily demonstrated, both conceptually and empirically. Conceptually, a belief that Jews are wealthier than other people may be accurate or inaccurate, but knowing that someone believes Jews are wealthier than other people does not indicate anything about whether they like or dislike Jews.

Because liking is irrelevant to accuracy (e.g., how accurate is your liking of Coca-Cola or intellectuals, or your distaste for olives or lawyers?), prejudice-triggered interaction sequences may not fulfill a strict definition of self-fulfilling prophecy (because there is not necessarily an initially inaccurate belief). Nonetheless, prejudice may trigger an interaction sequence that results in targets' behaving in a manner that seems to justify stigmatizing them or their group. In this sense, prejudice may indeed trigger self-fulfilling prophecies.

Prejudice/Affect Interpretations of Some Classic Studies. Several of the classic studies in the expectancy confirmation area may be interpreted as evidence of affect-triggered self-fulfilling prophecies rather than stereotype-triggered self-fulfilling prophecies. For example, the classic Word et al. study (1974, described previously) never actually assessed Whites' beliefs about Blacks. However, a pilot study did assess Whites' *attitudes* toward Blacks and did indeed find evidence of White prejudice. Furthermore, the behaviors that mediated self-fulfilling prophecies in this study (physical distance, speech errors, interview duration) seem more likely to represent nonverbal manifestations of dislike or discomfort than to represent inaccurate stereotype-based expectations.

The classic Snyder et al. (1977) study can be interpreted similarly. Independent of any stereotypes about the personality traits associated with attractiveness, the college-age men in the study may have liked attractiveness per se. That is, the men might have been more interested in and friendly toward the supposedly more beautiful targets because they enjoyed, valued, and liked their attractiveness. They might have found the prospect of getting to know the more attractive targets better or getting a date with them appealing in itself, regardless of the targets' personalities.

Teacher Expectations. The teacher expectation work, too, is consistent with an affective interpretation of some self-fulfilling prophecy effects. Teacher expectations may also be associated with teacher affect: Teachers may, on average, like high-expectancy students more than they like low-expectancy students. This seems especially plausible if one can assume that most teachers value education; presumably they would also often prefer students who appear motivated and committed to education.

In addition to this speculative analysis, results from the teacher expectation research are consistent with this interpretation. The biggest factor mediating self-fulfilling prophecies in the classroom is "climate"—the extent to which teachers provide a warm and supportive environment for their students (Harris & Rosenthal, 1985). Indeed, Rosenthal (1989) has proposed an affect–effort theory to account for this pattern. The main idea is that teachers like their high-expectancy students more, and then exert more effort in teaching them. This interpretation fits results from the tracking literature showing that teachers often spend more time preparing for, and are more interested in, their high-track classes (e.g., Evertson, 1982); it also fits the results from Rist (1970) showing that early elementary school teachers spent disproportionate amounts of time and attention on the students they believed to be more capable.

Recent Work. Several recent studies further suggest that the role of affect in driving "expectancy" effects may be greater than once believed. The Harris et al. (1992) study (described earlier) found that children were less warm, friendly, and involved when playing with other children who were stigmatized with the ADHD label. These behaviors would seem to reflect disliking at least as much as low expectations.

A few years ago, a series of studies in our laboratory directly examined the relative roles of stereotypes (beliefs) and prejudice (liking–disliking) in perceivers' judgments of targets (Jussim, Nelson, Manis, & Soffin, 1995). In three experiments, perceivers evaluated the sanity of targets who were given either a stigmatized label ("child abuser") or nonstigmatized label ("rock performer"). Bias occurred in all three studies: In all cases, child abusers were seen as more mentally ill than were rock performers. However, the main purpose of this study was not to demonstrate bias; it was to test alternative models of the role of stereotypes/beliefs and prejudice/affect in mediating this bias. The greatest support was found for the model assuming that prejudice/affect entirely mediated the bias; little support was found for the model assuming that stereotypes/beliefs entirely mediated the bias. The fourth study used the same procedures to examine another stigmatized label, "gay male." Results were more mixed, providing some support for both the prejudice/affect mediation model and the stereotype/belief mediation model.

Another recent study (Chen & Bargh, 1997) showed that a priming manipulation could trigger a self-fulfilling prophecy. First, the researchers subliminally presented to perceivers either African American or White faces. Perceivers and targets (all of whom were White) were then placed into different rooms where they played a game without seeing one another (they communicated through microphones and headphones). These interactions were tape-recorded. Two coders then rated the tape-recorded interactions for hostility.

The priming manipulation produced a self-fulfilling prophecy: Perceivers primed with an African American face were rated as more hostile, and targets interacting with more hostile perceivers reciprocated with greater hostility themselves. Chen and Bargh (1997) interpreted the pattern as demonstrating a self-fulfilling effect of an automatically activated stereotype. Although this is certainly possible, it is also possible that, rather than activating racial *beliefs* (stereotypes), the priming manipulation activated *affect* (prejudice or dislike toward African Americans). This seems especially likely because the behavioral outcomes involved hostility (which was operationally defined as frustration, raised voice volume, insults, etc.) These outcomes seem to be manifestations of negative affect more than they are manifestations of unflattering beliefs.

Prejudice as Trigger: Conclusions. Our analysis must remain somewhat speculative, because we know of no research that has directly examined the role of prejudice/affect in triggering self-fulfilling prophecies. Instead, prejudice/affect seems to provide a plausible alternative interpretation for many of the studies once interpreted as demonstrating self-fulfilling effects of stereotypes or teacher expectations. The one study that did directly examine the role of affect in expectancy effects (Jussim, Nelson, et al., 1995) focused on evaluative biases, rather than behavioral confirmation, as an outcome. Nonetheless, this research at least raises the possibility that prejudice may drive some expectancy effects—both biases and self-fulfilling prophecies.

Target-Initiated Self-Fulfilling Prophecies

Thus far, we have reviewed evidence showing how the expectations or prejudices of perceivers (or potential stigmatizers) may lead to self-fulfilling prophecies. This is important because perceiver-initiated self-fulfilling prophecies represent a sort of "classic" view of stigma: Stigmatizers hold nasty beliefs about or attitudes toward a group of people, and act in such a way as to reinforce the target group's inferior status.

However, stigmas may lead to self-fulfilling prophecies even in the absence of nasty perceivers. Sometimes the beliefs and expectations held by the targets (the potentially stigmatized persons) may lead to self-fulfilling prophecies. This is because targets' beliefs that other persons stigmatize them, even when these beliefs are erroneous, may lead the *targets* to initiate an interaction process in which they ultimately fulfill the stereotypic expectations associated with their stigma.

For example, one of the early classics in stigma research was a study of the interactions of people who were led to believe that others thought they had epilepsy, a gruesome facial scar, or an allergy (Kleck & Strenta, 1980). Each person then interacted with a confederate (this interaction was videotaped). Compared to those who thought their partners believed they had an allergy , those who thought their partners stigmatized them thought the confederates were more tense and patronizing and were less attracted to them. Observers who viewed only the confederates' portions of the tapes, however, did not detect any differences between the behavior of the confederates interacting with "scarred" or "allergic" subjects.

These results demonstrate some pernicious effects of simply *believing* that one is stigmatized. However, they stop short of demonstrating a self-fulfilling prophecy because, although there was considerable evidence that this belief affected subjects' perceptions, there was no evidence that this belief actually affected their behavior. However, several studies have indeed demonstrated that simply believing one is stigmatized is sufficient to produce self-fulfilling behavior.

For example, Zanna's sexist-interviewer studies (von Baeyer et al., 1981; Zanna & Pack, 1975), described earlier, provide evidence of target-initiated self-fulfilling stereotypes. Many of the dependent variables (how much makeup and accessories the women wore, their performance on a test, etc.) were all assessed prior to the interview (which, in the case of Zanna & Pack [1975], never took place). Thus these studies show that *women's beliefs* regarding how they are viewed by others can at least sometimes lead them to act in ways fulfilling sex stereotypes.

Similarly, believing that others view oneself as mentally ill can actually evoke more rejection from those others. In an ingenious series of studies, targets were led to believe that perceivers viewed them as mentally ill, even though perceivers were actually unaware of targets' mental health status (Farina, Allen, & Saul, 1968; Farina, Gliha, Boudreau, Allen, & Sherman, 1971). Results showed that targets actually evoked more rejection from those perceivers.

This pattern may be quite common. The recently developed notion of "rejection sensitivity" captures the idea that some people are particularly vigilant at seeking signs of rejection from others (e.g., Downey & Feldman, 1996). Furthermore, high rejection sensitivity may become a self-fulfilling prophecy (Downey, Freitas, Michaelis, & Khouri, 1998). When one person involved in a romantic relationship is hypervigilant for signs of rejection, that person is more likely to find such signs. This leads the person to become hurt and resentful, triggering hostility and angry outbursts; these lead the other person to be more likely to reject the hypervigilant partner.

This analysis—especially when combined with some of the classic stigma research (Farina et al., 1968, 1971; Kleck & Strenta, 1980)—strongly suggests that at least some people from stigmatized social groups enter at least some interactions with what, in colloquial terms, would be called a major chip on their shoulders. They may have heightened sensitivity to the possibility that others dislike, reject, and patronize them. By looking harder for rejection, they may be more likely to find it. If perceivers simply respond to this target-generated hostility, they are likely to distance themselves from targets, thereby fulfilling and reinforcing the stigma.

Dyadic Expectancy Effects: Powerful and Pervasive?

An impressive number of studies conducted in a wide variety of laboratory and field settings and addressing a wide variety of potential stigmas (race, sex, SES, various physical attributes, mental illness, etc.) has demonstrated the potentially self-fulfilling nature of many stigmas. Thus the self-fulfilling effects of stigmas are pervasive, in the sense that they can happen at almost any time to almost anyone possessing a stigmatizable characteristic.

In addition, reviews of expectancy effects, self-fulfilling prophecies, and behavioral confirmation appeared in the social-psychological literature in the 1980s and early 1990s, all of which emphasized the widespread power of erroneous beliefs to create social reality (e.g., Fiske &

Taylor, 1984; Jones, 1990; Miller & Turnbull, 1986; Snyder, 1984). It appeared, therefore, that stigmas were likely to be powerfully self-fulfilling—and, therefore, that self-fulfilling prophecies constituted a major social process serving to maintain and exacerbate many stigmatizing conditions.

Unfortunately for this view, however, a series of meta-analyses and reviews conducted between 1978 and 1996 all concluded that self-fulfilling prophecy effect sizes are typically not very large. The first meta-analysis of expectancy effects (Rosenthal & Rubin, 1978) concluded that although self-fulfilling prophecies were real phenomena, nearly two-thirds of the studies examining effects of erroneous expectations failed to find significant evidence of self-fulfilling prophecies. In addition, the average effect size of erroneous expectations was fairly small—about .2.

These conclusions were later reaffirmed in a meta-analysis focusing exclusively on effects of teacher expectations on student IQ (Raudenbush, 1984), which found that even the most powerful expectancy effect sizes were typically only about .2. In addition, reviews that explicitly examined the power of self-fulfilling prophecies in the laboratory, in the classroom, and in other field settings consistently concluded that such effects were on average typically quite small—.1 to .2 in terms of correlation or regression coefficients (e.g., Brophy, 1983; Jussim, 1991; Jussim & Eccles, 1995; Jussim et al., 1996).

Thus, although stigmas may be self-fulfilling, the reviews emphasizing the modest nature of the effects have seemed to undermine the idea that self-fulfilling prophecies provide a major contribution to the maintenance of social stigmas. Such reviews, however, have only concluded that average expectancy effects are not particularly large. It therefore remains possible that under some conditions, self-fulfilling prophecies are much larger than average—large enough to make substantial contributions to the maintenance and exacerbation of some stigmas. Next, therefore, we review research addressing moderators of self-fulfilling prophecies.

Moderators of Self-Fulfilling Prophecies

However, even small effects may be more powerful under certain conditions and among certain targets. One of the challenges for researchers who study self-fulfilling prophecies, therefore, has been to identify when self-fulfilling prophecies are especially powerful. In this spirit, researchers have identified two broad classes of factors that influence the power of self-fulfilling prophecies and that may help us understand stigma: (1) characteristics of the perceiver; and (2) characteristics of the target.

Perceiver Characteristics

Goals. Perceivers often enter social interactions with specific goals (Hilton & Darley, 1991) that can influence the power of self-fulfilling prophecies. For example, self-fulfilling prophecies are more likely to occur when perceivers desire to arrive at a stable and predictable impression of a target (Snyder, 1992), when perceivers are more confident in the validity of their expectations (Jussim, 1986; Swann & Ely, 1984), and when they have an incentive for confirming their beliefs (Cooper & Hazelrigg, 1988). Self-fulfilling prophecies are less likely when perceivers are motivated to develop an accurate impression of a target (Neuberg, 1989), when perceiver outcomes depend on the target (Neuberg, 1994), and when perceivers' main goal is to get along in a friendly manner with targets (Snyder, 1992). These findings raise the following question: When are perceivers likely to be motivated by accuracy or a desire to get along in a friendly manner, and when are they likely to be overconfident in their beliefs or motivated by desires to reach a particular conclusion?

Prejudice, Cognitive Rigidity, and Belief Certainty. Prejudiced individuals seem especially unlikely to be motivated by either accuracy concerns or the desire to get along with members of the group they dislike. Instead, they seem likely to desire to reach the particular conclusion that members of the stigmatized group have negative, enduring attributes (Pettigrew, 1979). People high in cognitive rigidity or belief certainty also may not be motivated to consider different viewpoints. Cognitive rigidity, which is usually construed as an individual-difference factor (e.g., Adorno, Frenkel-Brunswik, Levinson, & Sanford, 1950; Allport, 1958; Harris, 1989), and belief certainty, which is usually construed as a situational factor (Jussim, 1986; Swann & Ely, 1984), are similar in that they describe people who may be unlikely to alter their beliefs when confronted with disconfirming evidence. Whether the source is prejudice, cognitive rigidity, or belief certainty (which may tend to co-occur within individuals—see Adorno et al., 1950), people who are overly confident in their expectations may be most likely to maintain biased perceptions of individuals and to create self-fulfilling prophecies (Babad, Inbar, & Rosenthal, 1982; Harris, 1989; Swann & Ely, 1984).

Target Characteristics

Goals. Considerable research has examined the role of targets' goals in moderating self-fulfilling prophecies. Although this research has rarely addressed stigma, it may provide at least some insights into the role of expectancy effects in maintaining or reducing stigma.

When perceivers have something targets want (such as a job), and when targets are aware of the perceivers' beliefs, they often confirm those beliefs in order to create a favorable impression (von Baeyer et al., 1981; Zanna & Pack, 1975). Similarly, when targets desire to facilitate smooth social interactions or feel they should defer to perceivers (Smith, Neuberg, Judice, & Biesanz, 1997) they are also more likely to confirm perceivers' expectations (Snyder, 1992). These motivations are likely to maintain and reinforce the stigma, because they lead targets to confirm perceivers' beliefs about them.

Targets, however, are rarely rudderless boats tossed about on the seas of others' expectations for them. When targets believe that perceivers hold a negative belief about them, they often act to disconfirm that belief (Hilton & Darley, 1985). Similarly, when their main goal is to defend a threatened identity, or to express their personal attributes, they are also likely to disconfirm perceivers' inaccurate expectations (Snyder, 1992). Thus, when targets believe perceivers stigmatize them, they may work particularly hard to disconfirm the stigma.

Demographics. For several reasons, we suspected that students from stigmatized social groups might be more vulnerable to expectancy effects (see Jussim et al., 1996, for more details on both the conceptual analysis and the empirical results). For African American students, students from lower-SES backgrounds, and girls (at least in math classes), school may not be a particularly friendly place (American Association of University Women, 1992; Lareau, 1987; Steele, 1992). When faced with negative teacher expectations, such students may be particularly likely to devalue the importance they place on achievement. Similarly, when they are faced with supportive and demanding (high-expectancy) teachers, this may feel like a breath of fresh air, thereby inspiring these students to new heights. This perspective may not be as Pollyanna-like as it sounds. In his influential article on African American disidentification with school, Steele (1992) described academic programs in which previously low-performing students (e.g., some with Scholastic Aptitude Test scores in the 300s) took on difficult honors-level work and outperformed their White and Asian American classmates.

Therefore, we (Jussim et al., 1996) assessed whether student demographics moderated relations between teacher expectations (assessed early in the school year) and students' subsequent achievement, in the context of a model that included many controls (previous achievement, motivation, etc.). We found virtually no evidence that student sex moderated expectancy effects; for both boys and girls, the standardized regression coefficients relating teacher expectations to future achievement were typically small (.1 to .2).

However, we found considerable evidence of moderation by ethnicity and by SES. Standardized coefficients relating teacher perceptions to future standardized test scores were .14 for White students, .37 for African American students, .11 for students from higher-SES backgrounds, and .25 for students from lower-SES backgrounds. These findings mean that for White and middle-SES students, the difference in achievement outcomes predicted by the highest and lowest teacher expectations was about 20 percentile points. But for African American students and students from lower-SES backgrounds, the difference in achievement outcomes predicted by the highest and lowest teacher expectations was about 50 percentile points.

That is a dramatic difference, and we found the same pattern when using grades as the achievement outcome. In addition, the effects of ethnicity and SES were independent: Excluding the African American students from analyses did not change the SES effects, and expectancy effects were just as powerful among middle-SES African American students as among less well-off African American students.

Prior Achievement. We wondered whether this pattern of greater susceptibility among students from stigmatized groups might also extend to students with histories of poor academic performance. Although low school achievement per se has rarely been discussed as a stigma, it clearly fits. Low-performing students are often placed into low-track classrooms, which has been compared to a caste system for maintaining inequalities (Oakes, 1985; Rist, 1970). Teachers often communicate negative expectations to lower-achieving students by criticizing them more often, interacting with them less often, and demanding Jess from them (Brophy, 1983). These types of behaviors may undermine these students' motivation, rendering them more susceptible to confirming negative expectations (Eccles & Wigfield, 1985). However, when teachers communicate positive expectations to lower-achieving students, their motivation for school may rise dramatically and inspire them to make substantial gains in their achievement (Eccles & Wigfield, 1985).

We know of only one study that has empirically examined whether students' prior achievement moderates expectancy effects (Madon et al., 1997). Our results mirrored the patterns that we found among African American and lower-SES students. Teachers' expectations predicted students' future achievement more strongly for students with lower previous standardized test scores than for students with higher previous standardized test scores. Thus it seems that students who are stigmatized, whether because of their demographic group membership or because of their history of achievement, are more vulnerable to expectancy effects.

Multiple Stigmas. We wondered whether the expectancy moderators we discovered were additive—for example, did teacher expectations predict students' future achievement more strongly among low-performing students from lower-SES backgrounds? They did. The relation (standardized regression coefficient, obtained in context of a model with all the controls) of teacher expectations to future achievement among low-performing students from lower-SES backgrounds was .62. This is one of the strongest relations between teacher expectations and student achievement ever obtained, especially in a naturalistic study. Unfortunately, however, because of the small number of African American students in the sample, we could not examine whether teacher expectations also more strongly predicted the future achievement of low-performing African American students.

Self-Fulfilling Prophecies: Harmful or Helpful?

The research on demographics, prior achievement, and multiple stigmas all shows that self-fulfilling prophecies are stronger among targets in low-status groups. This pattern might appear consistent with the long-held assumption that self-fulfilling prophecies help to create and maintain social problems and inequalities (Merton, 1948; Rist, 1970; Rosenthal & Jacobson, 1968b; Snyder, 1984; Word et al., 1974). It would be tempting to conclude, therefore, that self-fulfilling prophecies function to further disadvantage individuals from these groups.

For that to be the case, however, self-fulfilling prophecies would need to mostly harm these students. If they mostly help these students, then self-fulfilling prophecies would be functioning more to reduce their disadvantage than to exacerbate it. However, we know of only three studies that seem to have addressed this issue, and all have focused on teacher expectations.

The first (Babad et al., 1982) examined the power of negative and positive self-fulfilling prophecies among students in gym classes who had either low-bias or high-bias teachers. Although there were no differences between high- and low-expectancy students' athletic performance with low-bias teachers, the high-expectancy students consistently performed more highly than did the low-expectancy students with high-bias teachers (a result demonstrating the occurrence of a self-fulfilling prophecy). However, a simple difference between high- and low-expectancy students is insufficient to determine whether self-fulfilling prophecies primarily helped or hurt students. A difference between these groups of students could occur if (1) high expectations helped students and low expectations had no effect; (2) low expectations harmed students and high expectations had no effect; or (3) high expectations helped students *and* low expectations hurt students.

Because there was no evidence of self-fulfilling prophecies among low-bias teachers, students' performance with low-bias teachers could be used as a sort of control group for determining whether self-fulfilling prophecies primarily helped or hurt students with high-bias teachers. Among students with high-bias teachers, if negative self-fulfilling prophecies were more powerful than positive self-fulfilling prophecies, then (1) low-expectancy students with high-bias teachers should consistently perform worse than such students with low-bias teachers; and (2) there should be little difference between the performances of high-expectancy students with high-bias or low-bias teachers.

This was not the case. There were three performance measures: sit-ups (for girls) and push-ups (for boys); distance jump; and speed. For sit-ups/push-ups, the power of negative and positive self-fulfilling prophecies was similar. The performance differences between low-expectancy students with low-bias and high-bias teachers were similar in magnitude to the performance differences between high-expectancy students with low-bias and high-bias teachers.

For the distance jump, negative self-fulfilling prophecies were more powerful than positive ones. Low-expectancy students with low-bias teachers jumped farther than such students with high-bias teachers, whereas high-expectancy students with high-bias teachers jumped the same distance as such students with low-bias teachers. For the speed measure, there was no evidence of self-fulfilling prophecies. The performances of low-expectancy students with low- and high-bias teachers were similar, indicating that negative self-fulfilling prophecies did not occur. High-expectancy students with high-bias teachers actually performed worse than such students with low-bias teachers, which may be an interesting effect of teacher bias, but does not represent a self-fulfilling prophecy.

Overall, therefore, Babad et al.'s (1982) results provide a decidedly mixed picture. Although they clearly did find evidence of negative self-fulfilling prophecies, they also found evidence of positive self-fulfilling prophecies. Their research provides no evidence that negative self-fulfilling prophecies are stronger than positive self-fulfilling prophecies.

There is a less frequently cited study that did test this hypothesis (Sutherland & Goldschmid, 1974). Their results indicated that negative expectations undermined the future IQ scores of high-IQ students, whereas positive expectations had no significant effects on the future IQ scores of low-IQ students. Although these results suggest that negative self-fulfilling prophecies are more powerful than positive ones, this study suffered from a serious methodological weakness: Specifically, negative expectations underestimated students more than positive expectations overestimated them. Thus the greater power of negative versus positive self-fulfilling prophecies that emerged may have reflected the greater inaccuracy of negative expectations in their particular sample, rather than any generally greater power of negative expectations.

Therefore, we recently reexamined the issue of whether negative or positive self-fulfilling prophecies are more powerful. Specifically, we examined this issue among students in sixth-grade math classes who had histories of either poor or good performance in school (Madon et al., 1997). Our results were quite provocative. In contrast to claims that self-fulfilling prophecies have mostly damaging effects on target outcomes, our results indicated that positive self-fulfilling prophecies were more powerful than negative ones. Positive teachers' expectations predicted greater improvements than negative expectations predicted decrements. Furthermore, these beneficial effects were most pronounced among students who were most highly stigmatized. Students with histories of poor performance actually improved more in response to positive expectations than did the performance of students with histories of high performance.

However, the news was not all good. When negative self-fulfilling prophecies did occur, they were more powerful among students with histories of poor performance than among student with histories of high performance. In fact, students with histories of high performance seemed to be inoculated against low teacher expectations: We had no evidence whatsoever of negative teacher expectations' undermining the future performance of such students. Thus, although self-fulfilling prophecies *on average* helped more than they hurt students, and although this pattern was particularly likely to benefit low achievers, it was also true that negative self-fulfilling prophecies were more likely to hurt low achievers than high achievers.

SOCIOLOGICAL SELF-FULFILLING PROPHECIES

Although self-fulfilling prophecies clearly occur in dyadic interactions, they may have only limited involvement in many of the deepest and most intractable social problems associated with stereotypes, prejudice, and discrimination. For example, the ghettoization of Jews in Europe, the Hindu caste system, American slavery, and South African apartheid could not have been maintained by the actions of a handful of individuals. In general, one private citizen, no matter how strong the stigma, cannot single-handedly force another to live in a ghetto unless there is considerable institutional support for such an action. Similarly, in dyadic interactions, if the target convinces perceivers to adopt a more accurate expectation, the potential for self-fulfilling prophecy is drastically reduced (Madon et al., 2000; Neuberg, 1989; Swann & Ely, 1984).

Because there has been little empirical research on self-fulfilling prophecies at the sociological level, this section of our chapter is neces-

sarily more discursive and speculative. However, we suspect that sociological self-fulfilling prophecies may be much more powerful and have
much more lasting effects than dyadic ones. Major institutions (government, businesses, churches, etc.) often do indeed have the power to "in-
stitutionalize" stigmas. For example, although slavery has been out-
lawed in the United States for 130 years, its after effects are still readily
apparent (segregation, wage disparities, etc.). Similarly, there is no longer apartheid in South Africa, but ethnic differences are still a major social problem for the country. Thus institutionalized stigmas often have
profound effects that last long after the institutional supports for those
stigmas have ended.

In fact, Merton's (1948) original article primarily discussed self-fulfilling prophecies as explanations for broad sociocultural patterns and
social problems. In this section, we review the limited empirical evidence
regarding sociocultural, institutional, and group-level self-fulfilling
prophecies. Even in the absence of hard scientific evidence, we attempt
to follow in Merton's (1948) original ground breaking footsteps by spec-
ulating on the potential involvement of self-fulfilling prophecies in some
broad social patterns and problems.

What Do We Mean by a "Sociological" or "Group" Level of Analysis?

The meaning of dyadic-level self-fulfilling prophecies is probably obvious: One person's initially erroneous beliefs lead to interactions with a
second person that evoke from that second person behaviors confirming
the first person's expectations. The nature of group-level self-fulfilling
prophecies may be less obvious (in this chapter, we use the terms
"group" and "sociological" to mean the same thing), especially because,
after all, groups are nothing but collections of many individuals. The
fundamental difference between the two is that self-fulfilling prophecies
at the sociological or group level require actions on the part of many
people (often in the form of cultural institutions). To help clarify this difference, we next present a few examples of sociological self-fulfilling
prophecies and discuss how they simply cannot be accounted for by
dyadic interactions.

Bank Failures

Some self-fulfilling prophecies require interactions between groups of
people (or between people and institutions). For example, let us assume
that Mary decides that the Last National Bank is having financial problems, when in fact the bank is perfectly solvent. Mary then removes all

her money (about $25,000) from Last National and places it in Suburban Bank of America. Because both these banks are huge and have assets in the billions, this one person's action has no effect on the solvency or profitability of either bank.

Now consider Merton's (1948) classic example of bank runs during the Great Depression. Somehow a false rumor starts that Small Town Bank is teetering on the brink of insolvency. Half of the depositors in Small Town then rush to remove their savings. Of course, like most profitable banks, Small Town does not keep half of its assets liquid. When the run starts, the bank is no longer able to pay its depositors, and it becomes insolvent. Note, however, that self-fulfilling this originally false rumor requires interaction between a mass of people and an institution.

Exclusion of African Americans from Unions

Consider another example—one closer to the focus of this chapter. Merton (1948) discussed how, in the early part of this century, most labor unions barred African Americans from membership. Union members often claimed that African Americans were strikebreakers and could not be trusted. This severely limited African Americans' job opportunities. When faced with a strike, companies often offered jobs to all takers, and African Americans often jumped at the chance for work. Thus the unions' beliefs about African Americans were confirmed. It is important to note, however, that if an individual union member, acting alone, held this stereotype of African Americans, it would have had no effect on African Americans' job opportunities.

Merton's (1948) examples involving bank failures and exclusion of African Americans from unions nicely illustrate the nature of sociological self-fulfilling prophecies, but they have little direct relevance to present-day American society. Do sociological self-fulfilling prophecies still contribute to social problems and the maintenance of social stigmas? Unfortunately, the empirical research addressing group-level self-fulfilling prophecies is extremely limited. Nonetheless, in the next section, we attempt to integrate research and theory from psychology, education, sociology, and. history in order to suggest that sociological self-fulfilling prophecies may be a powerful force in the maintenance of some social stereotypes.

Sociological Self-Fulfilling Prophecies and Stigma

School Tracking

"School tracking" refers to the policy of segregating students into different classes according to their ability. For example, smart students may be assigned to one class, average students to another, and slow students to a third. Tracking represents institutional justification for believing that some students are smart and others are not. Due to cultural beliefs regarding the meaning of low ability, particularly in math and science, it essentially provides students and teachers with an explanation for the students' low skill level that absolves both the students and the teachers of responsibility for continued learning. Thus it may lead to the types of rigid teacher expectations that are most likely to evoke self-fulfilling prophecies and perceptual biases (Eccles & Wigfield, 1985; Jussim, 1986, 1990).

In addition, poor-quality instruction may occur in at least some low-track courses. In part, this is a consequence of student characteristics. These classes are harder to manage, and traditional teaching techniques are not likely to be successful. But teachers' expectations can also exacerbate the poor environment. If teachers think that low-skill children cannot learn or do not want to learn, they may reduce their teaching efforts (Allington, 1980; Evertson, 1982)—which is exactly one type of behavior that often leads to self-fulfilling prophecies (Harris & Rosenthal, 1985). Thus tracking has been accused of creating a caste-like system that oppresses minorities and students from lower-SES backgrounds (Oakes, 1985; Rist, 1970).

We recently addressed these issues in a study of sixth-grade public school math classes (Smith et al., 1998). We examined whether self-fulfilling prophecies were more powerful for students in low tracks. Our results demonstrated that teachers' expectations were self-fulfilling primarily among students in low-ability groups. In addition, we also found that the achievement gap between students in low- and high-ability groups (within classrooms) increased over the course of the school year. Furthermore, teacher perceptions almost completely mediated this pattern of increasing differences. Our results suggest that expectancy effects may contribute to exacerbating the achievement gap between students in low- and high-ability groups.

However, the role of tracking in leading to such injustices is less clear than it might appear. Tracking is often intended to be a prosocial intervention. By putting students with similar capacities together, teachers have the opportunity to tailor their lessons in such a way as to maximize those students' learning and achievement. Furthermore, conclusions reached in several meta-analyses show that ability grouping generally has a positive effect on student attitudes and achievement. Although these meta-analyses demonstrate that high-ability groups benefit most from grouping programs, they also document positive effects of such programs for students from all ability levels (Feldhusen & Moon, 1992; Kulik & Kulik, 1982, 1987, 1992). Thus identifying whether tracking primarily helps students, or primarily leads to a caste system through institutional self-fulfilling prophecies, is an important question for future research.

Socioeconomic Status and Funding of Public Education

In many states throughout the United States, public schools are funded through local property taxes. This policy often leads to greater spending per pupil in upper-middle-class and wealthy areas than in working-class and poor areas (e.g., Firestone, Goertz, Nagle, & Smelkinson, 1994). Increased spending improves schools in several ways: It reduces the ratio of students to teachers; it allows schools to hire more highly qualified teachers; and it increases the number of professional support staff available to teachers and students, such as psychologists, counselors, and social workers (Bidwell & Kasarda, 1975). When the ratio of teachers to students is lower, and when teachers' qualifications are higher, students actually score higher on standardized achievement tests (Bidwell & Kasarda, 1975). It seems, therefore, that funding schools through property taxes creates a socioeconomic self-fulfilling prophecy at the sociological level: Students from lower-SES areas receive an education inferior to that received by students from middle- and upper-SES areas. The lower standardized test scores that result from lower spending will confirm socioeconomic stereotypes and reduce the chances that students from lower-SES backgrounds will be accepted into high-quality colleges. This in turn will reduce their occupational opportunities, thereby perpetuating their lower SES.

Stereotype Threat

Cultural stereotypes may take on a (self-fulfilling) life of their own. Even in the absence of individual racist or sexist perceivers, negative cultural stereotypes may become self-fulfilling: Their mere existence (or even perceived existence) may undermine the motivation and accomplishments of members of traditionally devalued groups. Steele (1992, 1997) has articulately argued that people who feel undervalued and "marked" by stigma are especially likely to feel threatened when faced with the prospect of being negatively stereotyped or evaluated in a stereotypic manner. Therefore, even if they do not fail more frequently than others, they are more likely to be psychologically devastated by such failures, leading them to "disidentify" with academic and occupational achievement. Next, therefore, we briefly review existing research on how negative cultural stereotypes may become self-fulfilling prophecies.

Women and Math. Several experiments have examined this process (called "stereotype threat"). One compared the performance of equally competent male and female college students on a difficult math test (Spencer & Steele, 1992). Participants were told either that the test usually reflected gender differences in math ability or that it did not. Presumably, the characterization of the test as reflecting gender differences would activate stereotype threat in female participants. Results showed that women and men performed equally well on the test when it was characterized as gender-neutral, but that women performed more poorly than men when the test was characterized as assessing skills at which males were better than females.

Race, Socioeconomic Status, and Intellectual Achievement. A recent series of studies examined the role of the stigma of African American intellectual inferiority in African American underachievement (Steele & Aronson, 1995). In one study, half the participants were informed that the test (which actually consisted of Graduate Record Examination study guide questions) was diagnostic of their "verbal ability." The other half were not given any diagnosticity information (they were told that the researchers were studying problem solving). Labeling the test as diagnostic of verbal ability was designed to activate the negative ability stereotype among African Americans. African Americans and Whites performed equally well when participants believed the test measured problem-solving skills, but African Americans performed more poorly than Whites when they believed the test measured verbal ability.

A nearly identical pattern occurred in another study, in which participants either did or did not indicate their race on another questionnaire before taking the test. A test difference between racial groups emerged only when participants wrote down their race. Another study showed that even a subtle activation of racial stereotypes (through a separate word completion task—see Steele & Aronson, 1995) aroused African American students' self-doubts and led them to avoid mentioning their race, but *only* when they believed the test was diagnostic of their ability.

The same pattern has been found in research using SES, rather than race, as the stigmatizing condition (Croizet & Claire, 1998). When researchers indicated that an exam tested intelligence, students from lower-SES backgrounds underperformed their middle-SES peers; when researchers indicated that the same exam tested problem solving, there was no SES difference in achievement.

Sometimes, however, activating stereotypes about one's group can be beneficial, at least if the stereotype is positive. Shih, Pittinsky, and

Ambady (1999) activated either the Asian or woman stereotype among a group of Asian women. They then administered questions from a standardized math test. Replicating Spencer and Steele (1992), they found that activating the female stereotype depressed these women's performance. Activating the Asian stereotype, in contrast, led to improved performance on the math test, presumably because of positive stereotypes regarding Asians and math.

Whites and the "Racist" Stigma. Although Steele's research has focused exclusively on African Americans and women, the stereotype threat notion may be applicable in a wide variety of domains and groups. As long as any particular group is stigmatized as possessing a negative attribute, individual members of that group may potentially be threatened by that stereotype.

For example, racism and prejudice have become increasingly socially undesirable over the last few decades. In short, racists have become stigmatized. We suspect that many Whites (even well-intentioned ones who are not racists in the classic sense) are aware of the history of their group's oppression of African Americans. Thus, when interacting with African Americans, many Whites may feel that they are under a cloud of "suspicion of racism." If not being racist is important to them, this suspicion may be highly threatening. It is at least possible that the tension and anxiety produced by this threat may then undermine the quality of their interactions with African Americans. When people in general are tense or anxious, they often appear less friendly, make more speech errors, and may end the interaction sooner (Stephan & Stephan, 1985). Thus when Whites who are most committed to not being racist find themselves in situations that raises the specter of racism, they may be particularly likely to show signs of coldness or hostility to African Americans (e.g., Weitz, 1972).

Of course, this is not to suggest that Whites cannot overcome the stigma and have warm and close relationships with African Americans. Just as there are many women who do succeed in math and science, and many African Americans who succeed in school, it is clear that the racist stigma need not necessarily undermine interracial interactions. But it is also likely that the racist stigma. adds yet another obstacle that needs to be overcome In Whites' interactions with people belonging to ethnic minority groups.

Stereotype Threat: Conclusions. One of the unique aspects of stereotype threat research is that it links cultural stereotypes with individual psychology. Indeed, one of Steele's (1997) articles is titled "A Threat in the Air," to capture the idea that the problem resides primarily in the culture that supports the negative stereotyping of some groups, rather than in the psyches of the victims. Neither Steele nor any of the other researchers engaged in stereotype threat research assume that the victims of stereotype threat necessarily *believe* in the validity of the negative stereotypes of their groups. Thus the problem is not that members of stigmatized groups subscribe to the negative views of their groups. The problem of reduced standardized test performance results from the damaging effects of the broader cultural stereotypes on those individuals.

CONCLUSION: ON THE POWER AND PERVASIVENESS OF STIGMA-INDUCED SELF-FULFILLING PROPHECIES

In this chapter, we have identified some of the ways that stigmas may lead to self-fulfilling prophecies. Most social-psychological research has focused on dyadic self-fulfilling prophecies—interactions between two individuals. Negative social stereotypes are one aspect of stigmas, and abundant research has demonstrated the self-fulfilling effects of a wide variety of social stereotypes in dyadic interactions, including those involving ethnicity, gender, SES, physical attractiveness, obesity, and ADHD. Similarly, much research at least suggests the possibility that prejudice, too, may at least sometimes trigger self-fulfilling interactions.

Nonetheless, we have also identified several important limitations of the role of stigmas in creating self-fulfilling prophecies. First, with the exception of gender, there has not been much empirical research on the self-fulfilling nature of specific social stereotypes. Because individual studies invariably have important limitations, and because only one or two studies have investigated particular stereotypes, whether most stereotypes regularly lead to self-fulfilling prophecies remains largely unknown.

Second, most of the naturalistic studies show that the self-fulfilling effect of stereotype-based expectations tends to be relatively small (about .2 or less, in terms of correlation and regression coefficients). Especially in conjunction with the considerable evidence showing that in general, perceivers judge targets far more on the basis of their personal characteristics than on the basis of their membership in social groups (for reviews, see Jussim, 1990, 1991; Kunda & Thagard, 1996), this suggests that the overall extent to which stigmas produce dyadic self-fulfilling prophecies is probably modest at best. The long-term maintenance of social stigmas probably involves factors considerably more powerful than dyadic self-fulfilling prophecies.

Self-fulfilling prophecies at the sociological level may be one such factor. Self-fulfilling prophecies involving political and institutional policies, and broad-based oppression of social-groups, may influence the educational and occupational opportunities of large numbers of people. We have suggested that school tracking may contribute to ethnic self-fulfilling prophecies; that funding schools through property taxes may contribute to SES self-fulfilling prophecies; and that some gender and racial stereotypes may be so threatening to many women and minorities, and so interwoven into the cultural fabric of present-day America, that they take on an often self-fulfilling life of their own.

Of course, empirical research on these types of sociological self-fulfilling prophecies is considerably more difficult than research on dyadic self-fulfilling prophecies. Consequently, the extent to which they serve to maintain and reinforce social stigmas may be unknowable. However, we suspect that at least sometimes such effects may be more powerful.

ACKNOWLEDGMENT

This research was supported by National Institute of Child Health and Human Development Grant No. 1 R29 HD28401-01A1 to Lee Jussim.

REFERENCES

Adorno, T., Frenkel-Brunswik, E., Levinson, D., & Sanford, R. N. (1950). *The authoritarian personality*. New York: Harper.

Allington, R. (1980). Teacher interruption behavior during primary grade oral reading. *Journal of Educational Psychology, 72,* 371–377.

Allon, M. (1982). The stigma of overweight in everyday life. In B. Wolman (Ed.), *Psychological aspects of obesity: A handbook* (pp. 130–174). New York: Van Nostrand Reinhold.

Allport, G. W. (1958). *The nature of prejudice.* Garden City, NY: Doubleday.

American Association of University Women. (1992). *How schools shortchange girls.* Washington, DC: American Association of University Women Education Foundation, National Education Association.

American Psychiatric Association. (1994). *Diagnostic and statistical manual of mental disorders* (4th ed.). Washington, DC: Author.

Anderson, S. M., & Bem, S. L. (1981). Sex typing and androgyny in dyadic interaction: Individual differences in responsiveness to physical attractiveness. *Journal of Personality and Social Psychology, 41,* 74–86.

Ashmore, R. D., & Del Boca, F. K. (1981). Conceptual approaches to stereotypes and stereotyping. In D. L. Hamilton (Ed.), *Cognitive processes in stereotyping and intergroup behavior* (pp. 1–35). Hillsdale, NJ: Erlbaum.

Babad, E., Inbar, J., & Rosenthal, R. (1982). Pygmalion, Galatea, and the Golem: Investigations of biased and unbiased teachers. *Journal of Educational Psychology, 74,* 459–474.

Bidwell, C. E., & Kasarda, J. D. (1975). School district organization and student achievement. *American Sociological Review, 40,* 55–70.

Brophy, J. (1983). Research on the self-fulfilling prophecy and teacher expecta-tions. *Journal of Educational Psychology, 75,* 631–661.

Brophy, J., & Good, T. (1974). *Teacher–student relationships: Causes and conse-quences.* New York: Holt, Rinehart & Winston.

Canning, H., & Mayer, J. (1966). Obesity: Its possible effect on college accep-tance. *New England Journal of Medicine, 275,* 1172–1174.

Chen, M., & Bargh, J. (1997). Nonconscious behavioral confirmation processes: The self-fulfilling consequences of automatic stereotype activation. *Journal of Experimental Social Psychology, 33,* 541–560.

Cooper, H., & Hazelrigg, P. (1988). Personality moderators of interpersonal ex-pectancy effects: An integrative research review. *Journal of Personality and Social Psychology, 55,* 937–949.

Crandall, C. (1991). Do heavyweight students have more difficulty paying for col-lege? *Personality and Social Psychology Bulletin, 17,* 606–611.

Crandall, C. (1995). Do parents discriminate against their heavyweight daughters? *Journal of Personality and Social Psychology, 21,* 724–735.

Crandall, C., & Biernat, M. (1990). The ideology of anti-fat attitudes. *Journal of Applied Psychology, 20,* 227–243.

Crocker, J., Major, B., & Steele, C. (1998). Social stigma. In D. T. Gilbert, S. T. Fiske, G. Lindzey (Eds.), *Handbook of social psychology* (4th ed., Vol. 2, pp. 504–553). New York: McGraw-Hill.

Croizet, J., & Claire, T. (1998). Extending the concept of stereotype and threat to social class: The intellectual underperformance of students from low socio-economic backgrounds. *Personality and Social Psychology Bulletin, 24,* 588–594.

Darley, J., & Fazio, R. H. (1980). Expectancy-confirmation processes arising in the social interaction sequence. *American Psychologist, 35,* 867–881.

Downey, G., & Feldman, S. (1996). Implications of rejection sensitivity for inti-mate relationships. *Journal of Personality and Social Psychology, 70,* 1327–1343.

Downey, G., Freitas, A. L., Michaelis, B., & Khouri, H. (1998). The self-fulfilling prophecy in close relationships: Rejection sensitivity and rejection by roman-tic partners. *Journal of Personality and Social Psychology, 75,* 545–560.

Doyle, W. J., Hancock, G., & Kifer, E. (1972). Teachers' perceptions: Do they make a difference? *Journal of the Association for the Study of Perception, 7,* 21–30.

Dusek, J., & Joseph, G. (1983). The bases of teacher expectancies: A meta-analy-sis. *Journal of Educational Psychology, 75,* 327–346.

Eagly, A., Ashmore, R., Makhijani, M., & Longo, L. C. (1991). What is beautiful is good, but . . . : A meta-analytic review of research on the physical attractive-ness stereotype. *Psychological Bulletin, 110,* 109–128.

Eagly, A., & Mladinic, A. (1989). Gender stereotypes and attitudes toward men and women. *Personality and Social Psychology Bulletin, 15,* 543–558.

Eccles, J., & Wigfield, A. (1985). Teacher expectations and student motivation. In J. Dusek (Ed.), *Teacher expectancies* (pp.185–226). Hillsdale, NJ: Erlbaum.

Elashoff, J. D., & Snow, R. E. (1971). *Pygmalion reconsidered.* Worthington, OH: Jones.

Evertson, C. (1982). Differences in instructional activities in higher and lower achieving junior high English and math classes. *Elementary School Journal, 82,* 329–350.

Farina, A. (1982). The stigma of mental disorders. In A. G. Miller (Ed.), *In the eye of the beholder: Contemporary issues in stereotyping* (pp. 305–362). New York: Praeger .

Farina, A., Allen, G., & Saul, B. (1968). The role of the stigmatized person in affecting social relationships. *Journal of Personality, 36,* 169–182.

Farina, A., Gliha, D., Boudreau, L. A., Allen, J. G., & Sherman, M. (1971). Mental illness and the impact of believing others know about it. *Journal of Abnormal Psychology, 77,* 1–5.

Feingold, A. (1992). Good-looking people are not what we think. *Psychological Bulletin, 111,* 304–341.

Feldhusen, J., & Moon, S. (1992). Grouping gifted students: Issues and concerns. *Gifted Child Quarterly, 36,* 63–67.

Firestone, W. A., Goertz, M. E., Nagle, B., & Smelkinson, M. F. (1994). Where did the $800 million go?: The first year of New Jersey's Quality Education Act. *Educational Evaluation and Policy Analysis, 16,* 359–373.

Fiske, S. T., & Taylor, S. E. (1984). *Social cognition.* Reading, MA: Addison-Wesley

Frieze, I. H., Olson, J. E., & Russell, J. (1991). Attractiveness and income for men and women in management. *Journal of Applied Social Psychology, 21,* 1039–1057.

Goffman, E. (1963). *Stigma: Notes on the management of spoiled identity.* Englewood Cliffs, NJ: Prentice-Hall.

Goldman, W ., & Lewis, P. (1977). Beautiful is good: Evidence that the physically attractive are more socially skillful. *Journal of Experimental Social Psychology, 13,* 125–130.

Goodman, N., Richardson, S., Dornbusch, S., & Hastorf, A. (1963). Variant reactions to physical disabilities. *American Sociological Review, 28,* 429–435.

Harris, M. J. (1989). Personality moderators of expectancy effects: Replication of Harris and Rosenthal (1986). *Journal of Research in Personality, 23,* 381–387.

Harris, M. J., Milich, R., Corbitt, E., Hoover, D., & Brady, M. (1992). Self-fulfilling effects of stigmatizing information on children's social interactions. *Journal of Personality and Social Psychology, 63,* 41–50.

Harris, M. J., Milich, R., Johnston, E., & Hoover, D. (1990). Effects of expectancies on children's social interactions. *Journal of Experimental Social Psychology, 26,* 1–12.

Harris, M. J., & Rosenthal, R. (1985). Mediation of interpersonal expectancy effects: 31 meta-analyses. *Psychological Bulletin, 97,* 363–386.

Hilton, J. L., & Darley, J. (1985). Constructing other persons: A limit on the effect. *Journal of Experimental Social Psychology, 21,* 1–18.

Hilton, J. L., & Darley, J. M. (1991). The effects of interaction goals on person perception. In M. P. Zanna (Ed.), *Advances in experimental social psychology* (Vol. 24, pp. 235–267). San Diego, CA: Academic Press.

Jacobs, J. E., & Eccles, J. S. (1992). The impact of mothers' gender-role stereotypic beliefs on mothers' and children's ability perceptions. *Journal of Personality and Social Psychology, 63,* 932–944.

Jones, E., Farina, A., Hastorf, A., Markus, H., Miller, D., & Scott, R. (1984). *Social stigma: The psychology of marked relationships.* New York: Freeman.

Jones, E. E. (1986). Interpreting interpersonal behavior: The effects of expectancies. *Science, 234,* 41–46.

Jones, E. E. (1990). *Interpersonal perception.* New York: Freeman.

Jost, J. T., & Banaji, M. R. (1994). The role of stereotyping in system-justification and the production of false consciousness. *British Journal of Social Psychology, 33,* 1–27.

Jussim, L. (1986). Self-fulfilling prophecies: A theoretical and integrative review. *Psychological Review, 93,* 429–445.

Jussim, L. (1990). Social reality and social problems: The role of expectancies. *Journal of Social Issues, 46,* 9–34.

Jussim, L. (1991). Social perception and social reality: A reflection-construction model. *Psychological Review, 98,* 54–73.

Jussim, L., Coleman, L., & Lerch, L. (1987). The nature of stereotypes: A comparison and integration of three theories. *Journal of Personality and Social Psychology, 52,* 536–546.

Jussim, L., & Eccles, J. (1995). Naturalistic studies of interpersonal expectancies. *Review of Personality and Social Psychology, 15,* 74–108.

Jussim, L., Eccles, J., & Madon, S. (1996). Social perception, social stereotypes, and teacher expectations: Accuracy and the quest for the powerful self-fulfilling prophecy. In M. P. Zanna (Ed.), *Advances in experimental social psychology* (Vol. 28, pp. 281–388). San Diego, CA: Academic Press.

Jussim, L., Madon, S., & Chatman, C. (1994). Teacher expectations and student achievement: Self-fulfilling prophecies, biases, and accuracy. In L. Heath, R. S. Tindale, J. Edwards, E. J. Posavac, F. B. Bryant, E. Henderson-King, Y. Suarez-Balcazar, & J. Myers (Eds.), *Applications of heuristics and biases to social issues* (pp. 303–334). New York: Plenum Press.

Jussim, L., McCauley, C. R., & Lee, Y. T. (1995). Why study stereotype accuracy and inaccuracy? In Y. T. Lee, L. Jussim, & C. R. McCauley (Eds.), *Stereotype accuracy: Toward appreciating group differences* (pp. 3–28). Washington, DC: American Psychological Association.

Jussim, L., Nelson, T., Manis, M., & Soffin, S. (1995). Prejudice, stereotypes, and labeling effects: Sources of bias in person perception. *Journal of Personality and Social Psychology, 68,* 228–246.

Jussim, L., Smith, A., Madon, S., & Palumbo, P. (1998). Teacher expectations. In J. Brophy (Ed.), *Advances in research on teaching* (Vol. 7, pp. 1–48). Greenwich, CT: JAI Press.

Kimball, M. M. (1989). A new perspective on women's math achievement. *Psychological Bulletin, 105,* 198–214.

Kleck, R., & Strenta, A. (1980). Perceptions of the impact of negatively valued physical characteristics on social interactions. *Journal of Personality and Social Psychology, 39,* 861–873.

Kulik, C., & Kulik, J. (1982). Effects of ability grouping on secondary school students: A meta-analysis of evaluation findings. *American Educational Research Journal, 19,* 415–428.

Kulik, J., & Kulik, C. (1987). Effects of ability grouping on student achievement. *Equity and Excellence, 23,* 22–30.

Kulik, J., & Kulik, C. (1992). Meta-analytic findings on grouping programs. *Gifted Children, 36,* 73–77.

Kunda, Z., & Thagard, P. (1996). Forming impressions from stereotypes, traits, and behaviors: A parallel-constraint-satisfaction theory. *Psychological Bulletin, 103,* 284–308.

Lareau, A. (1987). Social-class differences in family–school relationships: The importance of cultural capital. *Sociology of Education, 60,* 73–85.

Larkin,J., & Pines, H. (1979). No fat persons need apply. *Sociology of Work and Occupations, 6,* 312–327.

Madon, S., Jussim, L., & Eccles, J. (1997). In search of the powerful self-fulfilling prophecy. *Journal of Personality and Social Psychology, 72,* 791–809.

Madon, S. J., Smith, A., Walkiewicz, M., Jussim, L., Eccles, J., & Palumbo, P . (2000). *A naturally-occurring battle of wills: Self-fulfilling prophecies versus self-verification in the classroom.* Manuscript submitted for publication.

Marger, M. N. (1991). *Race and ethnic relations* (2nd ed.). Belmont, CA: Wadsworth.

McCauley, C., & Stitt, C. L. (1978). An individual and quantitative measure of stereotypes. *Journal of Personality and Social Psychology, 36,* 929–940.

Merton, R. K. (1948). The self-fulfilling prophecy. *Antioch Review, 8,* 193–210.

Miller, C., Rothblum, E., Barbour, L., Brand, P., & Felicio, D. (1990). Social interactions of obese and nonobese women. *Journal of Personality, 58,* 365–380.

Miller, D. T., & Turnbull, W. (1986). Expectancies and interpersonal processes. *Annual Review of Psychology, 37,* 233–256.

Millman, M. (1980). *Such a pretty face: Being fat in America.* New York: Norton.

Neuberg, S. L. (1989). The goal of forming accurate impressions during social interactions: Attenuating the impact of negative expectancies. *Journal of Personality and Social Psychology, 56,* 374–386.

Neuberg, S. L. (1994). Expectancy-confirmation processes in stereotype-tinged social encounters: The moderating role of social goals. In M. P. Zanna & J. M. Olson (Eds.), *The Ontario Symposium: Vol. 7. The psychology of prejudice* (pp. 103–130). Hillsdale, NJ: Erlbaum.

Oakes, J. (1985). *Keeping track: How schools structure inequality.* New Haven, CT: Yale University Press.

Palardy, J. M. (1969). What teachers believe—what children achieve. *Elementary School Journal, 69,* 370–374.

Pettigrew, T. F. (1979). The ultimate attribution error: Extending Allport's cognitive analysis of prejudice. *Personality and Social Psychology Bulletin, 5,* 461–476.

Raudenbush, S. W. (1984) Magnitude of teacher expectancy effects on pupil IQ as a function of the credibility of expectancy inductions: A synthesis of findings from 18 experiments. *Journal of Educational Psychology, 76,* 85–97

Rist, R. (1970): Student social class and teacher expectations: The self-fulfilling prophecy in ghetto education. *Harvard Educational Review, 40,* 411–451.

Rist, R., & Harrell, J. E. (1982). Labeling the learning disabled child: The social ecology of educational practice. *American Journal of Orthopsychiatry, 52,* 146–160.

Rosenhan, D. (1973). On being sane in insane places. *Science, 179,* 250–258.

Rosenthal, R. (1974). *On the social psychology of the self-fulfilling prophecy: Further evidence for Pygmalion effects and their mediating mechanisms.* New York: MSS Modular.

Rosenthal, R. (1989, August). *Experimenter expectancy, covert communication, and meta-analytic methods.* Invited address presented at the 97th Annual Convention of the American Psychological Association, New Orleans, LA.

Rosenthal, R., & Jacobson, L. (1968a). *Pygmalion in the classroom: Teacher expectations and student intellectual development.* New York: Holt, Rinehart & Winston.

Rosenthal, R., & Jacobson L. (1968b). Teacher expectations for the disadvantaged. *Scientific American, 218,* 19–23.

Rosenthal, R., & Lawson, R. (1964). A longitudinal study of the effects of experimenter bias on the operant learning of laboratory rats. *Journal of Psychiatric Research, 2,* 61–72.

Rosenthal, R., & Rubin, D. B. (1978). Interpersonal expectancy effects: The first 345 studies. *Behavioral and Brain Sciences, 3,* 377–386.

Ross, L. (1977). The intuitive psychologist and his shortcomings: Distortions in the attribution process. In L. Berkowitz (Ed.), *Advances in experimental social psychology* (Vol. 10, pp. 173-220). New York: Academic Press.

Rothblum, E., Brand, P., Miller, C., & Oetjen, H. (1990). The relationship between obesity, employment discrimination, and employment-related victimization. *Journal of Vocational Behavior, 37,* 251–266.

Rowe, D. C. (1995, Jan. 2). Intervention fables. *New York Times,* p. A25.

Shih, M., Pittinsky, T. L., & Ambady, N. (1999). Stereotype susceptibility: Identity, salience, and shifts in quantitative performance. *Psychological Science, 10,* 80–83.

Sibicky, M., & Dovidio, J. (1986). Stigma of psychological therapy: Stereotypes, interpersonal reactions, and the self-fulfilling prophecy. *Journal of Counseling Psychology, 33,* 148–154.

Skrypnek, B. J., & Snyder, M. (1982). On the self-perpetuating nature of stereotypes about women and men. *Journal of Experimental Social Psychology, 18,* 277–291.

Smith, A., Jussim, L., Eccles, J., Van Noy, M., Madon, S., & Palumbo, P. (1998). Self-fulfilling prophecies, perceptual biases, and accuracy at the individual and group level. *Journal of Experimental Social Psychology, 34,* 530–561.

Smith, D. M., Neuberg, S. L., Judice, T. N., & Biesanz, J. C. (1997). Target complicity in the confirmation and disconfirmation of erroneous perceiver expectations: Immediate and longer term implications. *Journal of Personality and Social Psychology, 73,* 974–991.

Snyder, M. (1984). When belief creates reality. In L. Berkowitz (Ed.), *Advances in experimental social psychology* (Vol. 18, pp. 247–305). New York: Academic Press.

Snyder, M. (1992). Motivational foundations of behavioral confirmation. In M. P. Zanna (Ed.), *Advances in experimental social psychology* (Vol. 25, pp. 67–114). San Diego, CA: Academic Press.

Snyder, M., Tanke, E. D., & Berscheid, E. (1977). Social perception and interpersonal behavior; On the self-fulfilling nature of social stereotypes. *Journal of Personality and Social Psychology, 35,* 656–666.

Sobal, J., & Stunkard, A. J. (1989). Socioeconomic status and obesity: A review of the literature. *Psychological Bulletin, 105,* 260–275.

Spencer, S. J., & Steele, C. M. (1992). *The effect of stereotype vulnerability on women's math performance.* Paper presented at the 100th Annual Convention of the American Psychological Association, Washington, DC.

Staffieri, R. (1967). A study of social stereotype of body image in children. *Journal of Personality and Social Psychology, 7,* 101–104.

Steele, C. (1992, April). Race and the schooling of Black Americans. *The Atlantic Monthly,* pp. 68–78.

Steele, C. (1997). A threat in the air: How stereotypes shape intellectual identity and performance. *American Psychologist, 52,* 613–629.

Steele, C., & Aronson, J. (1995). Stereotype threat and the intellectual test performance of African Americans. *Journal of Personality and Social Psychology, 69,* 797–811.

Stephan, W., & Stephan, C. (1985). Intergroup anxiety. *Journal of Social Issues 41,* 157–175.

Sutherland, A., & Goldschmid, M. L. (1974). Negative teacher expectation and IQ change in children with superior intellectual potential. *Child Development, 45,* 852–856.

Swann, W., Jr., & Ely, R. (1984). A battle of wills: Self-verification versus behavioral confirmation. *Journal of Personality and Social Psychology, 46,* 1287–1302.

vonBaeyer, C. L., Sherk, D. L., & Zanna, M. P. (1981). Impression management in the job interview: When the female applicant meets the male (chauvinist) interviewer. *Personality and Social Psychology Bulletin, 7,* 45–51.

Wadden, T., Foster, G., Brownell, K., & Finley, E. (1984). Self-concept in obese and normal-weight children. *Journal of Consulting and Clinical Psychology, 52,* 1104–1105.

Wadden, T., & Stunkard, A. (1985). Social and psychological consequences of obesity. *Annals of Internal Medicine, 103,* 1062–1067.

Weitz, S. (1972). Attitude, voice, and behavior: A repressed affect model of interracial interaction. *Journal of Personality and Social Psychology, 24,* 14–21.

Williams, T. (1976). Teacher prophecies and the inheritance of inequality. *Sociology of Education, 49,* 223–236.

Wineburg, S. S. (1987). The self-fulfillment of the self-fulfilling prophecy. *Educational Researcher, 16,* 28–37.

Word, C. O., Zanna, M. P., & Cooper, J. (1974). The nonverbal mediation of self-fulfilling prophecies in interracial interaction. *Journal of Experimental Social Psychology, 10,* 109–120.

Zanna, M. P., & Pack, S. J. (1975). On the self-fulfilling nature of apparent sex differences in behavior. *Journal of Experimental Social Psychology, 11,* 583–591.

14

The Social Consequences of Physical Disability

MICHELLE R. HEBL
ROBERT E. KLECK

Early in one of our seminar courses on stigma, a White male student stated that he was lucky because he would never have to deal with a stigma and its terrible social consequences. After a few weeks in the course, however, he recognized his potentially erroneous thinking. There was a very strong likelihood that at some point in his life, he would gain firsthand experience with the consequences of being stigmatized: He would probably someday join the ranks of physically limited or disabled individuals. Even if he were able to dodge diseases and avoid traumas and accidents during the majority of his life, he would at least experience the negative attitudes and discriminatory behavior associated with old age in this society (Jette, 1996; see also Zebrowitz & Montepare, Chapter 12, this volume). In short, many of the social dynamics discussed in this volume will confront most of us at some point in our lives (see McNeil, 1993), even though we currently may not be members of a minority group or "marked" (Jones et al., 1984) by a characteristic that our culture devalues.

This chapter considers the stigmas associated with the various forms of physical limitations and disabilities that either do or will confront many of us, and that influence our social interactions and outcomes. Although the traditional symbol of physical disability in Western society is a person in a wheelchair, this stigma category is actually very broad. As Karp (1999) points out, even those who use a wheelchair do so for a wide range of reasons, including amyotrophic lateral sclerosis, amputations, Friedrich's ataxia, cerebral palsy, muscular dystrophy, myasthenia gravis, polio, rheumatoid arthritis, spina bifida, spinal cord injury, spinal muscular atrophy, a stroke, traumatic brain injury, age-related mobility impairment, and temporary impairment (e.g., a broken leg). Furthermore, one caveat that must be entered at the outset is the need for caution in generalizing across specific forms of physical disabilities. As we will see later, the important social-psychological consequences of any particular type or form of disability may depend upon how visually obvious the disability is, the degree to which visibility draws attention, the perceived conditions of onset of the disability, and the amount of effort disabled individuals must devote to overcoming their physical limitations. Given the current state of empirical research on physical disability, we know less concerning these moderating factors than we would like to, and much of what we do know is limited to persons who use wheelchairs.

In this chapter we begin by discussing the nonequitable and dysfunctional interaction outcomes that have been observed to occur for physically disabled individuals. In addition to discussing dyadic-level interactions and outcomes, we discuss the societal constraints (e.g., biased terminology) and environmental constraints (e.g., no ramps, no curb cuts) that influence the life outcomes of physically limited individuals but are largely perceived as irrelevant by those in our society who do not share those physical limitations. Next, we discuss how social outcomes are influenced by the specific dimensions associated with a given physical disability. For instance, those who have visible stigmas may be more negatively affected both in social interactions and in societal-level functioning than those who have nonobvious or invisible stigmas may be. We then consider people's attributions and theories concerning stigmas from the perspectives of both disabled and nondisabled individuals, who interact together in what Goffman (1963) termed "spoiled interactions." Finally, we will discuss a number of possible strategies for "unspoiling" disabled–nondisabled social interactions. In this chapter, we do not exhaustively review the physical disabilities literature, but rather use selected elements of this body of research for illustrative purposes.

NONEQUITABLE/DYSFUNCTIONAL INTERACTION OUTCOMES

Autobiographical memoirs and extensive empirical research show strong, consistent evidence that individuals with physical disabilities experience social interactions that are problematic on a number of dimensions. Poignant first-person accounts suggest that people without disabilities stare at, laugh at, direct jokes toward, overcompensate their dislike with feigned hospitality toward, or (perhaps worst of all) simply ignore people who have physical disabilities (Charlton, 1998; Goffman, 1963; Hockenberry, 1995; Karp, 1999; Kleege, 1999). One behavior that is particularly disturbing to those with physical limitations is the tendency for others to want to assist them in various situations without being asked. Hockenberry (1995), a news correspondent and journalist who is partially paralyzed, has described how insulting this can be. Although others believe they are helping, such "helpful" actions remove an individual's autonomy and are frequently associated with expressions of pity and nervousness. Similarly, Karp (1999) wrote that those with disabilities often feel as if being helped is synonymous with being the target of someone's "good deed for the day." Furthermore, when one pushes the wheelchair of another person, for example, the normal physical context of the interaction between two people is disrupted. Rather than walking abreast, two friends become a "helper" and a "helpee"; eye contact and reciprocity of nonverbal behaviors are lost; and the nature of the interaction can change dramatically, often to the disadvantage of the person in the wheelchair.

First-person accounts and casual observations have obvious limits as methods for analyzing the nature of the social lives of physically limited individuals and of stigmatized persons generally. These accounts do tell us a great deal concerning how such persons perceive their interactions, but they neglect the transactional nature of stigmatizing processes. In our view, a full understanding of the nature of these processes is greatly facilitated through a careful analysis of what actually transpires when stigmatized people interact with nonstigmatized people (see Archer, 1985, for a similar point of view).

Empirical studies conducted on such mixed interactions also provide consistent evidence of the nonequitable/dysfunctional outcomes. For instance, in one of the earliest studies on social interactions involving physical disability, Kleck, Ono, and Hastorf (1966) examined the behavior of individuals interviewing a confederate who either did or did not use a wheelchair. The findings revealed that participants were more physiologically aroused during the interaction, took a longer time deciding what interview questions to ask, terminated the interview sooner, and showed more behavioral inhibition when interacting with a physically disabled versus a nondisabled individual. In addition, participants were more likely to distort their own personal opinions in a direction consistent with the opinions thought to be held by the other individual if that individual was physically disabled rather than nondisabled.

Further studies in this program of research revealed similarly biased and avoidant behaviors toward individuals with physical disabilities. In-dividuals who were not disabled exhibited reduced motoric behavior (Kleck, 1968b), displayed reduced gestural behavior (Kleck, 1968a), and stood at greater speaking distances (Kleck, 1969; Sigelman, Adams, Meeks, & Purcell, 1986) when interacting with a physically disabled versus a nondisabled individual. Similarly, parents with children tended to stand closer to their children, seemingly in a protective gesture, when interviewing with a physically disabled versus a nondisabled individual (Sigelman et al., 1986). Finally, perhaps the most important finding of this research was that if their motives could go undetected, nondisabled individuals chose to avoid interactions with physically disabled individu-als altogether (Snyder, Kleck, Strenta, & Mentzer, 1979).

If mixed interactions cannot be avoided, however, severe communi-cation difficulties may result. Gouvier, Coon, Todd, and Fuller (1994) examined language directed toward either a physically disabled or a nondisabled individual who requested information from strangers. Indi-viduals with disabilities were addressed in simpler language, more ap-propriate to interactions with children. Additional content analysis in another study revealed that individuals with disabilities were evaluated more stringently for poor task performance (Russell et al., 1985). Fur-thermore, they received inaccurate verbal feedback and were accorded personality impressions that were overly positive (Hastorf, Northcraft, & Picciotto, 1979). Although this pattern of behavior is consistent with a "be kind to the handicapped" norm and may initially seem supportive and helpful to disabled individuals (see Siller, 1986), the inaccurate na-ture of the social feedback leaves them with false impressions and may be competence-debilitating.

One particularly interesting set of results in this early interaction re-search yielded a consistent discrepancy between the verbal and nonver-bal behaviors of individuals interacting with physically stigmatized oth-ers. For instance, in a combined person perception and interactional study (Kleck, 1969), able-bodied participants taught origami (Japanese paper folding) to a person who did or did not use a wheelchair. Though participants reported very positive impressions of the physically disabled learner and of her performance, they at the same time displayed nonver-bal behavior suggesting anxiety and avoidance. This inconsistency led Kleck and his colleagues to advance a two-factor theory to account for such discrepancies (Kleck et al., 1966; Kleck, 1969). On the one hand, behaviors readily under the control of a nondisabled individual (e.g., speech content) tended to conform to the normative pressure to be "kind" to physically disabled individuals. On the other hand, overt non-verbal behaviors tended to be unresponsive to this norm, presumably be-cause many such behaviors are not under voluntary control or are not being as carefully monitored as are verbal statements (see Heinemann, Pellander, Vogelbusch, & Wojtek, 1981).

There are a number of reasons why these more "automatic" behaviors are negatively connoted. First, they may reflect an underlying negative affective disposition toward physically disabled individuals that cannot be masked as easily as it is in the case of verbal statements (see Dovidio, Kawakami, Johnson, Johnson, & Howard, 1997, for a related distinction between implicit and explicit measures). Second, the behaviors may reflect an anxiety and uncertainty that is not based in social rejection, but rather stems from the uncertainty felt by nonstigmatized individuals as a consequence of limited interaction experience with physically disabled people (e.g., Langer, Fiske, Taylor, & Chanowitz, 1976). Third, people simply may be curious about physical variations in others, particularly those they do not encounter frequently (Zebrowitz-McArthur, 1982). Their desire to stare at or visually examine a disabled person may be at odds with the learned behavioral norm of not treating an individual with a disability differently from a nondisabled one. Whatever the reason, the important point is that expressed attitudes toward physically limited individuals and the nature of the behavior displayed toward them do not readily map onto one another. Whether physically stigmatized persons detect these inconsistencies and, if so, what meaning they attribute to them are neglected issues in this line of research. Further empirical research is necessary to better understand the implications of these discrepancies.

It could be argued that the use of an experimental paradigm in which confederates play the role of physically disabled persons seriously distorts what happens in everyday encounters between such persons and nondisabled individuals. It would be reasonable to expect that over time the stigmatized individuals would develop ways of overcoming the sorts of biases they confront in social interactions. Early research by Comer and Piliavin (1972) suggests that this is in fact unlikely. When truly disabled individuals were observed in interactions with a physically able confederate, they also terminated the interview sooner, were more inhibited in their motor movements, and engaged in less eye contact than when they interacted with an interviewer in a wheelchair. Thus, rather than displaying compensatory behaviors that might serve to "normalize" the interaction, the stigmatized individuals engaged in behaviors that would appear to exacerbate its dysfunctional nature. We return later in the chapter to the issue of whether there are interactional strategies that physically stigmatized individuals can adopt to mitigate unwanted social outcomes.

The research literature specifically focusing on interaction outcomes for those with physical disabilities is admittedly small. However, what has been done does confirm that these outcomes are less than optimal, at least in initial encounters, and that physically stigmatized individuals do not readily display interactional strategies to overcome the dysfunctional aspects of such interactions. Not only do physically disabled people show a lack of compensatory behavior in social interaction, but they also show a tendency to perceive even neutral behaviors displayed by nondisabled individuals as discriminatory actions against their stigmatized status. Kleck and Strenta (1980), for example, had individuals who had had cosmetic scars applied to their faces interact with another subject. Unbeknownst to the "scarred" individuals, the scars were actually removed prior to the interaction under the pretext that the experimenter was putting the final touches on the makeup job. When asked to interpret the interactants' responses, those who believed they had scars were much more likely to report behavioral discrimination and negativity than were the control individuals who never had such scars applied in the first place.

Similarly, Strenta and Kleck (1985) had nondisabled and physically disabled participants view a videotape of a person supposedly in a wheelchair interacting with a nonstigmatized individual. They were asked to describe whether and to what extent the disability affected various aspects of the behavior of the nonstigmatized individual. Unknown to the perceivers, the videotapes were constructed in such a way that both participants in the interaction were physically normal and holding a spontaneous conversation. Both paraplegic perceivers and those without a disability believed that the presence of a disabled individual in the interaction had a significantly debilitating effect on the social interaction. In particular, they perceived the nonstigmatized individual as being more tense, liking the interactant less, finding the interactant less attractive, and behaving in a more patronizing manner than when they presumed that neither individual was physically stigmatized. In short, perceivers readily found evidence to confirm negative reactions to a stigma when no such reactions could exist. Thus, although in many cases negative reactions do occur, this study showed that individuals' presumptions about what is happening in a social interaction may contribute to interactional difficulties and may lead to a social reality all their own (see Snyder, Tanke, & Berscheid, 1977; see also Jussim, Palumbo, Chatman, Madon, & Smith, Chapter 13, this volume).

SOCIETAL AND ENVIRONMENTAL CONSTRAINTS

One of the most basic societal constraints that physically disabled individuals experience is the very nature of the language our society uses to describe them. These labels typically depict them as second-class citizens who are tainted, sick, and less than whole. For instance, they are described as being "afflicted," "stricken," "deformed," or "invalids." Even "disabled" suggests an inability to measure up to some appropriate level—that is, being "not able." The commonly used dichotomy of "handicapped" and "normal" starkly denotes mutual exclusiveness, in that "handicapped" people are *not* "normal." Euphemisms such as "differently able" and "physically challenged or limited" are hardly better, and people with disabilities do not prefer these labels to others. There is no general answer as to how best to treat the language problem, except to address individuals less in terms of their disabilities and more in terms of their personhood (for a fuller discussion of this "naming" issue, see Johnson, 1994). That is, individuals are sometimes simply referred to as "the disabled" or "the handicapped," and tend to be identified by their stigmas rather than as people who have many behavioral and physical features, only one of which happens to involve using a wheelchair or otherwise being physically different. A statement by an individual with cerebral palsy, as quoted by Karp (1999), particularly identifies how language constrains those with disabilities:

> My name is not cerebral palsy. There's a lot more to me than my disability and the problems surrounding it. That's what I call the disability trap. This country has a telethon mentality toward disability that thinks disabled people are not supposed to talk about anything but their disabilities. (p. 165)

If the language used by physically able others serves to constrain and one-dimensionalize disabled individuals, so also does a physical environment constructed largely without thought given to the physical limitations of many of its inhabitants. As described by Pelka (1997), some of the most limiting environmental constraints for mobility-impaired people include the fact that in many public places there are no elevators, chairs at tables are often immobile, thresholds between rooms are raised too dramatically for passage, tables are placed too closely together, and the access to restroom facilities is blocked. Furthermore, there are contrasting lips on doorways; a general lack of sidewalk curb cuts; an absence of accommodating ramps; and a lack of adequate clearance space in doors, halls, and entryways. Similarly, a short venture around the block often leads to an encounter with automobiles parked on the street blocking access to curbside ramps or the entire sidewalk, or with snow-embanked sidewalks left unshoveled by homeowners.

Although federal regulations have resulted in a dramatic reduction of these unwitting constraints, which serve as constant reminders that one is physically different, "disability" is in many respects still as much a function of the environment as it is a function of the capabilities of those who inhabit it. From a social-psychological perspective, an environment that is not readily accessible, or that requires unusual amounts of energy, thought, or preparation to navigate, becomes an environment that exacerbates one's self-awareness of the disability and a general sense of incompetence. Social psychology has been remiss for not more carefully examining the ways in which simple architectural barriers may contribute to the stigmatizing effects of physical disabilities of all sorts. At the very least, architectural barriers seriously inhibit physically limited individuals from pursuing a more active social life. Furthermore, such barriers may facilitate psychological dynamics in such individuals that heighten a focus on their shortcomings rather than their competencies.

DIMENSIONS OF DISABILITY STIGMAS

The interaction outcomes and environmental constraints that we have discussed thus far are obviously not constant across all sorts of physical disabilities and all social contexts (see Jones et al., 1984). A woman who has lost her leg in a car accident that she caused but who has a very realistic-looking and functional prosthesis, for example, may be in a very different physical and psychological situation than is a man who was born without the use of his limbs and must use his mouth to ambulate his wheelchair. These two instances differ on a variety of dimensions, but here we focus on three that appear to be particularly influential in determining the daily interaction outcomes and social lives of physically disabled individuals.

First, whether a stigma is immediately "visible" or "invisible" has long been recognized as important in determining the outcomes associated with a particular mark. Goffman (1963) divided individuals who possess stigmas into those with "discrediting" (visible) and those with "discreditable" (invisible) stigmas. Discrediting conditions include, for example, having facial scars, port-wine birthmarks, or physical deformities. According to Goffman, these stigmas are difficult to manage because their possessers live in "glass houses," so to speak; that is, something very personal and potentially self-defining is immediately known to others in any face-to-face interaction. The "discreditable" stigmas are also difficult to manage, but for very different reasons. These individuals must decide to whom, when, and how they should disclose information about their stigmas. They report risking rejection when the moment of revelation comes and hence are often motivated, in Goffman's (1963) terms, to "pass," or to keep their stigmas a secret and act as though they do not possess them. Examples of these conditions include homosexuality, epilepsy, and wearing a colostomy bag. Several researchers (e.g., Crocker & Major, 1994; Jones et al., 1984; Kleck, 1968c) have noted the importance of the visibility–invisibility dimension in predicting interaction outcomes, self-esteem, and overall social functioning. The empirical results consistently point to the conclusion that disabled individuals with invisible or hidden stigmas have less problematic or anxiety-provoking social interactions than do those with visible stigmas (but see Smart & Wegner, Chapter 8, this volume, for some of the "hidden costs" associated with the former).

A second important dimension of stigma is whether the disability is perceived as "controllable" or "uncontrollable." Research by Weiner and colleagues (Weiner, 1995; Weiner, Magnusson, & Perry, 1988) reveals that physical disabilities are largely thought to be uncontrollable—a perception that results in nonstigmatized people's according positivity, sympathy, and empathy to the bearers of such stigmas. This is in contrast to stigmas perceived to be controllable (e.g., child abuse, obesity, homosexuality), toward which people tend to feel more hostility and negativity. Even within physical disabilities, we (Hebl & Kleck, 2000) have shown that when a disability can be attributed to factors beyond a disabled individual's control (e.g., a doctor's mistake), much more positive affect, personality attributes, and skills are accorded to the individual than when the individual is perceived to have brought on the condition him- or herself. Such findings replicate those obtained in AIDS research. For example, people who contract AIDS through sexually promiscuous and controllable behaviors are reacted to less positively than those who contract it through less controllable circumstances such as having blood transfusions (Graham, Weiner, Giuliano, & Williams, 1995).

The controllability dimension is strongly related to the social theories of entitlement that people develop around the issue of stigmas. For instance, beliefs in the Protestant work ethic (Weber, 1904–1905) affirm the notion that people get what they deserve and deserve what they get. If a disabled individual is perceived to have brought on the condition him- or herself, it is generally easier to attribute the presence of the disability to something he or she deserved. There is more dissonance in people's minds if the individual is perceived as not responsible for the disability onset, and people often continue to create or attach some blame on the disabled individual's part.

A third feature to consider is the extent to which the disability is mobility-impairing. In our earlier example, the woman with the prosthetic leg can maneuver herself almost anywhere. She is not limited by the absence of curb cuts, ramps, and elevators, as is the quadriplegic individual. The ease of mobility has not only physical ramifications but psychological and social consequences. A person with severe mobility constraints typically needs to plan well in advance, because going out for a simple meal or running an errand may turn into an all-day ordeal. In addition, in every encounter the person is faced with the challenge of other people staring, questioning, and wondering, and of thus being constantly reminded of the stigma.

ATTRIBUTIONS AND THEORIES ABOUT STIGMAS

Both stigmatized and nonstigmatized individuals tend to have expectations concerning their interaction partners and perceptions of the roles they themselves play in mixed interactions. However, these expectations and perceived roles differ across the two perspectives. For nonstigmatized perceivers, a large focus of their attention is placed on defining or redefining their own sense of identity. An individual with a physical disability often experiences a change of personhood (Riches, 1996; Wright, 1983), and this is particularly true if the individual has not had the disability for his or her entire life. As disability psychologist Carol Gill (qtd. in Karp, 1999, p. 162) states, "When you become a member of the group that you have previously felt fear of or pity for, you can't help but turn those feelings on yourself." It is little wonder that many individuals wish to retain their old identities and reject the acceptance offered by other individuals who are disabled. Part of the difficulty may be that the psychological and physical adjustments are suddenly thrust onto an individual, who must all too quickly develop strong coping skills. But, typically, those with disabilities first go through a range of strong emotions—including denial, anger, depression, grief, suicidal feelings, hope, and finally acceptance. On a more positive note, Schontz (1990) states that people are notoriously adaptive and can live with all sorts of difficulties and discomforts if they feel there is a good reason for doing so. If physically disabled people focus less rigidly on their disabilities and resulting body image problems, their lives do not necessarily become narrowed and restricted. Adjustment is possible, and people may even derive a number of benefits (e.g., increased meaning in life, self-assuredness, compassion, and awareness) from having a physical disability (Elliott, Witty, Herrick, & Hoffman, 1991; Taylor, 1983).

For nonstigmatized perceivers, their perspective may involve the elicitation of stereotypes and stigma schemas. Such cognitive heuristics may be particularly likely when little else is known about a person with a disability, relative to when a great deal is known. One particular set of expectations and behaviors that nonstigmatized people fall prey to is called "self-fulfilling prophecies," whereby the expectations that they have for disabled individuals actually cause them to treat disabled individuals in ways that create the expected social reality (see Merton, 1948). For instance, people may perceive disabled individuals to be childlike and naive. This expectation may lead people to treat disabled individuals in ways that a parent might teach a child; for instance, they may speak with more authority and dominance, and may be overly patient and responsive. As a result, the disabled individuals may come to need more direction, allow more invasions of privacy, ask more questions, and require more help. In essence, the disabled individuals are unwittingly conforming to the beliefs held by the nondisabled perceivers. Although research has not specifically addressed the role of self-fulfilling prophecies with respect to physical disabilities, the phenomenon has been identified with other stigmatizing conditions (see Rosenthal & Jacobson, 1968, and Jussim et al., Chapter 13, this volume).

STRATEGIES FOR "UNSPOILING" DISABLED–NONDISABLED INTERACTIONS

A number of interpersonal strategies can serve to "unspoil" interactions between disabled and nondisabled individuals. These strategies apply both to the dyadic, interactional level and to a more global, societal level. A few of the dyadic strategies that we specifically address include tactics such as "passing," acknowledging a disability, and requesting a favor within the context of an interaction. We also discuss the societal-level strategies of altering media portrayals of physically limited individuals and of improving environmental accommodations to persons with limited physical abilities.

Passing

Often disabled individuals try to hide or downplay their disabilities, or to "pass" as nondisabled. Goffman (1963) described such behaviors as one of the main motivations of stigmatized individuals, and passing no doubt works under various conditions and in various contexts. Nonoptimal interaction outcomes are avoided, and a semblance of interaction and relationship ease may be experienced. However, as Goffman notes, disabled individuals can take the goal of passing to such an extreme that they behave in ways that are actually self-damaging. For instance, a person may continue to use prosthetic devices for cosmetic reasons only, when those devices actually impair the physical competence of the individual. Goffman hypothesized, and later research has confirmed, that the tactic of concealing stigma-related information may result in a pervasive interpersonal strategy of concealing important personal and social information not related to the stigma (Kleck, 1968c).

Acknowledging

Another strategy that physically disabled individuals can adopt is to acknowledge their stigmas to interactants. Anecdotal evidence suggests that acknowledgments help both sides of a mixed interaction. The case of Morrie Schwartz—the Brandeis professor whose battle with amyotrophic lateral sclerosis is told in Mitch Albom's 1997 bestseller, *Tuesdays with Morrie*—serves as a good example. Morrie advised, "Talk openly about your illness with others who'll listen. It will help them cope with their own vulnerabilities as well as your own" (qtd. in Schwartz, 1996, p. 77).

One function of an acknowledgment is to move the interaction away from a focus on the disability. In the absence of a direct mention of the disability, it can remain a covert focus of everyone's attention. A stigmatized individual may realize that a nonstigmatized individual is looking at him or her and wondering how the disability was acquired or what its exact nature is. In turn, the nonstigmatized individual may realize that he or she is giving overt evidence of this curiosity. This "I know that you know that I know" interplay can readily subvert a spontaneous, contingent interaction (see Kelly & Kahn, 1994; Smart & Wegner, 1999).

A potential strategy for a disabled person, then, is to acknowledge at the outset of the interaction the existence of the stigmatizing characteristic. For example, an individual using a wheelchair might say, "As you can see, I use a wheelchair." Although seemingly obvious in content, statements like these may be profound in impact, serving to help individuals with overt stigmas "break through" more quickly or be viewed with something other than disdain, pity, and contempt (Davis, 1961; see also Weiner, 1995). In essence, breaking through, according to Davis, occurs when stereotypes begin to fall by the wayside and people see a person, not a stigma. The strategy of acknowledging a stigma may work to reduce stereotypy by straightforwardly addressing the source of the tension underlying a social interaction and allowing interactants to get beyond it sooner than might otherwise occur without the acknowledgment. An acknowledgment may also lead a nonstigmatized individual to infer or attribute particular personality characteristics to the acknowledging stigmatized individual.

Empirical research by Hastorf, Wildfogel, and Cassman (1979) supports this line of reasoning. They found that individuals with physical disabilities who acknowledged their stigmas were viewed as more per-

ceptive, open, empathic, well-adjusted, and/or willing to discuss normally sensitive issues than were individuals who did not acknowledge
their stigmas. In more recent research, we (Hebl & Kleck, 2000) examined how physically disabled individuals might benefit from the use of
an acknowledgment strategy in an interview setting. Consistent with the
research of Hastorf, Wildfogel, and Cassman, we found that individuals
who acknowledged their physical disabilities were accorded more positivity than those who did not acknowledge. Moreover, a follow-up
study revealed that individuals with physical disabilities were even more
likely to benefit from the acknowledgment if they revealed that their
condition was uncontrollable (e.g., the result of a medical mistake)
rather than controllable (e.g., the result of opting not to obtain suggested medical treatment). This latter result is consistent with Weiner's
(1995) assertions concerning the role of perceived causality in the perception of stigmatizing conditions, and it may be very important to
remediating the discrimination that disabled individuals face in the employment context (for a review, see Stone, Stone, & Dipboye, 1992).

    In addition to the acknowledgment itself, the specific interpersonal
manner (e.g., stereotype-congruent vs. stereotype-incongruent, depressed
style vs. socially appropriate style) that a physically disabled individual
adopts in a given social interaction has also been shown to influence a
nondisabled individual's behaviors (Elliott & MacNair, 1991; Elliott,
MacNair, Herrick, Yoder, & Byrne, 1991). Specifically, a socially appropriate, nondepressed interpersonal style adopted by a physically disabled individual significantly corresponded with an enhanced amount of
conversation, eye gazes, and positivity in social evaluations from nondisabled interactants.

Requesting Favors

One of the goals of acknowledgment is to ease social interaction. But
this obviously cannot happen if nondisabled individuals altogether avoid
interacting with the disabled. A social tactic disabled people can use to
overcome this interaction avoidance is to request a favor (Belgrave &
Mills, 1981; Belgrave, 1984; Mills, Belgrave, & Boyer, 1984). Making a
request for help seems to provide a natural context for mixed interactions: Nonstigmatized individuals are initially drawn in by a plea for assistance, which forces them to address rather than to ignore persons with
physical limitations. Thus disabled individuals who ask for help in
sharpening a pencil because "there are just some things you can't do
from a wheelchair" are liked better and rated more positively than disabled individuals who do not make such requests. One caveat to this
strategy is that it may directly reinforce the often restricting stereotype

that individuals with disabilities are dependent and need to be treated like children. If so, requests for favors can readily become "awkward moments" (see Hebl, Tickle, & Heatherton, Chapter 10, this volume), particularly for disabled individuals.

Advocating Changes in Media Portrayals

While dyadic-level strategies may serve to improve the outcomes of specific individuals in specific situations, interventions at a societal level could obviously be much more robust in improving the social outcomes of all persons with physical limitations. It is now taken as a truism that mass media portrayals of minority groups play an important role in shaping both how the majority views members of these groups and how they view themselves. Rather than being an agent for positive change, however, all forms of media for most of the 20th century appear to have been part of the problem (for a well-documented indictment of the film industry on this score, see Norden, 1994). One aspect of their problematic nature is what they did not do: They simply neglected to portray persons with disabilities as part of the normal fabric of this society. A particularly egregious example of this was the media treatment of President Franklin D. Roosevelt (see Maney, 1998). During his four terms in office, dramatic efforts were exerted by the media to hide the fact that he needed to use a wheelchair or could stand only with the aid of braces (the sequela of polio). Even political cartoonists honored the tacit agreement not to portray him as physically limited in any way (Nelson, 1994).

Over the last 20 years, among the few regular television portrayals of disabled individuals have been "Jerry's kids," who are shown on the annual Jerry Lewis telethons for muscular dystrophy. These disabled children evoke pity, sympathy, and emotions of guilt and sorrow from viewers—a technique that is apparently successful in persuading viewers to open their pocketbooks and donate money. However, these depictions narrowly define those with disabilities, restricting their portrayal to those who are completely dependent, are "unwhole," and who are living very disrupted lives. This is captured in a statement by Lewis, in which he adopted what he believed to be the perspective of the physically disabled individual: "I realize my life is half, so I must learn to do things halfway. I just have to learn to try to be good at being half a person" (qtd. in Pelka, 1997, p. 301). A few years later, when the telethon was again about to air, various groups of physically disabled persons actively protested what they saw as the dehumanizing nature of such appeals (Nelson, 1994); such protests continue to the present day. Pelka (1997) has proposed that the Jerry Lewis telethons undermine all that the disability rights movement tries to do, and actually reinforces the stigmas associated with physical disabilities. Furthermore, he argues that many people's reaction to the telethons is to feel that such individuals need no further help because organizations and charities (such as the one Lewis represents) take care of those with physical disabilities.

Bogdan, Biklen, Shapiro, and Spelkoman (1990), in a recent general review of how disability is treated in the media, have argued that disabled people are frequently portrayed as "dangerous" or "monstrous" persons. They suggest that such depictions both perpetuate existing stereotypes and stimulate the continued social exclusion of these individuals. Their analysis is consistent with that of Norden (1994), who argues that the most common cinematic portrayals of physically disabled individuals

> include extraordinary (and often initially embittered) individuals whose lonely struggles against incredible odds make for what it considers heart-warming stories of courage and triumph, violence-prone beasts just asking to be destroyed, comic characters who inadvertently cause trouble for themselves or others, saintly sages who possess the gift of second sight, and sweet young things whose goodness and innocence are sufficient currency for a one-way ticket out of isolation in the form of a miraculous cure. (p. 3)

It could be argued that a noteworthy exception to this trend in media presentations of persons with disabilities involves the many recent television appearances of Christopher Reeve. Whether he is raising funds for spinal research, giving an interview to Barbara Walters, or presenting an Academy Award, Reeve is raising America's consciousness concerning physical disabilities. Reeve's case is a particularly interesting one to follow, in that he could be breaking new ground in "normalizing" severe physical disability (in his case, quadriplegia). Yet, at the same time, he is not unanimously well received among individuals with physical disabilities. Instead, his professed motivations have elicited a great deal of controversy. Many persons are outraged by his singular goal of shedding, rather than accepting, his new identity. His "I will overcome" attitude may actually reinforce many societal myths (consonant with those portrayed in the Jerry Lewis telethons) about the controllability of physical limitations and the single-minded goal of overcoming such limitations. The most recent controversy involving Reeve as of this writing—the debate over depicting him as "walking" in a television commercial that aired during the 2000 Super Bowl—illustrates both sides of the issue very clearly.

For the same reasons that the media may have historically been part of the problem, they can also be part of the solution. Indeed, some authors (e.g., Nelson, 1994) take the view that film and television portrayals of physically limited individuals have moved toward reversing or undermining the negative attitudes and stereotypes associated with disabilities. In particular, Nelson points to the progress that has resulted from the influence of the Media Access Office in Hollywood, which was organized in 1978. This group, which is made up of hundreds of actors and actresses with various disabilities, has been actively lobbying the film and television industries for more realistic and more "normal" portrayals of people with disabilities. The problem, of course, lies in deciding what constitutes realism and normality, and in moving from what is to what ought to be the case. To portray "realistically" the social outcomes of persons with physical limitations would require the inclusion of all the forms of discrimination and bias they currently experience.

Modifying the Environment

Environmental modification is another possible answer to "unspoiling" social and societal outcomes for physically disabled individuals. As noted earlier, the environment that humans have constructed for themselves has unwittingly "disabled" those with various sorts of physical limitations. The Americans with Disabilities Act of 1990 (ADA) (1993) has had a dramatic impact on improving disability access under federal law, and a great deal of interdisciplinary attention is being given to how environments can be designed to be enabling rather than "dis"-abling (e.g., Steinfeld & Danford, 1999). Titles II and III of the ADA are particularly relevant, as they prevent discrimination in public services and in public accommodations. The effects are clearly seen in mass transit, where new buses must conform by having lifts, drivers must announce key stops, and bus and railroad stations must be accessible. Although private clubs and religious organizations are exempt, the law prevents discriminating in public accommodations, thus allowing persons with disabilities to have greater access to places such as parks, libraries, schools, stores, hotels, and restaurants.

In spite of this progress, there is growing discontent concerning both the public accommodations that have not been made and the loopholes in the ADA that exempt certain organizations from conforming to the standards. One example is that owners of old buildings are required to make only "reasonable modifications" and may be exempt from even this if "undue burden" would result. Moreover, private single-family homes are completely exempt from ADA restrictions. Finally, some mandated accommodations, such as convenient parking places for mobility-impaired individuals, depend upon compliance by able-bodied individuals. Research suggests that both willing compliance by the public and legal enforcement of the mandate are well below optimal levels (e.g., Fletcher, 1996).

On a positive note, many advances in technology are greatly assisting those with disabilities. For instance, wheelchair design has advanced to the level where an individual is being fitted to an ideal chair, with desires for specifications such as chair weight, wheel size, seat fabric, and chair size taken into account. In addition, cushion technology has resulted in a significantly lower level of sores and ulcers. Given such advancements, however, one can expect to pay anywhere from $2,000 up to and beyond $30,000 for a chair.

Those who use wheelchairs are becoming more and more competitive and successful in the job market. Furthermore, many architectural firms—even without being required to do so by the federal government—are beginning to build homes that are adaptive environments or have "universal designs." Features of such homes include building stoves and kitchen surfaces at a slightly lower level, designing doorless showers without tubs, lowering the light switches throughout the home, creating level rather than raised entrances, and designing wider doorways. In addition, "visitability" standards (making private homes accessible to persons with physical limitations) are rare, but are becoming mainstream in sections of Atlanta, Georgia, and Austin, Texas.

CONCLUSION

This chapter has attempted to heighten our understanding of the many social-interactional difficulties and challenges that physically disabled individuals face. In addition, it has considered potential remediation strategies at both personal and societal levels that may function to destigmatize physical disability. Research that would serve to guide the development of such remediation strategies is clearly in its infancy. The fact that most of us will be disabled or otherwise stigmatized during our lifespan should induce us to place a high priority on such research.

To conclude on a positive note, never before has our society witnessed more physically disabled individuals leaving their homes and entering public places, the workforce, and society generally. We attribute this advance in part to the strides that the ADA has helped make (especially its regulations mandating access), as well as to an increase in the motivation of physically disabled individuals to participate fully and actively in society. Research on stigmatization (e.g., Archer, 1985) shows that some physically distinctive features lose their stigmatizing quality over time. We hope that our society will continue to become a more accessible place for physically disabled individuals; that the sheer frequency of mixed interactions will increase; that our media will more accurately depict physically disabled persons; and that more stigma research will be devoted to understanding the psychological, social, and environmental factors involved in mixed interactions. As a result of such advances, physical disabilities will increasingly be viewed as variations in the human condition, and not as justifications for social exclusion.

REFERENCES

Albom, M. (1997). *Tuesdays with Morrie*. New York: Doubleday.

Americans with Disabilities Act of 1990, 42 U.S.C.A. § 12101 *et seq*. (West 1993).

Archer, D. (1985). Social deviance. In G. Lindzey & E. Aronson (Eds.), *Handbook of social psychology: Vol. 2. Special fields and applications* (3rd ed., pp. 743–804). New York: Random House.

Belgrave, F. Z. (1984). The effectiveness of strategies for increasing social interaction with a physically disabled person. *Journal of Applied Social Psychology, 14*, 147–161.

Belgrave, F. Z., & Mills, J. (1981). Effect upon desire for social interaction with a physically disabled person of mentioning the disability in different contexts. *Journal of Applied Social Psychology, 11*, 44–57.

Bogdan, R., Biklen, D., Shapiro, A., & Spelkoman, D. (1990). The disabled: Media's monster. In M. Nagler (Ed.), *Perspectives on disability* (pp. 138–142). Palo Alto, CA: Health Markets Research.

Charlton, J. I. (1998). *Nothing about us without us: Disability oppression and empowerment*. Berkeley, CA: University of California Press.

Comer, R. J., & Piliavin, J. A. (1972). The effects of deviance upon face-to-face interaction: The other side. *Journal of Personality and Social Psychology, 55*, 33–39.

Crocker, J., & Major, B. (1994). Reactions to stigma: The moderating role of justifications. In M. P. Zanna & J. M. Olson (Eds.), *The Ontario Symposium: Vol. 7. The psychology of prejudice* (pp. 289–314). Hillsdale, NJ: Erlbaum.

Davis, F. (1961). Deviance disavowal: The management of strained interaction by the visibly handicapped. *Social Problems, 9*, 120–132.

Dovidio, J. F., Kawakami, K., Johnson, C., Johnson, B., & Howard, A. (1997). On the nature of prejudice: Automatic and controlled process. *Journal of Experimental Social Psychology, 33*, 510–540.

Elliott, A. J., Witty, T. E., Herrick, S., & Hoffman, J. T. (1991). Negotiating reality after physical loss: Hope, depression, and disability. *Journal of Personality and Social Psychology, 61*, 608–613.

Elliott, T. R., & MacNair, R. R. (1991). Attributional processes in response to social displays of depression. *Journal of Social and Personal Relationships, 8*, 129–132.

Elliott, T. R., MacNair, R. R., Herrick, S. M., Yoder, B., & Byrne, C. A. (1991). Interpersonal reactions to depression and physical disability in dyadic interactions. *Journal of Applied Social Psychology, 21,* 1293–1302.

Fletcher, D. (1996). Illegal parking in spaces reserved for people with disabilities: A review of the research. *Journal of Developmental and Physical Disabilities, 8,* 151–165.

Goffman, E. (1963). *Stigma: Notes on the management of spoiled identity.* Englewood Cliffs, NJ: Prentice-Hall.

Gouvier, W. D., Coon, R.,C., Todd, M. E., & Fuller, K. H. (1994). Verbal interactions with individuals presenting with and without physical disability. *Rehabilitation Psychology, 39,* 263–268.

Graham, S., Weiner, B., Giuliano, T., & Williams, E. (1995). An attributional analysis of reactions to Magic Johnson. *Journal of Applied Social Psychology, 23,* 996–1010.

Hastorf, A. H., Northcraft, G. B., & Picciotto, S. R. (1979). Helping the handicapped: How realistic is the performance feedback received by the physically handicapped? *Personality and Social Psychology Bulletin, 5,* 373–376.

Hastorf, A. H., Wildfogel, J., & Cassman, T. (1979). Acknowledgment of handicap as a tactic in social interaction. *Journal of Personality and Social Psychology, 37,* 1790–1797.

Hebl, M. R., & Kleck, R. E. (2000). *To mention or not to mention: Acknowledgment of a stigma by physically disabled and obese individuals.* Unpublished manuscript, Rice University

Heinemann, W., Pellander, F., Vogelbusch, A., & Wojtek, B. (1981). Meeting a deviant person: Participative norms and affective reactions. *European Journal of Social Psychology, 11,* 1–25.

Hockenberry, J. (1995). *Moving violations: War zones, wheelchairs, and declarations of independence.* New York: Hyperion.

Jette, A. M. (1996). Disability trends and transitions. In R. H. Binstock & L. K. George (Eds.), *Handbook of aging and the social sciences* (4th ed., pp. 94–116). San Diego, CA: Academic Press.

Johnson, M. (1994). Sticks and stones: The language of disability. In J. A. Nelson (Ed.), *The disabled, the media, and the information age* (pp. 25–43). Westport, CT: Greenwood Press.

Jones, E. E., Farina, A., Hastorf, A. H., Markus, H., Miller, D. T., & Scott, R. A. (1984). *Social stigma: The psychology of marked relationships.* New York: Freeman.

Karp, G. (1999). *Life on wheels: For the active wheelchair user.* Beijing: O'Reilly.

Kelly, A. E., & Kahn, J. H. (1994). Effects of suppression of personal intrusive thoughts. *Journal of Personality and Social Psychology, 66*(6), 998–1006.

Kleck, R. E. (1968a). Physical stigma and nonverbal cues emitted in face-to-face interaction. *Human Relations, 21,* 19–28.

Kleck, R. E. (1968b). The role of stigma as a factor in social interaction. In *Perspectives on human deprivation: Biological, psychological and sociological* (NICHD Task Force Report). Washington, DC: U.S. Department of Health, Education and Welfare.

Kleck, R.E. (1968c). Self-disclosure patterns of the nonobviously stigmatized. *Psychological Reports, 23,* 1239–1248.

Kleck, R.E. (1969). Physical stigma and task oriented interactions. *Human Relations, 22,* 53–60.

Kleck, R. E., Ono, H., & Hastorf, A. H. (1966). The effects of physical deviance upon face-to-face interaction. *Human Relations, 19,* 425–436.

Kleck, R. E., & Strenta, A. (1980). Perceptions of the impact of negatively valued physical characteristics on social interaction. *Journal of Personality and Social Psychology, 39,* 861–873.

Kleege, G. (1999). *Sight unseen.* New Haven, CT: Yale University Press.

Langer, E. J., Fiske, S., Taylor, S. E., & Chanowitz, B. (1976). Stigma, staring, and discomfort: A novel-stimulus hypothesis. *Journal of Experimental Social Psychology, 12,* 451–463.

Maney, P. J. (1998). *The Roosevelt presence: The life and legacy of FDR.* Berkeley, CA: University of California Press.

McNeil, J. M. (1993). *Americans with disabilities: 1991–1992* (Current Population Reports No. P-70-33). Washington DC: U.S. Government Printing Office.

Merton, R. K. (1948). The self-fulfilling prophecy. *Antioch Review, 8,* 193–210.

Mills, J., Belgrave, F. Z., & Boyer, K. M. (1984). Reducing avoidance of social interaction with a physically disabled person by mentioning the disability following a request for aid. *Journal of Applied Social Psychology, 14,* 1–11.

Nelson, J. A. (1994). Broken images: Portrayals of those with disabilities in American media. In J. A. Nelson (Ed.), *The disabled, the media, and the information age* (pp. 1–17). Westport, CT: Greenwood Press.

Norden, M. F. (1994). *The cinema of isolation: A history of physical disability in the movies.* New Brunswick, NJ: Rutgers University Press.

Pelka, F. (1997). *The disability rights movement.* Santa Barbara, CA: ABC-CLIO.

Riches, V. (1996). *Everyday social interaction: A program for people with disabilities.* Baltimore: Brookes.

Rosenthal, R., & Jacobson, L. (1968). *Pygmalion in the classroom: Teacher expectations and pupils' intellectual development.* New York: Holt, Rinehart & Winston.

Russell, D., Lenel, J., Spicer, C., Miller, J., Albrecht, J., & Rose, J. (1985). Evaluating the physically disabled: An attributional analysis. *Personality and Social Psychology Bulletin, 11,* 23–31.

Schontz, F. C. (1990). Body image and physical disability. In T. F. Cash & T. Pruzinsky (Eds.), *Body images: Development, deviance, and change* (pp. 149–169). New York: Guilford Press.

Schwartz, M. (1996). *Morrie: In his own words.* New York: Dell.

Sigelman, C. K., Adams, R. M., Meeks, S. R., & Purcell, M. A. (1986). Children's nonverbal responses to a physically disabled person. *Journal of Nonverbal Behavior, 10*(3), 173–186.

Siller, J. (1986). The measurement of attitudes toward physically disabled individuals. In C. P. Herman, M. P. Zanna, & E. T. Higgins (Eds.) *The Ontario Symposium: Vol. 3. Physical appearance, stigma, and social behavior* (pp. 245–288). Hillsdale, NJ: Erlbaum.

Smart, L., & Wegner, D. (1999). Covering up what can't be seen: Concealable stigma and mental control. *Journal of Personality and Social Psychology,* 77(3), 474–486.

Snyder, M. L., Kleck, R. E., Strenta, A., & Mentzer, S. J. (1979). Avoidance of the handicapped: An attributional ambiguity analysis. *Journal of Personality and Social Psychology, 37,* 2297–2306.

Snyder, M. L., Tanke, E. D., & Berscheid, E. (1977). Social perception and interpersonal behavior: From social perception to social reality. *Journal of Personality and Social Psychology, 35,* 656–666.

Steinfeld, E., & Danford, G. S. (Eds.). (1999). *Enabling environments: Measuring the impact of environment on disability and rehabilitation.* New York: Kluwer Academic/Plenum Press.

Stone, E. F., Stone, D. L., & Dipboye, R. L. (1992). Stigmas in organizations: Race, handicaps, and physical unattractiveness. In K. Kelley (Ed.), *Issues, theory, and research in industrial/organizational psychology* (pp. 385–457). New York: Elsevier.

Strenta, A. C., & Kleck, R. E. (1985). Physical disability and the attribution dilemma: Perceiving the causes of social behavior. *Journal of Social and Clinical Psychology, 3,* 129–142.

Taylor, S. E. (1983). Adjustment to threatening events: A theory of cognitive adaptation. *American Psychologist, 38,* 1161–1173.

Weber, M. (1904–1905). *The Protestant ethic and the spirit of capitalism.* New York: Scribner.

Weiner, B. (1995). *Judgments of responsibility: A theory of social conduct.* New York: Guilford Press.

Weiner, B., Perry, R. P., & Magnusson, J. (1988). An attributional analysis of reactions to stigmas. *Journal of Personality and Social Psychology, 55,* 738–748.

Wright, B. (1983). *Physical disability: A psychological approach* (2nd ed.). New York: Harper.

Zebrowitz-McArthur, L. (1982). Judging a book by its cover: A cognitive analysis of the relationship between physical appearance and stereotyping. In A. H. Hastorf & A. M. Isen (Eds.), *Cognitive social psychology* (pp. 149–211). New York: Elsevier.

Index

and negative ethnic stereotypes,
380–381
and physical attractiveness, 386–
388
and school tracking, 405–407
sociological level, 375, 403–404,
410–411
stereotype trigger, 99–100, 102,
107, 379
and stigma maintenance, 374, 376
target initiated, 395–396
teacher expectation studies, 384,
393
Self-inference processes, 185–186,
199–200, 260
and attributional analysis of
behavior, 204–205
impact of public behavior on, 200–
202, 208
behavior vs. existing beliefs,
202–203
evaluative anchors, 203–205
mediated by "episodic construal,"
190, 193
Self-presentation, 194,210
attunements, 195
contextual cues and different social
pasts, 194–195, 196
extra effort requirements, 326–327
stereotype confirmation/
disconfirmation response
choice, 253–255
Social Darwinism, 133
American, 133–134
and group stigmatization, 136–
137
modern, 134–135
Social dominance orientation (SDO),
135
Social role theory, and gender
stereotypes, 93
Social token, 20, 186–187
disengagement, 208–209, 351–352
and self-inference processes, 185–
186, 189–190, 199
sense of representativeness, 188–
189, 203, 205
sense of social scrutiny, 185, 198,
200–201, 205–206, 255, 289
behavioral inhibition, 207–209
cognitive effects, 206–207

compensatory communication
goals, 209–210
and state of reflective expectancy,
187–188, 195, 199, 209–210
Sociality, biologically based human
characteristic, 35
Spencer, Herbert, and social
Darwinism, 133
Stereotype development theories, 63
consensus, 69–73
alteration, 72
and communication/social exchange, 69–70
and imperfect agreement, 72–73
and social norms, 70–71, 80
functional, 67–68, 111, 136
motivational factors
flattering self-image, 91
as just-world belief, 91
maintaining advantageous status
quo, 91
perceptual, 68
accentuation theories, 69
belief creation theories, 68–69,
396
Stereotype reduction
approaches
alternative cognitive approach,
108–109
conversion model, 109
"exemplar-based" models, 109
positive intergroup contact, 110,
297–298
"subtyping" model, 109
effort, 320
limitations in stigma reduction
stereotypes resulting from stigmas, 109
stigmas without stereotypes, 109
Stereotype threat hypothesis, 166–
167, 325, 350–351, 407
cultural stereotypes and individual
psychology links, 409–410
and effort requirements of mixed
interactions, 326–327
experiments, 408–409
and role of deep activation, 226
Stereotyping, 88, 379
affective reactions, 95–96, 308
and cognitive limitations, 2, 67,
89, 95

CPSIA information can be obtained
at www.ICGtesting.com
Printed in the USA
BVHW031955181021
619253BV00006B/54